The Gynecological Sourcebook

M. Sara Rosenthal

Foreword by Suzanne Pratt, M.D., F.A.C.O.G.

Lowell House
Los Angeles

Contemporary Books
Chicago

In memory of Monica S. Burg

Library of Congress Cataloging-in-Publication Data

Rosenthal, M. Sara.
The gynecological sourcebook / by M. Sara Rosenthal ; with a foreword by Suzanne Pratt.
p. cm.
Includes bibliographical references and index.
ISBN 1-56565-331-9
1. Gynecology—Popular works. I. Title.
RG121.R76 1994
618.1—dc20 94-6010
CIP

Publisher: Jack Artenstein
General Manager, Lowell House Adult: Bud Sperry
Text design: Mary Ballachino/Merrimac Design

Manufactured in the United States of America
10 9 8 7 6 5 4 3 2 1

Contents

Acknowledgments

If it weren't for the commitment, hard work, and guidance of the following people, this book would never have been written: Suzanne Pratt, M.D., F.A.C.O.G., who served as medical adviser; my research assistant, Ellen Tulchinsky, B.A., M.L.I.S.; my editorial assistant, journalist Laura Tulchinsky, B.A.; my editor, Bud Sperry; and my copyeditor, Dianne J. Woo.

Special thanks to the physicians and health practitioners who donated their time and expertise: Jerald Bain, M.D., F.R.C.P.(C); Jane Bell, B.Sc.PHM.; Susan R. George, M.D., F.R.C.P.(C), F.A.C.P.; Christine Herbert, B.Sc.PHM.; Masood A. Khatamee, M.D., F.A.C.O.G.; Debra Lander, M.D., F.R.C.P.(C); Matthew Lazar, M.D., F.R.C.P.(C), F.A.C.P.; Michelle Long, M.D.; Kelly S. MacDonald, M.D., F.R.C.P.(C); Sandy Mesner, M.D.; Michael Policar, M.D., F.A.C.O.G.; and Daniel Rappaport, M.D., F.R.C.P.(C).

Finally, in the moral support department—my husband, Gary S. Karp, and all the relatives and friends who cheered me on.

Foreword

In the last twenty years, many physicians have come to realize that their patients deserve and can understand much more information about health and illness than was previously believed. This willingness on the part of the patient to become a partner in the therapeutic relationship rather than just a passive recipient can have a tremendous beneficial effect on the outcome. For example, diabetics who monitor their own blood sugars and adjust insulin doses to compensate for changes in diet and activity during the day can possibly lower their risk of long term complications of their diabetes.

The purpose of *The Gynecological Sourcebook* is to provide you with the information you need to become an active participant in your own gynecologic health care.

In the following pages, you will find discussions of normal physiology, infectious diseases (including AIDS, herpes, and other sexually transmitted diseases), hysterectomy (and how to determine when it is indicated), pregnancy, contraception, and other issues of common interest. In addition, sources are provided for further study and contacts for support groups for those with particular concerns. Armed with the appropriate information, there is much the contemporary woman can do to protect and preserve her reproductive health.

You are encouraged to find a physician you can trust and with whom you can establish an ongoing dialogue concerning your own unique situation. Personality conflicts can occur, even with a practitioner who is thoroughly knowledgeable and competent. You should never be afraid to seek a second opinion concerning a diagnosis or recommended therapy. Even in the context of malignancy there is sometimes more than one alternative course of treatment. It is your right to have all alternatives presented clearly and in language you can understand. Physicians have access to an abundance of patient instructional materials, including not only written but often video tape formats, which make this process easier and can provide the basis for your true informed consent to treatment.

It is your responsibility to provide your physician with an accurate personal history. This can contain important clues to current diagnosis. Any new doctor should be aware of medication allergies, medications you are currently taking, and any ongoing medical condition for which you are being treated. What you tell your doctor is confidential, and it is hazardous to withhold information.

Finally, remember that the treatment you choose be the one that is right for you, not necessarily for your sister, best friend, or coworkers. New technology increases your options, but you and your doctor may decide that the best for you is not necessarily the newest.

So do your homework (Sara Rosenthal will help you get started), and if you have any questions, ask your doctor!

Suzanne G. Pratt, M.D., F.A.C.O.G.
The Three Rivers Gynecology, P.C.
909 North Fifth Avenue
Rome, GA 30165

INTRODUCTION

All the Headlines in One Place

When *Our Bodies, Ourselves,* the woman's "bible," was first published, I was 11 years old; it had been given as a gift to my mother for her 35th birthday. I would often read the book in my mother's bedroom. I was fascinated with the diagrams and pictures and tried to absorb as much information as I could. When I was older, I got my own copy, a revised edition that became known as "the green one." (There is now a "red one," revised for the 1990s.) It's the kind of book you read for years, becoming more interested in sections you thought you'd never "grow into."

Growing up as a woman requiring gynecological care in a post–*Our Bodies, Ourselves* era is an entirely different matter. For one thing, women's health issues and attitudes about sexuality have radically changed over the past two decades. Issues that never existed in the 1970s are now at the forefront, and women are far more knowledgeable about gynecological issues than they were in the late 1980s. This is partly because of AIDS (acquired immunodeficiency syndrome), but in general, women are reclaiming their own gynecological "territory."

Amazingly, the field of gynecology was considered a "male" profession until as recently as the 1970s. Since then, the profession has been flooded with women. As a 30-year-old woman in 1970, you had little choice but to see a male gynecologist for an internal exam; today, women can choose from a variety of men and women gynecologists, while midwifery is a legalized profession once again. We're also more informed about routine procedures, are more apt to question non-routine procedures, and are becoming more vigilant about *mis*treatment. But more important, the *world* we live in is a different place. Very few women stay home anymore, not because it is viewed unfavorably, but because of economic necessity. In 1973 it was considered a "luxury" to have a career; today, my husband and I argue over which of us will be *lucky* enough to stay home when we have children.

Attitudes toward issues in women's health care have changed considerably. PMS and breast cancer, taboo subjects in the 1970s, are openly discussed and regularly covered in the media. Most women routinely do breast self-examinations (BSE). The openness regarding breast cancer has led to a new debate: breast implants. Although many women seek implants for cosmetic reasons, hundreds of thousands of women get them for reconstructive purposes after a mastectomy procedure. The health risks regarding implants are *still* unknown, and women are openly expressing their anger regarding the lack of initial research that went into the implants. Pregnancy and contraception were never discussed on television in the '70s the way they are today. Condoms, home pregnancy test kits, and home ovulation test kits are on the market in abundance. AIDS has entirely changed the way most women think about sex, bringing virginity and abstinence back in vogue. As we "tail-end" baby boomers enter our childbearing years, pregnancy and infertility issues are hot topics and "front-end" baby boomers are entering menopause and demanding more information. Finally, some issues have only *gained* momentum. The abortion issue, for example, has never been more heated than it is today.

There are many other gynecological issues that are still not openly discussed. Materials are scarce when it comes to cervical dysplasia, viruses, vaginal infections, fibroids, hormones and medications, endometriosis, tumors, ovarian and cervical cancers, pregnancy loss, infertility, menopause, and how dieting and eating disorders affect the reproductive organs. There are basic questions that no one feels comfortable asking: "What is being checked in my pelvic exams?" "What's a colposcopy?" "What's the difference between safe sex and contraception?" "Do I really need this hysterectomy or should I get another opinion?"

This book is specifically designed to address the gynecological issues of *this* era. Who is the reader I'm targeting? In some ways she's more savvy and technically up-to-date when it comes to gynecological issues than women in past decades, but she often feels lost when she's forced to deal with basic issues she thinks she *should* know or an issue unpopular with the media. It's an all-too-familiar feeling. When was the last time uterine prolapse, yeast infections, urinary tract infections, or fibroadenomas were discussed on

"Oprah"? When was the last time someone explained how a menstrual cycle *really* works—without using diagrams? How many of us have wanted to fire our gynecologists but didn't know how? How many of us have watched our friends get pregnant while we've been struggling? How many of us have had three miscarriages in a row and can't even *look* at a pregnant woman anymore? How many of us have read conflicting articles about premenstrual syndrome (PMS), nutrition, or menopause issues and are left *so* confused we don't know *what* to believe? How many of us have tried to look up something in a reference book only to discover the topic wasn't covered?

The Gynecological Sourcebook is designed for the late '90s and beyond. Consider it the New Testament on gynecological health issues. In writing this book, I've interviewed gynecologists and obstetricians in a variety of subspecialties as well as endocrinologists, pediatricians, family practitioners, oncologists, social workers, radiologists, and psychiatrists. Dozens of medical articles and reports—not intended for the lay public—have been researched. The book also contains a valuable Appendix that suggests materials for further reading and places to go for more information on every subject covered in the text.

Chapters 1 and 2 help you "brush up" on your gynecological knowledge by explaining the female reproductive system and menstrual cycle in a new way. In these chapters, you'll find all the latest information on the *true* functions of estrogen, progesterone, luteinizing hormone and follicle stimulating hormone, and you will learn how the reproductive organs respond to too much or too little of each hormone, and how our reproductive organs react and interact in the presence of disease or infection. Chapter 2 provides the latest information on how emotional health affects a menstrual cycle, as well as updated information on PMS and endometriosis.

Chapter 3, "Finding a Plumber: A Woman's Guide to Gynecological Care," highlights gynecologist-patient relationships. You'll learn the right way and wrong way to "use" a gynecologist, what to expect in a pelvic exam, what you should know about the Pap test, and more.

Chapter 4 discusses the differences between contraception and safe sex and points out which devices protect you from pregnancy and which protect you from sexually transmitted diseases (STDs). It contains the most current information on the newest prophylactic and contraceptive products such as the female condom, Norplant, and Depo-Provera. You'll also find answers to all those embarrassing questions, including how to use a diaphragm, how to use a cervical cap, and the correct way to use a condom.

Women and AIDS are the focus of chapter 5. There are several unique physical and emotional issues that affect women living with either human immunodeficiency virus (HIV) or AIDS and women who wish to get tested for the HIV virus.

Chapter 6 deals with the "other" viruses and infections that nobody seems to talk about anymore: "traditional" venereal diseases such as herpes, gonorrhea, and syphilis, as well as chlamydia, one of the most insidious and common STDs among the 18–30 population and currently the number-one cause of infertility in women. Also discussed are the range of vaginal infections women are prone to, such as trichomoniasis and yeast, and the human-papillomavirus, which can predispose you to cervical dysplasia and condyloma, and which occurs at epidemic rates in sexually active women between the ages of 18 and 35.

In chapter 7 the focus is on fibroids and hysterectomies, both necessary and unnecessary! Symptoms, diagnosis, and treatment options for fibroids are covered in detail. Varieties of hysterectomy procedures and oophorectomies and the postoperative side effects of each are also discussed.

Chapters 8 and 9 are devoted to tumors and cancer. You'll learn the differences between benign and malignant lumps in the breasts and on the ovaries, and other benign conditions such as endometrial hyperplasia and the mythical fibrocystic breast disease. The diagnostic journey of determining whether a tumor is benign or malignant is fully discussed. Chapter 9, "When They Tell You It's Cancer," explains the different kinds of cancers that exist and discusses realistic treatment options, surgery, and radiation therapies.

No gynecological sourcebook would be complete without a chapter on pregnancy. Separated into three sections—first trimester, second trimester, and third trimester—chapter 10 provides everything you need to know on pregnancy in the 1990s. Complete sections on miscarriage are included, as well as updated information on prenatal testing,

Chapter 11, "The Right to Know," is devoted solely to abortion. The chapter contains information on where you can go for counseling or a therapeutic abortion, appropriate and outdated procedures, postoperative side effects and complications, and what you can do if you *don't* want an abortion.

Chapter 12 covers infertility and fertility awareness. It outlines fertility awareness techniques, the differences between infertility and sterility, and the causes of each. There's also a complete section on the female infertility workup, fertility drugs, assisted-conception techniques, and ways to parent without pregnancy.

In chapter 13, "Menopause 101," you'll find all the latest information on the emotional and physical changes associated with both surgical and natural menopause, the benefits and risks of hormonal replacement therapy or unopposed estrogen (HRT or ERT), and a complete discussion of the long-term effects of estrogen loss: osteoporosis, skin changes, vaginal changes, and so on. Also included are details on common gynecological post-menopausal problems, such as urinary incontinence and uterine prolapse, and the postmenopausal pelvic exam.

The Gynecological Sourcebook is packed with information for a reason. As we enter the 21st century, scientific knowledge and technological improvements are constantly on the rise. More than ever, women need—and deserve—to know how their bodies work, what their health care options are, and how they can use this knowledge to enhance their quality of life. This is *your* sourcebook. Enjoy it, learn from it, and grow *with* it.

ALSO BY M. SARA ROSENTHAL:

The Thyroid Sourcebook

The Pregnancy Sourcebook

The Fertility Sourcebook

The Breastfeeding Sourcebook

CHAPTER 1

Meet Your Reproductive Team

This may be an odd way to start a book on gynecology, but I'm going to begin with a set of assumptions. Just as a software manual takes it for granted that you have a certain amount of memory in your hard drive, I'm going to assume you already have a certain amount of knowledge about female anatomy and human sexuality. So let's assume that:

- you know all about menstruation;
- you know the correct physiological names for most of your major sexual parts, within reason (it's OK, for example, if you don't know what a *coccygeus muscle* is or what your *pelvic muscles* do, but if you don't know what a *hymen* or a *clitoris* is, you should find out before you continue);
- you know where your vagina is located and know the difference between it and your vulva;
- you know how to use a tampon;
- you have had sexual intercourse or know what *happens* during sexual intercourse;
- you have an idea of where your cervix, uterus, ovaries, and fallopian tubes are (a refresher course may be helpful for old times' sake, though!); and
- you've examined your breasts—occasionally—for lumps.

Let's also assume that at least half of the women reading this book:

- are sexually active;
- have masturbated;
- practice contraception;

- practice safe sex if they're not monogamous;
- have had children, been pregnant before, or are trying to get pregnant;
- have had a Pap smear;
- know what a diaphragm is;
- know what menopause is; and
- visit a gynecologist regularly.

In the 1970s, making these assumptions would have been unreasonable because most women knew very little about their bodies. This is where the book *Our Bodies, Ourselves* broke tremendous ground. For the first time, women were encouraged to explore their bodies and sexuality and were able to learn about the burning health issues of that time. Now, information that was once taboo is a basic element in women's health care.

The purpose of this chapter is to refresh your memory on the basics, to provide you with an understanding of how your reproductive organs work and interact during childbearing years, and to outline the kind of infections, viruses, and diseases these organs are prone to. The chapter delves into the origins of gynecological myths, explaining how the uterus, in particular, was perceived by the medical community throughout history. You will also be referred to other areas in the book that discuss all these issues in far more detail.

The Hysterical Connection

The uterus has a rich history. Because every human being develops in the womb, uncovering its mystery has been a preoccupation of male physicians for centuries.

Interestingly, the word *hysteria* comes from the Greek word *hystera*, meaning "womb." This is where the term *hysterectomy* is derived from, which refers to the removal of the uterus. (Hysterectomy procedures are discussed in detail in chapter 7.)

The Wandering Womb and Other Theories on Hysteria

There is a 4,000-year-old tradition of viewing hysteria as a disease of the womb. Written medical documents from Egypt date back to 1900 B.C. The oldest of these documents deals specifically with the subject of hysteria and describes it as a disease of women caused by "starvation of the uterus or by its upward dislocation with a consequent crowding of the other organs." The cure was to nourish the hungry organ or return it to its original home; you see, the womb was believed to have "wandered." The Greeks retained this association and named this peculiar condition after the word *womb*, and the legacy remains. The word *hysteria*, then, actually means "wandering uterus."

Why did the womb wander? It was believed at that time that when the womb was barren, it became vexed and aggravated. It would therefore wander throughout the body, blocking respiratory channels and causing bizarre behavior. Hysteria was viewed as a normal physiological reaction that occurred when the uterus was out of sync. Sexual factors, especially abstinence, were considered to be the predominant cause of hysteria, and sexual indulgence was the treatment of choice.

With the onset of Christianity, sexuality became associated with sin. Sexual abstinence was now seen as a virtue, not as the cause of a disease. In the Middle Ages, disease in general was thought to be a manifestation of evil, rooted in original sin. The hysteric was no longer perceived as a patient in emotional and physical distress, but as a victim of bewitchment or someone who was possessed. This was the true beginning of witch hunts; women suspected of being hysterics and witches were persecuted and burned.

In the meantime, physicians were dealing with hysteria through the more traditional Greco-Roman practices of diagnosis and treatment. The Swiss physician Paracelsus was one of them. He rejected the wandering-womb theory. Instead, he proposed that the cause of hysteria had to do with the fact that the womb ceased to "nourish" itself internally, and that hysteria resulted when the womb destroyed itself. He compared the process to wine's fermenting into vinegar.

Then there was the "suffocation" theory. In 1603 Edward Jorden published the first English-language work on hysteria, based on his experience as an "expert" medical witness in a witchcraft trial. In that trial he had proposed that the victim was suffering from a hysteria brought on by "natural causes." Amazingly, he believed that the afflicted womb caused suffocation. The womb gave off noxious vapors throughout the body that caused the victim to choke to death! (The "vapors" could have been anything: hormonal secretions or even an odorous discharge from a vaginal yeast infection.)

Later, in the 17th century, the focus on the origins of hysteria shifted from the uterus to the brain. Hysteria graduated to a disease of the mind and was considered a behavioral and psychological disorder. It never lost its sexual roots, though. Physician William Harvey maintained that hysteria was caused by a sexual overabstinence when "the passions are strong." Philippe Pinel, considered a psychiatric "innovator" in the 18th century, described hysteria as one of the "genital neuroses of women." Slowly, the theory of sexual abstinence evolved into a theory of sexual repression. By the 19th century, just before Freud's time, the medical community felt it was experiencing an "epidemic" of hysteria. Wilhelm Griesinger, a German doctor, insisted that "all local diseases of the uterus, ovaries, and vagina are likely to be followed by hysteria, which then may gradually progress into insanity." Freud then advanced the theory to far more sophisticated levels, proposing that repressed memory of traumatic experiences was the origin of hysterical behavior.

In the 1990s (a century after Freud) there is no such thing as a diagnosis of "hysteria" per se. Although psychiatrists recognize that there is a wide assortment of disorders linked to sexual dysfunction that are related to sexual abuse in childhood and other factors, "hysterical" symptoms are understood on a far deeper and more sophisticated level. On the other hand, however, sexual dysfunctions are often related to psychiatric disorders. For example, if a woman is depressed, her sexual drive may suffer as a result. Post-traumatic stress disorder, which has received much press lately, is known to occur in almost every woman who has been raped. Because of these connections, it's all the more crucial to understand how our gynecological parts really work.

Teamwork at its Best: The Female Reproductive Organs

To grasp how the female reproductive organs and hormones work, imagine the structure of a re-engineered manufacturing workplace. All job functions are team-based, the structure is horizontal rather than vertical, and when one team member is out of sync, the overall performance of the group suffers. No single team member takes credit for a job well done; instead, the entire team is rewarded. In other words, there is an *interdependency* at work.

The product this particular manufacturer makes is a baby. In order to function, of course, this manufacturer needs product from another supplier: the male. Before the female system accepts the male product, it puts the product through a vigorous quality control check. We all know that out of the millions of sperm that enter the reproductive system, only one makes it to the egg. One reason is because the vagina is a hostile, acidic environment, and the other is because the sperm literally have to swim against the flow of the fluids inside the vagina, uterus, and fallopian tubes assisted by uterine contractions that propel the sperm upward. As a result, the female system always gets the best of the bunch.

The male product is manufactured as needed. Because of this, the male doesn't need a disposal system for any unused product. There is no "male menstruation" wherein seminal fluid is shed once a month. (Gloria Steinem, in a 1992 appearance on "Donahue," discussed how different society would be if men *did* menstruate. Flow would suddenly become a macho thing. The amount of a man's flow would determine how masculine he was, and pads would become trendy, high-status things.)

Obviously, the female system is radically different from the male system. Even when there is no male supplier in place, the female reproductive system continues to manufacture the byproducts necessary to make a baby; it's always prepared to start production at any moment. There is no such thing as supply and demand here; the female reproductive system operates on a cyclical basis.

At the end of the cycle, when the system realizes that the male product isn't present, it throws away everything it makes. This is done through a reliable disposal system that goes to work once a month. The female reproductive system is therefore an extremely organized and intelligent system. The problem most women have is trying to figure out who's in charge. Although many of us feel as though we are slaves to our reproductive organs and hormones, the truth is quite the opposite: They are slaves to *us*.

The Key Players

The Pituitary Gland

The CEO of your reproductive company is the pituitary gland (also called the master gland), which is situated in the brain. The pituitary gland keeps track of your age, begins your reproductive cycle at puberty, controls your body during pregnancy, and ends your cycle at menopause. All this requires a multitude of parts and hormones that work together. Think of each organ as the hardware and each hormone as the software that make the system run. In a nutshell, here's how it works:

The hormone that jump-starts the entire reproductive process is called *follicle stimulating hormone* (FSH). FSH is similar to DOS on a computer; nothing will work until it's installed. For women, FSH installation begins at puberty when the pituitary gland starts releasing the hormone. FSH then stimulates the growth of little capsules, or follicles, containing the eggs. As they grow, they produce the hormone estrogen. When estrogen levels are high, the pituitary gland shuts off FSH and turns on *luteinizing hormone* (LH). When LH peaks, you ovulate. Technically, this means that the follicle bursts and spits out an egg; the follicle is now an empty sac, and the egg travels through the fallopian tube, awaiting fertilization.

But this is not the end of the follicle. Once empty, it transforms into something called the *corpus luteum* and starts producing a hormone called *progesterone,* formerly referred to as *luteum,* hence the name *luteinizing hormone.* In Latin, *luteus* means "yellow." When the follicle bursts, it grows larger in size and turns yellow, becoming luteinized. In fact, *corpus luteum* literally means "yellow body." Meanwhile, progesterone is often referred to as the pregnancy hormone, and it's the hormone responsible for preparing the lining of the uterus for pregnancy; it literally means "pro-pregnancy." An excess of progesterone is known to increase appetite and fatigue, lower libido, and cause acne.

If the egg happens to get fertilized, it produces *human chorionic-gonadotropin* (HCG)(the root word here is *gonad).* We'll learn more about this in chapter 10. HCG makes sure that progesterone levels are kept high until the placenta takes over the production. By this time, a baby is well in the making.

If the egg doesn't get fertilized, the progesterone levels drop off, the uterus sheds its lining and disposes of all that "product", and the whole cycle starts over again. More information on the menstrual cycle is provided in chapter 2.

The Breasts

Normally, when we think of gynecology, we think only of our pelvic contents, which consist of the uterus, fallopian tubes, and ovaries. But the breasts are an integral part of our reproductive system. The sole, technical purpose of breasts is to produce milk to feed a baby. In fact, the breasts define our biological class: The word *mammal* comes from the term *mammary glands.* Although mammals' breasts vary in size and number, we are the only biological group that breastfeeds. However, the difference between human females and other animals is that we are the only ones who develop full breasts long before they're needed for breastfeeding. This has to do with our sexual behavior. Since primates are also the only kind of animal that engages in sex when they are not necessarily fertile, the breasts serve a very important sexual purpose as well.

Human breast tissue begins to develop in the sixth week of fetal life. The "milk ridge," a line from the armpit all the way down to the groin, develops at this point. By the ninth week in most cases, the milk ridge reaches the chest area, where the nipples develop. But some women can develop accessory nipples and even breast tissue all the way down to the groin. Other mammals retain the milk ridge, which is why they have multiple nipples. When you're born, you already have breast tissue. Because your mother's sex hormones have been circulating through the placenta, you're born with little breasts. Infants may even have nipple discharge. This is known as "witch's milk" and goes away in a couple of weeks as the infant is weaned from its mother's hormones. Between 80 and 90% of newborns have this discharge the second or third day after birth.

For women, nothing much happens to the breast until puberty, when the pituitary gland starts the entire reproductive and development cycle. FSH, estrogen, and progesterone trigger puberty. Pubic hair begins to grow, which can precede or follow breast development. Breasts begin to develop at this point, and their development consists of five stages. The *prepubertal* stage is when the nipple becomes slightly more prominent; the *breast bud* stage marks the beginning of breast development. The third stage, *breast elevation*, is when the breast is formed and more erect; the fourth stage, the *areolar mound*, is when the areola enlarges in circumference. At the last stage, the *adult contour*, the breast is mature enough to produce milk. Breasts are considered mature when they are capable of breastfeeding. The first menstrual period is usually the "finale" of the breast's development.

The breasts are prepared for pregnancy each month. Estrogen causes an increase in ductal tissue in the breast, while progesterone causes an increase in lobular tissue. The result is swollen, sometimes painful breasts, which subside as the menstrual cycle comes to an end.

During pregnancy, breasts enter their final, mature stage of development. The breasts enlarge rapidly and become firm. The little glands around the areola (the dark skin surrounding the nipple) become darker and more prominent. These glands are known as *Montgomery's glands*. The areola itself darkens even more, and the nipples become larger and more erect, preparing themselves for future milk production. Two main hormones are responsible for milk production: *prolactin* and *oxytocin*. Both these hormones are released by the pituitary gland, which is in turn stimulated by an area of the brain known as the hypothalamus. Prolactin is sometimes called the "mothering hormone" and is crucial for breastfeeding; without it, you can't make milk. Prolactin goes to work around the eighth week of pregnancy, and its levels rise for the next seven months, peaking at your baby's birth. At this point your body is also producing high levels of estrogen and progesterone, which block some of the prolactin receptors and inhibit milk production. If it weren't for this, milk would be spurting out of you uncontrollably. Once the baby is born, your levels of estrogen and progesterone drop quickly, while the prolactin levels drop at a far slower almost unnoticeable rate. You begin to produce milk, and breastfeeding is now possible. At first, a pre-milk substance known as *colostrum* comes out, which nourishes the baby until the actual breast milk comes. But many women will leak colostrum during pregnancy.

Your baby would not get enough milk if it weren't for *oxytocin*. Oxytocin is responsible for milk delivery. The baby's sucking not only brings out the milk, but also sends a message to the pituitary gland—via the nipple's nerve endings (the thoracic nerves) and the hypothalamus—to send down the milk. The pituitary gland responds by manufacturing oxytocin, which makes the tiny muscles lining your breasts contract and squirt milk from the nipple. While some milk is actually sucked out by the baby, a lot of it is simply squirted down the baby's throat. Breast milk is about the only part of the reproductive system that works on supply and demand. The suckling triggers more milk; the lack of regular suckling inhibits milk production.

In the days of wet nurses, aristocratic mothers would not breastfeed because it was seen as undignified. Instead, a wet nurse would breastfeed the baby. These women stayed "wet" by continually breastfeeding after they themselves had children. In effect, one could conceivably breastfeed for years; as long as the suckling is there, the breast milk will continue. For the complete story on breastfeeding, please consult my book *The Breastfeeding Sourcebook.*

The Pelvic Players

The Ovaries

Situated on either side of your uterus, about five inches below your waist, the ovaries are organs about the size and shape of an actual small chicken egg. If you drew the capital letter Y, the base of the Y would be your uterus, and the arms of the Y would be your fallopian tubes. If you drew a circle behind each arm of the Y, toward the top, that would be where your ovaries are located. The ovaries have two functions in life: to make eggs (encased in follicles) and to make hormones. The ovaries report directly to the pituitary gland, in the way a senior manager might report to a CEO. Under the ovaries' supervision are the follicles. When the pituitary gland sends FSH to the ovary, the follicles start "growing" and, in turn, begin pouring estrogen into the bloodstream.

Estrogen does more than simply nourish the ovulation cycle. It's responsible for developing and maintaining the female sexual organs and for generally aiding in the growth of tissue. For example, it stimulates cellular division, especially in the base layers of the mucous membrane of the mouth, skin, nose, urethra, vagina, and breasts. Estrogen is also responsible for the retention of water and salt, hence weight gain. It makes the secretion of the sebaceous glands more fluid, which helps to prevent acne. (Testosterone, on the other hand, helps trigger acne!)

An important point is that while your ovaries are in a unique position to "job share," they don't take turns, as many women assume. Ovulation may occur from the same ovary in successive cycles. When an ovary is removed, the other one takes up the slack, and you'll get regular periods. In addition, your ovary can produce, as we all know, more than one egg every month. If more than one egg is fertilized, you'll have a multiple pregnancy. The hormonal relationship between your ovaries and your brain is indeed complex. Chapter 2 discusses this in more detail.

The Fallopian Tubes

Fallopian tubes don't really *do* anything except connect your ovaries to your uterus. Think of them as a chauffeur or shuttle service. When the follicles on the ovary burst and release the egg, the egg jumps down the tube and takes advantage of the shuttle service. Peristaltic (wavelike) contractions of the tube help the egg down. If the egg is fertilized in the outer third of the fallopian tube—the section nearest the ovaries—the fertilized egg will continue down the tube and implant itself in the lining of the uterus. This is pregnancy. Sometimes the egg doesn't quite make it to the uterus. It gets confused and starts to grow inside the fallopian tube. This is called a *tubal* or *ectopic* (misplaced) pregnancy. If this happens, the tube can burst, which is very dangerous. Although the tube would need to be removed in this case, with today's technology many ectopic pregnancies are diagnosed prior to rupture and the tube can be salvaged. The remaining fallopian tube will then service only one ovary. Ectopic pregnancy is covered in more detail in chapter 10.

The egg's fallopian tube journey takes about six and a half days. Pregnancy can occur only if the sperm meets the egg at precisely the right moment. If the sperm misses the egg at the entrance of the fallopian tube, that's it. It can't fertilize the egg once the egg hops off the tube into the uterus.

The fallopian tubes don't solely exist to chauffeur the egg from the ovary to the uterus; they also chauffeur sperm from the uterus to the ovary, where the egg is presumably waiting at the top. The sperm will swim up both fallopian tubes, forced to guess which ovary is active that particular month. That's another reason why there are so many millions of sperm each time. Half of them die swimming up the wrong tube!

The Uterus

The uterus, or womb, is more like a vessel or receptacle than an organ. In the past, it was believed that the uterus didn't produce any hormones at all, although it was 100% controlled by them. But current research suggests this isn't the case. The most important aspect of the uterus is its lining, called the endometrium. (This is where the disease *endometriosis* gets its name, discussed in detail in chapter 2.)

The endometrium is in a constant state of flux. At each stage of the menstrual cycle, the endometrium is also at a different stage. When estrogen is first produced at the beginning of the ovulation cycle, the endometrium grows, thickens, and forms glands that will secrete embryo-nourishing substances. These glands also increase the uterine blood supply. This happens when progesterone is secreted by the corpus luteum after ovulation. At this point the environment of the endometrium changes to one that is *secretory* (meaning nourishing, or filled with secretions). It is only in this kind of environment that a fertilized egg can survive.

Basically, the endometrium's function is to prepare itself as a shelter for a fertilized egg, just in case there is one. It never knows when a fertilized egg is on the way, so it's always ready. Estrogen and progesterone are produced only for about 12 days. If conception doesn't occur, the estrogen and progesterone levels will drop, and the arteries and veins in the uterus pinch themselves off. The nourishment to the endometrium is cut off, and the endometrium sheds. The bottom third of the endometrium lining remains intact and forms a new lining. Then the whole cycle starts again.

The Cervix

The cervix is perhaps the most forgotten organ, but it's an extremely important pelvic player. It is located deep inside the vagina and is actually the neck of the uterus. In fact, the word *cervix* clinically means "neck." The entrance into the uterus through the cervix is very small, about the diameter of a very thin straw. No tampon, finger, or penis can possibly go through it. Yet it is capable of expanding enough to allow a baby to pass through!

When a woman is not pregnant, the best way to describe the cervix is as the "gatekeeper" to the reproductive organs. If you've never had children, the "virginal" cervix will feel like the tip of your nose. If you've had children, it will feel more like the tip of your chin. The cervix, however, has gained more importance as a vital gynecological organ in the last 20 years and will become a widely discussed piece of gynecological equipment in the 1990s.

As the gatekeeper, the cervix fields all visitors wanting access into the uterus. It greets sperm, bacteria, and viruses alike. It's therefore the part most vulnerable to hostile visitors: sexually transmitted diseases (STDs) such as HIV. Certain STDs, among a host of other things, can cause the cells on the lining of the cervix to change, which can lead to cervical cancer. However, a Pap smear can help detect precancerous changes on the cervix before they do any damage. The Pap smear is now a routine procedure regularly performed during an annual pelvic exam. It's discussed in detail in chapter 3.

Barrier contraception methods such as the diaphragm and the cervical cap are rising in popularity (see chapter 4), and since masturbation is accepted more openly these days, sexual aids may be used more frequently.

Since the 1980s, cervical dysplasia and condyloma in particular have been occurring at epidemic proportions in sexually active women ages 18–35. There are several reasons for this. Detection has improved because of updated technology and equipment, and women in this age group have multiple sexual partners. The average woman in North America will have about five sexual partners until she marries or finds a long-term relationship. This is simply the norm. Despite the popularity of safe sex and abstinence in the age of AIDS, few people continue to practice safe sex even when they are in a long-term relationship. Many of these long-term relationships end and the couple moves on to other partners.

The unfortunate truth is that women are at risk of developing cervical cancer as soon as they become sexually active. In fact, women are considered to have a higher-than-average risk if they first had sexual intercourse *before* age 20 or have had two or more sexual partners. So, virtually *all* women fall into a high-risk category. As a result, there has been a dramatic increase in the incidence of precancerous conditions (abnormal cells on the surface of the cervix that precede cervical cancer). This condition is known as cervical intraepithelial neoplasia (CIN). CIN is usually seen in women aged 20–29, and in almost all cases there is a strong association with one particular STD: the human papillomavirus (HPV), otherwise known as genital warts. CIN is discussed in detail in chapter 3; cervical cancer is covered in chapter 9.

The cervix is not just an orifice. It also produces regular secretions of mucus that bathe and lubricate the vaginal walls. The amount of cervical secretions is affected by hormonal changes during the menstrual cycle. We can monitor these occurrences to help us read our cycles more accurately and hence plan or prevent pregnancy. This fertility awareness method is discussed in chapter 12. Although the cervix changes after pregnancy, it changes only in shape, not function (see chapter 10.)

The Vagina

If the cervix is the gatekeeper, the vagina is the gateway. This gateway is actually a balanced ecosystem. It is an efficient, self-maintaining environment with built-in protective devices that keep it healthy, moist, and clean. The two most important devices the vagina has are its acid-base balance and cervical secretions. A healthy vagina is lightly acidic, ranging from about 4 to 5 on the pH scale (1 is most acidic, 14 is most alkaline). The vagina's acidity discourages infections by bacteria and other organisms. Friendly bacteria called *Lactobacillus acidophilus* help keep the vagina acidic and resistant to infection.

Mucus secretions that come from the cervix wash and lubricate the vaginal walls. The vagina also produces its own secretions during sexual excitement. Normal vaginal secretions have a mild, slightly musky odor and fluctuate between a clear, egg-white consistency during ovulation to a creamy, milky-white consistency after ovulation.

The vagina has three functions: to fend off unwanted bacteria, to play host to the penis, and to expel the contents of the uterus, which consist of the uterine lining and a baby. To do this, the vagina, like the endometrium, is in a continuous state of flux. Its environment changes to accompany circumstances such as sexual activity, hormonal levels (as in menopause), labor, and menstruation.

The Vulva

The vulva refers to your outer genitals: everything you can actually *see*. Many women think the vulva is *one* of the many outer genitals, such as the vaginal lips. But it is simply a general term that refers to a whole collection of other parts.

On your vulva you'll find the *mons* (the area above your genitals that is covered with pubic hair), the *clitoris* (a sexual organ made of erectile tissue that, when stimulated, leads to orgasm), the *urinary opening*, the *outer* and *inner lips* of the vagina, the *vaginal opening*, the *perineum* (the area of skin that separates your anus from your vagina), and finally the *anus*. In the same way that your face is a collection of parts—eyes, nose, mouth, and so forth—your vulva is a *genital face*.

The Bladder and Urethra

In previous years, the bladder and uretha were not considered *gynecological* in nature. However, when women suffer from afflictions such as urinary incontinence or urinary tract infections their overall gynecological health can suffer as a result. Conversely, when women develop gynecological infections or are not practicing good gynecological hygiene, bladder infections can result.

The urethra is a tube that connects the bladder to the outside. The main function of the urinary tract in women is to transport urine (the body's liquid waste) from the kidneys and safely out of the body. Urine travels from the kidneys to the bladder, which is a collapsible bag for holding urine which functions like a holding tank. The urine flows from the bladder through the urethra to the outside. Little girls often make the common mistake of thinking that they're "peeing" out of their vaginas.

A woman's urethra is 2 inches long, while a man's is 10 inches long. Obviously, this creates huge differences between male and female urology. The woman's urethra is like a corrugated tube with a large surface area that can stretch and flatten out during childbirth to allow the baby's head to pass through the vagina. Women have a muscle, or sphincter, located in the wall along the whole length of the urethra that acts like an on/off valve. This muscle allows control over the timing of urination. Urologists used to think that women didn't have this external sphincter and unknowingly ruptured this muscle when they performed urethral dilations to stretch open the urethra. (This operation is rarely performed now.)

When a woman urinates, the urethra is positioned perfectly so that the urine flows out over the outer and inner vaginal lips, over the area between the vagina and rectum, and finally over the rectum itself. The problem with this setup is that the urethra, vagina, and rectum share a very small space. So, bacteria that normally inhabit the rectal and vaginal areas can gain access to the urethra and make their way into the bladder. When this happens, you develop a bladder infection.

Bladder infections are nasty. They are often not caught or are misdiagnosed. They are often caused by normal intercourse, but can also be caused by high-risk sexual behavior (for example, anal intercourse immediately followed by vaginal intercourse); see chapter 4. Other causes include pelvic surgery, such as a hysterectomy (discussed in chapter 7) and diaphragms. Bladder infections and urinary tract infections are discussed more thoroughly in chapter 6.

You, the Shareholder

Our reproductive players are at work 24 hours a day for about 30 years until they retire. Every woman is born with about 2 million potential eggs in her ovaries. That number dwindles throughout her childhood and over the 30 years that she menstruates. Any eggs that are left dissolve into the ovarian tissue. It is at this point that women officially enter menopause.

It's important to remember that during this complex activity from the time of puberty to menopause, all our parts are in service for *us*. We own the shares in this reproductive company, and ultimately we control it. Control means that we make choices. We know how to prevent pregnancy, we know how to plan pregnancy, and some of us will choose to terminate pregnancy. And as more advancements are made in reproductive technology, many of us will cross the reproductive "picket line" and *create* our own fertility, even though we may be infertile or lack the male supplier we need to make a successful product.

We must understand that our reproductive workers need our respect. This system, like everything else in our body, is delicate. Improper hygiene, poor health habits, or high-risk behavior can bankrupt the company. If we take care of it and watch out for it, it will take care of us. The choices are ours to make.

Things that Can Go Wrong

. . . *in the Vagina*

This time we'll work our way *up*—like sperm. Basically, what goes wrong in the vagina usually has to do with what goes *in* it! This includes a long list of garden-variety bacteria that can come from just about anywhere: fingers, vibrators, or penises that are already carrying an infection or are fresh from the anus after anal intercourse. Toilet habits are also a source of bacteria. For example, if you wipe from back to front, you could introduce fecal material into your own vagina. Using a wash cloth on your vagina can transfer germs from your wash cloth to your vagina.

Perfumed tampons, colored toilet paper, vaginal sprays, and chemicals (such as hair care products) that you use in the shower can cause an irritation in the vaginal area. But most often, a vaginal infection is present. These infections range from yeast infections (diet often predisposes certain women to yeast infections) to bacterial infections such as bacterial vaginosis and parasitic infections such as trichomoniasis. Symptoms vary from unusual discharge and odors to itching, redness, and burning. Treatments also vary depending on what you have. Oral antibiotics are usually prescribed and antifungals can be given in the form of creams or ointments. Diagnosis (examination and swabbing) and treatment of vaginal infections, viruses, and STDs are covered in detail in chapter 6. HIV is discussed in chapter 5.

Insufficient amounts of hormone can cause vaginal dryness and irritation (see chapters 6 and 13). Like any other organ or body part, the vagina is also vulnerable to cancer. Incidence of vaginal cancer is low compared to that of other kinds of cancers. Tumors and cancer are discussed in chapters 8 and 9.

. . . *on the Cervix*

The cervix is most vulnerable to sexually transmitted diseases and infections that cause the cells on the lining of the cervix to change and become cancerous. See chapter 3 for more information on diagnosis and treatment of precancerous cervical cell changes and chapter 9 for more information on cervical cancer.

Sometimes a cervical disorder is of a structural nature, as is the case with an "incompetent cervix." An incompetent cervix is a weak cervix that is unable to support a fetus. Women with an incompetent cervix usually suffer from a series of miscarriages or premature deliveries. This is discussed in more detail in chapters 10 and 12.

Finally, postcoital bleeding from the cervix can occur, which is a sign that something is wrong.

The problem with certain bacterial infections is that when left untreated, they can spread to your cervix and wreak havoc on your pelvic organs, sometimes causing a condition known as pelvic inflammatory disease (PID)(discussed briefly below and in chapter 6), subsequent infertility (discussed in chapter 12), or bladder infections (also discussed in chapter 6).

. . . *in the Uterus*

A common problem that originates in the uterus is fibroids. Fibroids are benign growths inside the uterus that cause extreme discomfort and are often the culprit behind heavy periods, hemorrhaging, clotting, and severe cramps. Often fibroids cause no symptoms and can coexist peacefully within your uterus. Symptoms, diagnosis, and treatment for both symptomatic and symptomless fibroids are discussed in detail in chapter 7. Endometrial hyperplasia (overgrowth of uterine lining), which can predispose you to uterine cancer, is probably next on the list (see chapters 8 and 9). Irregular bleeding and bleeding after menopause can also take place, which is a warning sign that something is wrong.

Chronic diseases such as endometriosis can also develop. Endometriosis occurs when tissue normally lining the uterus grows in parts of the body where it doesn't belong. Usually, this misplaced tissue ends up in the pelvic region; for example, on the ovaries, tubes, or the outside surface of the uterus. It can be very painful and causes a host of health problems, including painful periods and infertility. Endometriosis is discussed in chapter 2.

Miscarriages (see chapter 10), abortion procedures (chapter 11), intrauterine devices (chapter 4), and surgical procedures such as a dilation and currettage or D & C (chapter 7) can irritate the uterine lining and cause other uterine problems.

. . . *in the Fallopian Tubes*

Cancer in the fallopian tubes is uncommon. The tube is susceptible to infection, particularly bacterial infections that can lead to PID (see below and chapter 6). Another tubal problem is that of an ectopic, or tubal, pregnancy.

In this case, the tube may need to be surgically removed but can often be salvaged (see chapter 10).

When certan STDs are left untreated, the tubes can take the worst beating, which can lead to infertility. See chapters 6 and 12 for more details.

Finally, there can be a structural problem with the tubes where the tubes are blocked or not hollow.

. . . on the Ovaries

Ovarian cysts, endometriosis, scarring, polycystic ovary disease, and ovarian cancer are usually the culprits when there's a problem with your ovaries. See chapters 8 and 9 for more details on diagnosis, treatment, and surgeries.

. . . with Breasts

As we are all too aware, breasts are extremely susceptible to cancer. Breast cancer is still a major cause of death for women; two-thirds of all breast cancer diagnoses are in women over 50. Breasts are also vulnerable to benign, or noncancerous, lumps, however, and there is an entire range of lumps that fall into the benign category. Currently, the best treatment for breast cancer is early detection through frequent breast self-examination (BSE). Breast lumps and cancer are covered in chapters 8 and 9.

There are also several distinct, benign breast conditions that have been labeled fibrocystic breast disease. This is a very general term that refers to a variety of unrelated breast disorders ranging from normal physiological changes, such as the minor tenderness, swelling, and lumpiness women can experience before menstruation, to a condition known as *mastalgia,* which is severe breast pain. See chapter 8 for more information.

. . . in General

PID is a chronic condition that refers to infection and inflammation of the pelvic organs. PID can originate in the uterus, fallopian tubes, or ovaries, but it usually localizes in the fallopian tubes. Symptoms include lower abdominal pain, painful bowel movements and urination, lower back pain, nausea and dizziness, fatigue, fever, bleeding, unusual discharge, and bloating. Diagnosis and treatment of PID are discussed in detail in chapter 6.

Hormonal imbalances or deficiencies can cause a range of physical symptoms and disorders that can contribute to infertility (see chapter 12), problems during pregnancy (chapter 10), or conditions that may predispose you to uterine cancer. Hormonal changes can also cause a range of normal premenstrual symptoms, which in extreme cases can cause premenstrual syndrome (PMS), a chronic hormonal condition characterized by both emotional and physiological changes (chapter 2). Normal hormonal changes before, during, and after menopause are covered in chapter 13. The powerful influence of estrogen and progesterone on our overall health is discussed throughout the book.

There are also problems that occur as a result of various procedures, medications, and birth control devices. These problems are preventable in some cases, remedied in other cases, and sometimes irreversible. They are discussed throughout the book.

Finally, each of our reproductive organs is vulnerable to structural disorders, usually congenital, which means they are present at birth. There is such a thing as an inverted nipple, for example, a *bifid* vagina or uterus (twin vaginas or uteri), and an *inperforate* hymen (impenetrable hymen). These congenital problems represent a tiny segment of the female population and are therefore not discussed in this book in order to make room for more widespread gynecological conditions. The Appendix contains a list of sources that can give you more information on some of these areas.

Many of the early mysteries of the womb had to do with hormones, which came to be understood only in the 20th century. The next chapter discusses the myths surrounding menstruation, the crucial role hormones play in the menstrual cycle, and the hormonal changes that take place during the menstrual cycle and menopause. Information on interpreting the uterine and ovulation cycle is provided, and the chapter explains how our overall health affects the menstrual cycle, and vice versa. Also explored is how our emotional state and diet affect the cycle. Finally, symptoms, diagnosis, and treatment of endometriosis and PMS are outlined in detail.

CHAPTER 2

The Menstrual Cycle

The first menstrual period, clinically known as *menarche,* is probably one of the most powerful psychological, sociological, and physiological occurrences in any woman's life. It is her rite of passage. Once we begin our menstrual cycle, we enter a completely different physiological phase: our reproductive years.

Even today, many young women don't understand what the menstrual cycle is. They feel shame, fear, anxiety, and depression about their first periods and have negative experiences as a result. Sometimes the negative experience of the first period has to do with painful periods and cramping, but often the negative experience is linked to false information about what the period actually is and what it means. The negativity of menstruation is then reinforced when we become sexually active. Many men are repulsed by the menstrual flow and refrain from petting or having intercourse with menstruating women.

In many cases this negativity is a culturally based. In Judaism, for example, orthodox women are forbidden even to sit beside their husbands during menstruation. If they are traveling in a car with them while they are having their periods, they must ride in the back seat. After their periods, they have to visit what is called a *mikvah,* or ritual bath, to cleanse themselves. They go to the mikvah seven days after clear discharge, and they are not allowed to have intercourse until they visit the mikvah. Conveniently, they end up having intercourse at the most fertile times of their cycles. In some cultures, the women go into a menstrual hut until their periods are over.

There is also a negative mythology about menstruation that can be traced all the way back to the book of Genesis. The term *the curse* comes from the story of Adam and Eve. Eve's punishment for biting the apple—the forbidden fruit from the Tree of Knowledge—was to be cursed with painful childbirth ever after. The historical and completely erroneous translation is that the period is a monthly reminder to women that it is *they* who caused man to be kicked out of paradise.

Unfortunately, the negative mythology and imagery associated with menstruation is both a cultural and patriarchal reaction. Until this century, very little was understood about the menstrual cycle, and nothing was known about hormones. Menstruation was thus seen as a mysterious enigma, and women's emotional state prior to menstruation was feared, branded as a kind of hysteria by the male medical profession. Since women have been living in a patriarchal society for so many centuries, they, too, have become quasibelievers in the "evils" of menstruation, believing that medicating and masking our cycles is appropriate. The purpose of this chapter is to cast menstruation in a different light by highlighting the facts on cycles and flows, premenstrual syndrome (PMS), endometriosis, hygiene, and how oral contraceptives affect the cycle.

In Tune with the Moon

There is a completely different and positive mythology that most women don't know. Interestingly, the only event in human life that corresponds to the lunar calendar is menstruation. Time itself was probably first measured by the phases of the moon. One of the problems with the current English calendar is that the months don't coincide exactly with the solar year. In our current system, the months have been made to fit by Pope Gregory XIII, who gave them an arbitrary number of days unrelated to the moon calendar. Our calendar actually puts us *out* of sync with the moon.

The word *menstrual* comes from the Latin word *mens,* meaning "month"; the word *month* comes from the root word *moon.* The Greek word for moon is *mene,* and *menstruation* actually means "moon-change." (In some dictionaries the root word for month and menstruation is *measure.)* The point of all this is simply to establish that a far more accurate and positive interpretation of menstruation was recorded in our history through language.

Countless other languages and cultures link menstruation to the moon. German peasants literally refer to menstruation as "the moon," while the French term for menstruation is *le moment de la lune* ("the moment of the moon"). The Mandingo, Susus, and Congo tribes also call menstruation "the moon." In parts of East Africa, menstruation is thought to be caused by the new moon. The Papuans believe that the moon has intercourse with girls, triggering their periods; the Maori call menstruation "moon sickness"; and the Fueginas call the moon "The Lord of the Women." Clearly, the belief that the lunar cycle is identical to the menstrual cycle is universal. There is even some remarkable physical evidence that further connects the moon to menstruation. The cervix, *metra* in Greek, refers again to the word *measurement* and is also called the "meter of a woman" because it changes color, size, and position during menstruation. In fact, when it is viewed with a speculum (an instrument doctors use to open up the vagina) the cervix has been said to resemble a globe. Even in pregnancy, the embryo is shaped like the moon; it starts out round and full, and as it becomes a fetus, it curves like a half moon.

All this evidence suggests that women are perhaps far more in tune with the natural rhythms of the universe than they think. Comprehending the similarities between the menstrual and lunar cycles is crucial in order to understand what a healthy, normal menstrual cycle really is.

The Normal Menstrual Cycle

It's more accurate to call a menstrual cycle a hormonal cycle because that is in fact what the menstrual cycle is. As discussed in the previous chapter, the menstrual cycle is driven by a symphony of hormones that trigger one another, stopping and starting, flooding and tapering in a regular rhythm each month. Every woman's hormones dance to a different tune, but rarely does this dance correspond to the English calendar. Women's cycles can even become "in tune" with each other on levels not understood. Some suggest that it may be pheromones, a sexual odor that we all produce and unconsciously smell. For instance, women with completely different cycles may even synchronize their cycles after living together for a time as roommates.

The Hormonal Cycle

Sex hormones are continuously produced at low levels during a woman's reproductive years. It is the continuous fluctuation of hormones that establishes the menstrual cycle and the understandable premenstrual symptoms.

The main organs involved in the cycle are the hypothalamus (a part of the brain), the pituitary gland, and the ovaries. The hypothalamus is like the omniscient figure, watching over the cycle and controlling the symphony of

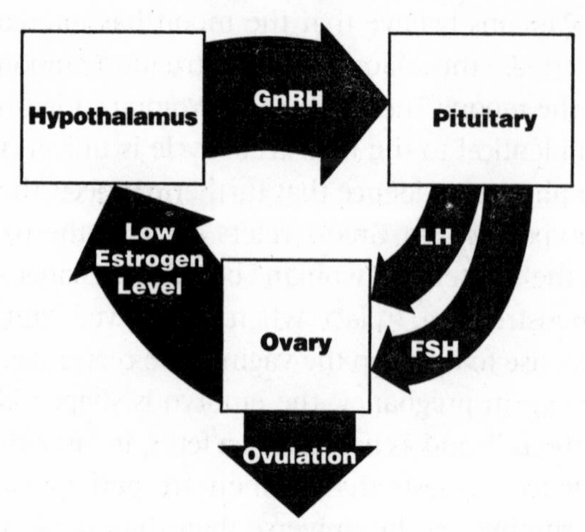

Figure 1.
Reprinted with permission of Serono Canada, Inc., 1994.

hormones. It tells the pituitary gland to start the hormonal process, which signals the ovaries to do their thing. The hypothalamus is sensitive to the fluctuating levels of hormones produced by the ovaries. When the level of estrogen drops below a certain level, the hypothalamus turns on GnRH (gonadotropin-releasing hormone), which stimulates the pituitary gland to release FSH. FSH triggers the growth of 10–20 ovarian follicles, but only one of them will fully mature; the others will start to degenerate sometime before ovulation. As the follicles grow, they secrete estrogen in increasing amounts. The estrogen affects the lining of the uterus, signaling it to grow. This is called the proliferatory phase.

When the egg approaches maturity inside the follicle, the follicle releases progesterone in addition to the estrogen. This progesterone/estrogen combination triggers the hypothalamus to secrete GnRH. This signals the pituitary gland to secrete FSH and LH. The FSH/LH levels peak and signal the follicle to release the egg (ovulation). To simplify this explanation, imagine a row of dominos standing on end. The hypothalamus, which sends out the GnRH, causes the first domino to fall; the second domino is FSH, which falls and touches the third domino, LH, and so on. When all the dominos have fallen, you menstruate (see Figure 1).

Under the influence of LH, the follicle changes its function. Now a corpus luteum, it secretes decreasing amounts of estrogen and increasing amounts of progesterone. The progesterone influences the estrogen-primed uterine lining to secrete fluids that nourish the egg. This is referred to as the secretory phase. Immediately after ovulation, FSH returns to normal or base levels, and LH decreases gradually as progesterone increases. If the egg is fertilized, the corpus luteum continues to secrete estrogen and progesterone to maintain the pregnancy. In this case, the corpus luteum is stimulated by human chorionic gonadotropin (HCG), a hormone secreted by the developing placenta. If the egg isn't fertilized, the corpus luteum degenerates until it becomes nonfunctioning. At this point it is called a *corpus albicans.* As degeneration progresses, progesterone levels decrease. The decreased progesterone fails to maintain the uterine lining, which causes it to shed. Then the whole cycle starts over again.

The first period usually starts around the middle of puberty, at 12 or 13 years of age. Prior to menarche there is a growth spurt. Pediatricians will measure a young girl's height and use it as an indicator of when she will get her first period. The first few periods are sporadic, and it's not uncommon for periods to be irregular for a couple of years. The periods continue until about 48 or 49 years of age and then start to get sporadic again, tapering off as menopause sets in. Few cycles are absolutely 28 days. Where does the number 28 come from? The figure is only an average; the cycle lengths of thousands of women are added together and divided by the number of women. It is therefore a statistical average, not a figure that refers to the typical number of days in a woman's cycle. Menstrual cycles range anywhere from 20 to 40 days, and the bleeding lasts anywhere from 2 to 8 days, 4 to 6 days being the average.

There's a big difference between your own cycle and a calendar month, however. Since your cycle length may be shorter or longer than the 30–31-day calendar month, the calendar date of your period may vary from month to month. That's why it's a good idea to keep a written record of your period. (Charting is discussed below.) Since each month has a different number of days, unless you were consistently irregular, you couldn't menstruate exactly on the 15th of each month.

It's important to count the first day of bleeding as day one of your cycle. Many women count the first day of clear discharge *after* their periods as day one, but this is not as accurate. What's the difference? First, since ovulation always takes place roughly 14 days before your period, 5 days off in your counting could radically interfere with your family planning. Second, if you're on the pill, the first day of bleeding is *always* counted as day one. If you're planning to go on or off the pill, your cycle is more accurately tracked by using the same counting method. Third, doctors always count the first day of bleeding as day one of the cycle.

Many of us wrongly assume that our menstrual flow is strictly blood. The menstrual fluid is composed of a variety of ingredients: cervical and vaginal mucus, degenerated endometrial particles, and blood. The fluid does not smell until it comes in contact with the bacteria in the air and starts to decompose.

Premenstrual Syndrome

PMS is a medical condition that affects about 40 percent of all women in their childbearing years. But because of the media circus surrounding PMS, women have been bombarded with misinformation about the condition.

To add to the confusion, the medical profession itself has lagged behind in recognizing PMS as a real biochemical hormonal condition that causes both physical and emotional symptoms. Ten doctors will have 10 different opinions about what PMS really is, and 10 PMS patients will have 10 different opinions on PMS as well. Some doctors deny that PMS exists at all; others treat it as a disease and medicate women with tranquilizers, water pills, or hormones. Still others are simply baffled or misinformed about the whole topic. (This is not surprising since nothing was taught about PMS in medical school until recently.)

To make matters worse, women's complaints about premenstrual symptoms have been viewed traditionally as either psychological or part of the biological lot of women. Women themselves may even be reluctant to admit they have PMS for fear of compromising their position in the workplace.

The unfortunate truth about PMS is that it's an extremely vague label. As a result, women who have *true* PMS have been lumped together with women who experience premenstrual symptoms that don't bother them or affect their ability to function on a daily basis. In fact, 90% of women who menstruate experience premenstrual symptoms of some sort. The remaining 10% experience *no* symptoms before their period. So clearly, not to experience premenstrual symptoms of some kind is extremely rare. Of the 90%, half will experience the more traditional PMS symptoms, such as breast tenderness, bloating, food cravings, irritability, and mood swings. For many women, these symptoms are welcomed because they indicate that all is well and that their period is on the way. These symptoms are the natural, outward signs for the remarkable fluctuations in hormone levels that a woman undergoes every month when she menstruates (or even after a hysterectomy if her ovaries are still in place.)

Of the remaining 45% who experience premenstrual symptoms, 35–40% suffer the same symptoms as the first group, but in a more severe form. They have breasts so sensitive they hurt if someone even lightly touches them; severe bloating, to the extent that they gain about five pounds before their periods; sudden voracious appetites instead of food cravings; and so on. Believe it or not, even these more severe symptoms are considered normal.

The remaining 5–10%, however, suffer from incapacitating symptoms. This group suffers from the kind of PMS symptoms the media has overreported. It might be more accurate to say that out of the 90% of women who experience some form of PMS, 80% experience premenstrual *symptoms*, and only 10% suffer from an actual premenstrual *syndrome* that has a real, negative affect on their lifestyle.

When doctors refer to *true* PMS, they are referring to both the severe premenstrual *symptom* group and the group that is incapacitated by their symptoms to the point where it becomes a true *syndrome*. Thus, PMS is a kind of umbrella term that refers to a cluster of physical and emotional symptoms that occur 1 to 14 days before the period, that significantly interfere with a woman's interpersonal relationships and daily activities, and that disappear at or during menstruation. The symptoms are diverse and affect almost every part of the body. The following symptoms are only a sample of what some women report:

- **Physical symptoms:** Breast swelling and tenderness, weight gain and abdominal bloating, constipation or diarrhea, headaches, acne or other skin eruptions, eye problems, joint and muscle pain, backache, sugar and salt cravings, increased appetite, fatigue, hoarseness, heart pounding, clumsiness or poor coordination, nausea, menopausal-like hot sweats and chills, shakiness, dizziness, changes in sex drive, sensitivity to noise, restlessness, insomnia, and even asthma and seizures.
- **Emotional symptoms:** The emotional symptoms of PMS often cause the most problems. They include sudden mood swings, melancholy, anxiety, irritability, emotional overresponsiveness, anger, rage, loss of control, depression, suicidal thoughts, nightmares, forgetfulness, confusion, decreased concentration, withdrawal, unexplained crying, inward anger, and physical or verbal aggression toward others.
- **Positive symptoms:** Some women report increased energy levels, increased sexual drive, and bursts of creativity. Even increased levels of anger and aggression can be used more constructively, particularly in business; for example, women may become more productive in their work.

A Look at Statistics

The menstrual cycle is a powerful force in our society. In the United States, billions of dollars are lost annually due to menstrual absenteeism, but it is PMS that is responsible for some of the most compelling statistics. There is a strong link between crime and PMS. Dr. Katharina Dalton, in her book *The Premenstrual Syndrome*, points out that at the time the book was published, 84% of violent crimes were committed by premenstrual women. One study showed that 50% of 156 newly convicted female prisoners committed their crimes when they were premenstrual; of 23 women who were autopsied after they committed suicide, 20 were premenstrual. Conversely, when the woman is the victim of a crime, she is more likely to be menstruating. For example, statistics show that most rapes are committed while the victim is menstruating.

What we can read from these statistics is how powerful the hormonal cycle drives our responses and reactions. In some otherwise docile women, there may be a fierce aggressiveness that explodes when she is premenstrual, causing her to literally take leave of her senses. And there may be a certain vulnerability women have while they're menstruating that is unconsciously picked up by an offender.

Charting Your Symptoms

If you menstruate, chances are you experience some of the physical and emotional symptoms associated with PMS. It is the emotional symptoms, however, that may wreak havoc on your personal life and are also more difficult to link to your periods. If you think that unexplained behavior and feelings may indeed be caused by PMS, the best thing you can do is *chart* your symptoms. Through charting, you'll become more aware of your body and emotions at various stages in the menstrual cycle. In fact, charting your symptoms is the only way your doctor can diagnose PMS. There isn't any blood test or diagnostic tool that can confirm the condition.

In a separate dayrunner or journal, write down how you feel every day for two or three months. The chart should begin on day one of your cycle, which is when you actually start bleeding. Invent your own system for charting your symptoms. For example, you may want to separate your physical symptoms from your emotional symptoms and designate a number ranging from 1 to 10 (1 being least severe) to chart the intensity of your symptoms. You should also note any unusual activities that might increase

Cycle Day: 12 **Calendar Date: 1/14/95**

Physical symptoms
Appetite = 5 (10 means voracious)
Cravings = 0 (10 means you have definite cravings)
Breasts = 3 (10 means they're extremely tender)
Bloat = 8 (10 means you're severely bloated)
Weight = 3 lb
Backache = 0 (10 means your back is extremely achy)

Emotional symptoms
Mood = 4 (1 means happy; 10 means sad, depressed, etc.)
Irritability = 6 (1 means calm; 10 means jumpy)
Energy = 7 (1 means low energy; 10 means high energy)
Sex drive = 7 (1 means low sex drive; 10 means high)
Stress = 6 (1 means low stress; 10 means high)

Special circumstances
Got into an argument with Lee again. The usual. I feel fine. Just a little miffed.

Cycle Day: 15 **Calendar Date: 1/17/95**

Physical symptoms
Appetite = 10
Cravings = 10 (chocolate!)
Breasts = 10
Bloat = 10
Weight = 6 lb (I'm a cow!)
Backache = 10

Emotional symptoms
Mood = 10!!!
Irritability = 10! 10! 10!
Energy = 0
Sex drive = 0
Stress = 10!

Special circumstances
I hate my life!

your stress levels, such as getting laid off, ending a relationship, getting married, moving, changing jobs, or fighting with a friend or family member. A sample appears on the following page.

If you compare the two charts, obviously there is more than just a change in numbers. In the first one some thought and logic appears to have gone into the charting. In the second chart, everything—whether real or imagined—is exaggerated. The woman was even irritated by her own chart! It's clear that the woman was in a significantly worse mood on January 17 than she was on January 14. On January 14, she was trying to be as accurate and scientific as possible; by January 17, however, she was filling out the chart hastily. Were her breasts really a 10, or were they in fact an 8.5? The point is, it doesn't matter. The second chart reveals a drastic change in her attitude and feelings—a definite indicator of how quickly her PMS symptoms overcame her and took hold of her lifestyle. Let's see how she felt after her period:

Cycle Day: 5 (bleeding—day 1 of the cycle—occurred on 1/30)
Calendar Date: 2/4/95

Physical symptoms
Appetite = 3
Cravings = 0
Breasts = 0
Bloat = 0
Weight = normal
Backache = 0

Emotional symptoms
Mood = 1 (feeling really great!)
Irritability = 0
Energy = 10 (I actually did the laundry!)
Sex drive = 8
Stress = 1

Special circumstances
I read my earlier charts—don't know what came over me a couple of weeks ago!

The woman is far happier on February 4 and is less stressed and more optimistic. She has even observed how different she was acting just 18 days ago, about 13 days before her period. (Indeed, not all women experience PMS *ex-*

actly 14 days before their period. It can vary.) A sample of a more clinical chart—the kind your doctor may have on hand—is shown in Figure 2. Charting helps you establish an awareness about your fertility, which is crucial for either planning or preventing pregnancy. (Fertility awareness is discussed in chapter 12.)

Natural Remedies

If you resemble the woman above, you probably do suffer from PMS. Before you resort to medication, however, there are a variety of steps you can take to reduce your symptoms. The most important step is nutrition.

Many doctors feel that a change in diet about 14 days before your period (again, this number may go up or down) can help alleviate symptoms. Experiment by reducing or eliminating sugar, salt, caffeine, and alcohol about two weeks before your period is due. Sugar and caffeine are stimulants, which may aggravate your PMS symptoms, and alcohol is a depressant, which may contribute to an already depressed mood during PMS. Salt causes you to retain water, so reducing your salt intake will help reduce bloating. Doctors also recommend eating small, frequent meals. This means eating three meals and three nutritious between-meal snacks. You should not go longer than three hours without eating. The kinds of foods you should stock up on around this time are grains and beans, fish, chicken, and fresh fruits and vegetables. Highly processed food and junk food, as well as dairy products, fat, and red meat, should be avoided. This is not so much a PMS diet as it is just adopting sensible eating habits. Doctors also recommend adding vitamin B_6 to your diet and taking between 50 and 200 mg. a day. Or, you can take a vitamin B complex pill containing all the B vitamins in equal amounts.

Another natural remedy is evening primrose oil, taken orally in capsule form. Women have found evening primrose oil particularly helpful for such symptoms as breast tenderness, depression, irritability, and bloating. The dosage begins at one or two capsules twice a day during the first two weeks of the cycle, increased to six capsules a day in the last two weeks of the cycle. Evening primrose oil is usually available in health food stores, and your doctor will know where it's available in your community.

To date, there isn't any proof that evening primrose oil is in fact helpful, and doctors tend to think that women who take it experience a placebo effect. Researchers from the University of Queensland, Australia, conducted an interesting study of PMS and evening primrose oil. Thirty-eight women with carefully documented PMS were given evening primrose oil capsules

DAILY SYMPTOM RECORD

START DATE

DAY OF CYCLE	1	2	3	4	5	6	7	8	9	10	11	12	13	14	15	16	17	18	19	20	21	22	23	24	25	26	27	28
BLEEDING																												
SYMPTOMS																												
Irritable																												
Fatigue																												
Inward anger																												
Moody																												
Depressed																												
Restless																												
Anxious																												
Insomnia																												
Lack of control																												
Swelling																												
Bloating																												
Breast tenderness																												
Bowels: const. (C) loose (L)																												
Appetite (↑,↓)																												
Sex drive (↑,↓)																												
Chills (C); Sweats (S)																												
Headaches																												
Crave sweets, salt																												
Feel unattractive																												
Guilt																												
Unreasonable behavior																												
Low self-image																												
Nausea																												
Menstrual cramps																												
LIFESTYLE IMPACT																												
Aggressive toward others																												
Wish to be alone																												
Neglect housework																												
Time off work																												
Distractable, disorganized																												
Clumsy																												
Uneasy about driving																												
Suicidal thoughts																												
Stayed at home																												
LIFE EVENTS																												
Negative experience																												
Positive experience																												
Social activities																												
Vigorous exercise																												
MEDICATIONS																												

Your doctor may ask you to keep a diary of symptoms and their severity by filling out a chart similar to this.

INSTRUCTIONS

1. Consider the first day of bleeding as DAY 1 of your menstrual cycle.
2. Record your symptoms each evening at about the same time.
3. BLEEDING: Indicate bleeding by shading the box; indicate spotting with an X.
4. Fill in the box corresponding to a symptom by indicating the degree of severity as follows:
   MILD: 1 (Noticeable but not troublesome)
   MODERATE: 2 (Interferes with normal activity)
   SEVERE: 3 (Temporarily incapacitating)
5. MEDICATIONS: List these and enter an X on bad days when you take them.

(Modified with permission from PRISM Calendar, by Reid and Maddocks)

Figure 2. Sample form used for charting PMS symptoms.

Reprinted with permission of Syntex, Inc., 1994.

over three menstrual cycles and identical placebo capsules for the next three cycles. These women reported the same improvement in symptoms during both trial periods. The study therefore concluded that the improvement the women experienced was a placebo effect. The bottom line, however, is that evening primrose oil certainly cannot hurt, and whether the effect is placebo based or not, some women may find it worth trying.

It has been proposed that PMS may be associated with a lack of vitamin E, and that vitamin E supplements can help reduce breast tenderness and other PMS symptoms. Some doctors report success with using vitamin E in doses of 200–800 I.U. Vitamin E should be taken with vitamin B_6 after meals. Again, the use of vitamin E treatment is controversial. Although some recent studies were conducted about the effectiveness of using vitamin E supplements to treat PMS symptoms, it's still considered an experimental treatment that is neither harmful nor helpful.

In addition, pampering yourself and learning various relaxation techniques helps relieve stress. Many women find talking to a counselor or social worker helpful when they are feeling moody and hopeless. Regular exercise is also key. Exercise releases endorphins in the brain that have a calming effect. Yoga is also recommended in helping to reduce PMS symptoms.

Alleviating PMS with Drugs

Although some women find relief from PMS through natural remedies, others don't. It is better to at least try natural remedies before you ask for drugs. Drugs are expensive, and natural remedies are less invasive. There are a variety of drugs that can successfully alleviate PMS symptoms.

Drugs that inhibit prostaglandins.

Recent evidence suggests that regular use of prescription drugs that inhibit body chemicals known as *prostaglandins* help reduce PMS symptoms. Prostaglandins are substances manufactured by the endometrium to help the uterus contract during and after labor. Shortly before your period starts, there is a sharp increase in the amount of prostaglandins produced. In fact, menstrual cramps may be a result of the presence of too much of the specific prostaglandin that causes contractions. Anti-inflammatory drugs, such as *naproxen sodium* (Anaprox), *mefenamic acid* (Ponstel), or *ibuprofen* (Motrin) help alleviate cramps. There is now evidence that when these drugs are taken during the last 7 to 10 days of the menstrual cycle, they can help decrease PMS symptoms as well.

Diuretics (water pills).

A diuretic helps you urinate excess water. Severe bloating may be alleviated by a diuretic called *spironolactone* (Aldactone), which preserves potassium in the body. Other diurectics can include *hydrochlorothiazide* (Hydrodiuril), *triamterene/hydrochlorothiazide* (Moduretic), or *furosemide* (Lasix). In general, other kinds of diuretics should be avoided unless they're natural. All of these diurectics are available only by prescription.

Natural progesterone suppositories.

Some doctors have found natural progesterone, in the form of rectal or vaginal suppositories, useful for treating severe PMS. These are very different from the synthetic progesterone found in oral contraceptives. They are still in an experimental stage of development, although a PMS clinic in England was set up that reports dramatic PMS relief with this therapy. Check with your doctor and ask about where this sort of therapy is available. Keep in mind that some studies have shown that this is not helpful, but ask your doctor about whether you should consider trying it anyway; it may help *you!*

Drugs you should avoid.

In 1969, a revolutionary book by Dr. Katharina Dalton called *The Menstrual Cycle*, introduced very advanced theories about PMS and painful periods. Dalton believed that painful periods and PMS symptoms were caused by a hormonal imbalance. This, as discussed above, *is* true, but we now know that it's all part of the normal, natural course of a woman's cycle. Being flooded with hormones is *normal* before a period. At the time, Dalton recommended treating PMS and painful periods with hormone therapy. In fact, hormone therapy was widely prescribed for PMS throughout the 1970s and 1980s, and many younger women are still put on oral contraceptives to help relieve painful periods and PMS symptoms. When it comes to PMS, though, hormonal therapy may not be necessary. Again, only about 5–10% of women who suffer from PMS find that they are incapacitated by it. And many women in this group *do* respond to a change in diet.

Warning: Some doctors in North America may prescribe *danazol* (Danocrine), a synthetic male hormone derivative that shuts down ovarian functions. The only real symptom that danazol helps is breast tenderness. However, treating this problem with danazol is inappropriate and will cause more problems than just living with PMS. The problem with PMS treatment is that what one doctor finds severe may be interpreted as moderate by another. The only time danazol should be used is if PMS is so severe that it causes true disaster in a woman's personal or professional life. So, unless your PMS symptoms drive you to murder, crime, or suicide, danazol is not a good idea. If you suffer from what you think is severe, incapacitating PMS, and this is the therapy your doctor suggests, by all means *get a second opinion.* (Dealing with doctors is discussed in chapter 3.)

Tender Boobs Affect Your Mood

As one primary care physician told me, if you take any male and fluctuate his hormone levels the way ours do before our periods, he would experience the same mood swings and variations in body temperature, appetite, and weight that we do. The important thing to remember about PMS symptoms is that most of them imitate the symptoms of pregnancy. Each cycle ends with your body deciding whether to shed or not to shed.

From the time your period starts in puberty, your body is waiting to get pregnant. All the hormones triggered during pregnancy are triggered before your period. This is normal. If you are among the 90% of women who do experience premenstrual symptoms, it's important to put your symptoms in perspective and realize that it's just you, not a syndrome or a disease. As one practitioner put it, "tender boobs affect your mood." In other words, when you're physically bloated and tender, you're not going to be in as good a mood as you normally are. Similarly, when you have a headache, your mood is also affected. Does this mean you have "headache syndrome?" No. You're just reacting normally to physical discomfort. So, in most cases, having PMS simply means you are a woman in your reproductive years. Our rush of hormones and premenstrual symptoms are like our own personal clocks, telling us what our reproductive organs are up to. In fact, women I've interviewed who are taking synthetic hormones in postmenopause (as a result of surgical or natural menopause) report how odd it feels to be even-tempered all the time.

PMS is a primary topic in women's health. For other sources of information, review the Appendix at the back of the book.

PMS and the Psychiatric Community

What does the psychiatric community have to say about PMS? Psychiatrists agree that there has been a lot of confusion and negative myths associated with PMS. Although many women will be sent for psychiatric evaluation for their premenstrual symptoms, psychiatrists report that it's actually quite rare to see a woman who has symptoms severe enough to be incapacitated by them.

In the 1980s, the psychiatric diagnostic "bible" suggested a more specific term for PMS: *late luteal phase dysphoric disorder* (*dysphoric* meaning "unhappy"—the translation being "women unhappy during the luteal phase of their cycles"). This meant that women needed to experience at least five of the following symptoms during their luteal phase: profound mood swings, sudden, unexplainable sadness, irritability, sudden or unexplainable anger, feelings of anxiety or being "on edge," depression, hopelessness, and self-deprecating thoughts. In addition, they would need to have some or all of the physical symptoms, including tender breasts, bloating, and so on. In order to be diagnosed with late luteal phase dysphoric disorder, these symptoms would then need to disappear once women entered the follicular phase of their cycles. In the psychiatric literature, even women with hysterectomies and oophorectomies (removal of their ovaries) were found to experience these symptoms. In the end, only 3–4% of women do meet these criteria, but nevertheless, more than 90% of all women will admit to suffering from it. In light of this, the psychiatric community criticized the label of "late luteal phase dysphoric disorder," arguing that women should not be branded as being at the whim of their hormones. Therefore, a new term has come to replace both late luteal phase dysphoric disorder and PMS: *premenstrual dysphoric disorder*. All this labeling can get a bit confusing, but what it boils down to is that women who do not have PMS symptoms during their luteal phase technically do not have PMS.

Symptoms of premenstrual dysphoric disorder will be considered the same as those of PMS, although psychiatrists believe that the literature and studies done on PMS so far have lacked scientific credibility. Currently, psychiatrists divide premenstrual changes into emotional, behavioral, and physical symptoms. Emotional symptoms include irritability, mood swings, anxiety, depression, decreased interest in usual activities, decreased libido, and the desire to be alone. Behavioral symptoms include increased appetite or food cravings, fatigue, insomnia, hypersomnia (oversleeping), agitation, poor concentration, and poor motor coordination. Physical symptoms include bloating, cramps, breast swelling, muscle aches, fluid retention, acne, and constipation.

Psychiatrists have found that women who *do* complain about these symptoms premenstrually, and believe they're suffering from some kind of premenstrual disorder, tend to have another major psychiatric illness, such as depression, or a psychotic disorder that is being exacerbated by premenstrual symptoms. Again, psychiatrists rely on charting the menstrual cycles to see if there is truly a link between the symptoms their patients report and their menstrual periods. Women suffering from a true menstrual disorder would see their symptoms vanish with the onset of their periods. In addition to charting, psychiatrists also feel it's crucial to rule out the possibility of another psychiatric disorder, such as major depression, panic disorders, or personality disorders. When the underlying psychiatric disorder is treated, the premenstrual symptoms often improve.

Finally, what do psychiatrists suggest as a treatment for premenstrual symptoms or even a premenstrual disorder? *Validation.* Women who feel they have severe premenstrual symptoms—whether real or imagined, or aggravated by another psychiatric disorder—respond well when they have a physician who validates their symptoms and feelings. In addition, these women have responded well to diet changes and lifestyle adjustments to accommodate their symptoms. (In other words, try not to schedule a board meeting or plan a dinner party for 40 before your period.) Although hormonal supplements and the medications discussed above have been known to help premenstrual symptoms, the psychiatric community doesn't recognize that any hormonal supplements such as danazol or even progesterone (the current fad) have been proven to have any value. Nevertheless, some antianxiety medications, such as alprazolam (Ativan) can be helpful in certain situations.

A 1995 study concluded that in cases of severe PMS, Prozac virtually eliminated the symptoms. It's important, however, that if your doctor does suggest Prozac for your PMS, you are truly suffering from the severe emotional symptoms associated with premenstrual syndrome, not just milder *physical* symptoms, such as tender breasts or bloating.

Irregular Cycles

One of the most common gynecological problems is an irregular menstrual cycle. But before you jump to the conclusion that you're irregular, it's important to remember that being regular doesn't mean your cycle is the same number of days each time. One month your cycle may be 29 days and the next month it may be 31 days. This is still considered the norm. It's also normal to have a light flow one month and a heavy flow the next. Another common misperception about irregular cycles is that unless you have a period every four weeks (again, the statistical average) you're irregular. This is not true. Some women menstruate every three weeks, which is normal for them; some menstruate every five weeks, which is also normal for them. The only time you should be concerned is if your period consistently yo-yos: for instance, three weeks, then four weeks, then five weeks, then three weeks. When this happens, it's usually a sign that you're not ovulating regularly. This is common in young girls after they first begin menstruating. If your period jumps around once or twice a year, there isn't anything to worry about. Occasional stress is usually the culprit when this happens.

Skipping a Period

Once in a while, women may skip a period and then experience a heavier flow with their next period. This is extremely common. Women who are trying to get pregnant, however, often fear that this is an early miscarriage—so mild it feels like a heavy period. This is usually not the case. Although it's possible for a pregnancy not to take and expel in the menstrual flow, it's rare and occurs in less than 1% of women. In most cases, skipping one period is caused by skipped ovulation, for reasons discussed below. The flow is heavier after a skipped period because the estrogen has been building up in the endometrium longer, and there is more lining than usual that needs to be shed. You would have built up two cycles' worth of lining, so the flow is naturally heavier than normal. That being said, you could have a lighter period or bleeding that fluctuates in duration or amount.

It's not unusual to skip one or two periods a year; it is unusual to skip more than that, however.

Causes of Irregular or Missed Cycles

The number one cause of a skipped period is pregnancy. Regardless of whether you've had sex, if you skipped a period, get a pregnancy test. If you're on oral contraceptives and have not missed a pill, the missed period is probably related to your dosage and can be remedied by adjusting the dosage. Another common cause of irregular or skipped periods is physical and emotional stress. One scenario is worrying that you might be pregnant and then actually missing your period *because* you're worried. Other stress-related situations revolve around career changes, job loss, a death in the family, going off to college, moving, exams, and stressful workloads. It's not really understood why stress can cause you to miss a cycle, but it is considered a protective mechanism, a sort of prehistoric parachute in the female body. The body senses the stress levels and somehow decides to stop ovulation for that month to prevent a "stressed" pregnancy.

Overdieting and overexercising can also affect your cycle. For example, sudden weight loss could cause you to miss your period or cause a long bout of irregular cycles. Overexercising can also cause you to miss your period. It's not unusual for female athletes to stop menstruating when they're in training.

Another cause of irregular cycles could be a thyroid disorder of some sort. The thyroid gland regulates your metabolism by secreting thyroid hormone. When the gland is overactive and secretes too much thyroid hormone, known as *hyperthyroidism,* or doesn't secrete *enough* hormone, known as *hypothyroidism,* this can interfere with your ovulation cycle. Thyroid problems occur in about 1 in 20 women and can be easily remedied. Once your thyroid problem is treated, your periods will simply return to normal.

Irregular cycles may be normal for your age. For example, it often takes young women several years before they establish a regular menstrual cycle, and some young women are put on oral contraceptives to regulate their periods. Women beyond 40 can begin menopause at any time, and irregular cycles may be a sign of perimenopause, discussed further in chapter 13. It's always a good idea to have a full pelvic and physical exam when you're experiencing irregular periods. There are a number of gynecological problems that can cause irregular bleeding, which are discussed throughout this book. You'll need to rule out "organic" causes, such as pregnancy, as well as hormonal causes and hypothalmic causes, in which things like stress and exercise interfere with your ovulation cycle.

Amenorrhea: The Absence of a Menstrual Cycle

There *is* such a thing as having no menstrual cycle. However, if you don't begin menstruating by the age of 16, there are some birth defects and potentially serious conditions that can prevent menstruation. It's important to diagnose these as soon as possible. There's usually a hormonal imbalance that is easily remedied with oral contraceptives or hormonal supplements. If you're menstruating regularly, and are between the ages of 20 and 40, it's unusual to simply stop menstruating. If this does occur, pregnancy, obesity (fat cells make more estrogen than your body needs, which interferes with ovulation), food refusal (anorexia nervosa), or vomiting/purging (bulimia) are common causes. When the problem is starvation-related, a protective mechanism is triggered in the body. When the female body is malnourished, it stops ovulating because it can't sustain a pregnancy. One doctor told me about an aboriginal tribe in Australia that demonstrates this unique protective mechanism. Women of that particular tribe menstruate only at certain times of the year, when the food cycle is abundant. Athletes, again, may experience amenorrhea, and either an overactive or underactive thyroid gland can cause it. Progesterone supplements will remedy it. If you skip periods, medication may be prescribed in either progesterone or oral contraceptive form.

The Need to Bleed

Today, women have to deal with more periods in their lifetime than women did in the past due to fewer pregnancies and a longer life cycle. Also, in the past century, women have experienced a radical change in diet, environment, stress levels, career, and family expectations. Understandably, the accumulated effect of all these factors has affected the hormonal cycle of women, which in turn, affects the menstrual cycle.

If you've missed more than two periods and know for certain that you're not pregnant (either confirmed by a pregnancy test or the absence of any sexual activity) then you need to see your doctor and have your period "induced." You'll be given a progesterone supplement, which will jump-start your cycle. It's dangerous to go longer than three months without a bleed; if the uterus isn't regularly cleaned out, the risk of uterine cancer increases (see chapter 8).

Menorrhagia: Extremely Heavy Flow

If you have an extremely heavy flow, it may be normal for you. A lighter flow can also slowly develop into a continuous heavy flow, or you may experience an isolated bout with it. In general, if you need to change your pad or tampon every hour, your bleeding may be unusually heavy. You'll need to get this checked out. There usually isn't anything to worry about. You should have your blood levels checked regularly (every six months), however, because consistent heavy flows could cause anemia. In fact, the number-one cause of anemia is a heavy menstrual flow. If this is the case, have a doctor evaluate you to uncover an underlying cause of your heavy bleeding. If no specific abnormality is found, the flow can be decreased with oral contraceptives. Nonsteroidal drugs such as ibuprofen, taken at the strength of 400 milligrams every four hours, can reduce your flow up to 40%. Even if ibuprofen doesn't work, this therapy is harmless at worst.

A Word About Clots

A clot looks like a tiny sample of raw liver or raw oyster, and often comes out with a heavy menstrual flow. Clots are normal and do *not* mean you're hemorrhaging and need to be rushed to the hospital. When you're sleeping during a heavy period, the blood will collect in clots and expel in the morning. The only time you need to worry about clots is if you're passing them after your period is over, during a prolonged period, in midcycle, or while you're pregnant. (Similarly, if you're bleeding at all during these times, you should see a doctor.)

Dysmenorrhea: Painful Periods

Primary dysmenorrhea means you've always had painful periods, ever since you started menstruating. *Secondary dysmenorrhea* means that your periods have become more painful with time. In either case, painful periods are common, and there are medications that can alleviate cramps. Cramps are caused by uterine contractions, which is how the lining is pushed out. Some uteri contract more than others. Taking an anti-inflammatory medication such as naproxen sodium (Anaprox) *before* your period starts can really help. If you're young, birth control pills can help. It's also important to distinguish normal cramping from unusual, debilitating pain. Endometriosis, a serious disease, is often the culprit behind severe pain during your period. After you read the section below, if you suspect your dysmenorrhea is a sign of something more serious, let your doctor know your suspicions and request a confirmation of diagnosis. If your pain is severe enough to cause you to miss work, school, or pleasurable activities, there's a 40% chance that you may be suffering from endometriosis, a condition discussed next.

Endometriosis

Endometriosis is a disease affecting women in their reproductive years. It was widely undiagnosed until recently. The name, as you've probably guessed, comes from the word *endometrium.* What happens is that endometrial tissue forms outside the uterus in other areas of the body. This tissue then develops into small growths, or tumors. (Doctors may also refer to these growths as nodules, lesions, or implants.) These growths are usually benign (noncancerous) and are simply a normal type of tissue in an abnormal location. Cancers that arise in conjunction with endometriosis appear to be very rare.

The most common location of these endometrial growths is in the pelvic region, which affects the ovaries, the fallopian tubes, the ligaments supporting the uterus, the outer surface of the uterus, and the lining of the pelvic cavity. Forty to 50% of the growths are in the ovaries and fallopian tubes. Sometimes the growths are found in abdominal surgery scars, on the intestines, in the rectum, and on the bladder, vagina, cervix, and vulva. Other locations include the lung, the arm, thigh, and other places outside the abdomen, but these are rare.

Since these growths are in fact pieces of uterine lining, they behave like uterine lining, responding to the hormonal cycle and trying to shed every month. These growths are blind—they can't see where they are and think they're in the uterus. This is a huge problem during menstruation; when the growths start "shedding," there's no vagina for them to pass through, so they have nowhere to go. The result is internal bleeding, degeneration of the blood and tissue shed from the growths, inflammation of the surrounding areas, and formation of scar tissue. Depending on where these growths are located, they can rupture and spread to new areas, cause intestinal bleeding or obstruction (if they're in or near the intestines), or interfere with bladder function (if they're on or near the bladder). Infertility affects about 30–40% of endometriosis sufferers, and as the disease progresses, infertility is often inevitable.

The most common symptoms of endometriosis are pain before and during periods (much worse than normal menstrual cramps), pain during or after intercourse, and heavy or irregular bleeding. Other symptoms may include fatigue, painful bowel movements with periods, lower back pain with periods, diarrhea and/or constipation with periods, and intestinal upset with periods. If the bladder is involved, there may be painful urination and blood in the urine with periods. Irregular menstrual cycles and heavier flows are also associated with endometriosis, but women with severe endometriosis usually continue to have regular, albeit painful, periods. Some women with endometriosis may have no symptoms at all.

It's important to note that the amount of pain is not necessarily related to the extent or size of the growths. Tiny growths, called *petechiae,* have been found to be more active in producing prostaglandins, which may explain the significant symptoms that seem to occur with smaller growths.

What Causes Endometriosis?

Nobody knows for certain what causes endometriosis, but currently environmental factors are identified as the chief cause. Recently, a laundry list of man-made chemicals, called organochlorines, have been found to be breaking down in the environment into a substance that mimics estrogen. These "environmental estrogens" as they're called, are being linked to an alarming increase in estrogen-dependent conditions such as endometriosis, fibroids, and a variety of reproductive cancers. Dioxins, in particular, have been linked to endometriosis. In a University of South Florida study, female monkeys fed very small amounts of dioxins went on to develop moderate to severe endometriosis within four years.

There are a few other worthwhile theories. One is the theory of *retrograde menstruation,* also known as the *transtubal migration* theory. During menstruation, some of the menstrual tissue backs up in the fallopian tubes, is implanted in the abdomen, and grows. Some researchers believe that all women experience some menstrual tissue backup, which is normally taken care of by their immune systems. An immune system problem or hormonal problem allows this tissue to take root and develop into endometriosis.

Another theory suggests that the endometrial tissue is distributed from the uterus to other parts of the body through the lymphatic system or blood system. A genetic theory suggests that it may be carried in the genes of certain families, or that certain families may be predisposed to the disease.

The most interesting theory proposes that remnants of the woman's embryonic tissue (from when she herself was an embryo) may later develop into endometriosis, or that some adult tissues retain the ability they had in the embryo *stage* to transform into reproductive tissue under certain circumstances.

Surgical transplantation of endometrial tissue has been cited as the cause in cases where endometriosis is found in abdominal surgery scars. This latter theory is certainly not possible if endometriosis occurs when surgery doesn't!

Diagnosis and Treatment

The only way to diagnose endometriosis is with an instrument called a laparoscope (a tubelike telescope with a light in it), used in a procedure known as laparoscopy. The procedure is a form of minor surgery. After a general anesthetic is administered, your abdomen is distended (expanded) with carbon dioxide gas to make the organs easier to see. A tiny incision is made, and a laparoscope is inserted into it. By moving the laparoscope around, your surgeon can check for any signs of endometrial tissue outside the uterus.

Although your doctor can often feel the endometrial growths during a pelvic exam, and your symptoms may be telltale signs of endometriosis, no competent physician would confirm the diagnosis without performing a laparoscopy procedure. The bottom line is that if you've been told you have endometriosis, but you haven't had a laparoscopy procedure done, insist that your doctor perform one, or get a second opinion. Often, the symptoms of ovarian cancer (discussed in chapter 9) are identical to those of endometriosis. If you've been misdiagnosed with endometriosis due to your doctor's failure to confirm it through a laparoscopy, he or she may miss an early diagnosis of ovarian cancer crucial for successful treatment.

A laparoscopy procedure also indicates the locations, extent, and size of the endometrial growths and will help your doctor better guide you in treatment decisions and family planning.

Treatment for endometriosis has varied over the years, and there is still no absolute cure. If you don't have any symptoms, and you're not planning to have any (more) children, then no treatment is necessary, just regular check-ups. If you have only mild symptoms, and infertility is not a factor, simple painkillers like *acetaminophen* (Tylenol) or ibuprofen may be all that's needed.

For severe symptoms, depending on where the growths are located and their size, your doctor may recommend a hysterectomy and removal of the ovaries. Before you decide whether this is indicated, get a few separate opinions from other doctors. Although hysterectomy is considered a definitive cure, research has shown that women who undergo a hysterectomy for endometriosis sometimes experience a recurrence of the disease. (See chapter 7 for details on hysterectomy and oophorectomy and chapter 13 for more information on surgical menopause.)

Conservative surgery involves removing the growths themselves, rather than any reproductive organs. One procedure, which was shown on The Learning Channel's "The Operation," is called operative laparoscopy. Through a laparoscope, surgery is done with a laser, a cautery, or small surgical instruments. Again, as with more radical surgery, recurrence is common after this procedure. Conservative surgery is the treatment of choice for women under 35 who are diagnosed with endometriosis in the early stages and who want to have children. About 40% of these women will go on to conceive. After conservative surgery, between 20 and 50% of endometriosis patients will need more radical surgery.

If you're infertile, or if you don't wish to get pregnant, a nonsurgical treatment that involves creating a "pseudopregnancy" with hormonal therapy can be used to stop ovulation. This *does* work for as long as you're taking the synthetic hormones, and sometimes the therapy can force endometriosis into remission for months or years after you go off the hormones. When you go off the hormones, the disease often comes right back, though. The hormonal recipe here can include estrogen and progesterone, progesterone alone, danazol (a testosterone derivative), and a new drug, Synarel, a gonadotropin-releasing hormone (GnRH) anologue, which creates a "pseudomenopause." But there are certain side effects associated with hormonal therapy.

Pregnancy as a cure.

Believe it or not, pregnancy does cause endometriosis to go into temporary remission, because you don't ovulate when you're pregnant. Furthermore, permanent remission of endometriosis has been known to occur after childbirth; the growths in this case shrink, and the pain associated with the disease stops. The problem is, the longer you have endometriosis, the greater your chance of becoming infertile. If you have been diagnosed with endometriosis, are planning to have children, and are in a *position* to have a family (that is, you have a supportive partner and are financially stable), then getting pregnant is a good idea. In other words, why wait? In addition, the disease may also worsen with time.

Pregnancy as a prescription is not feasible in many cases. Infertility may have already set in, while many women don't have the means in place to have a child. Even under the best of circumstances, women with endometriosis have a higher risk of ectopic pregnancy and miscarriage. One study found that full-term pregnancies and labor are more difficult when the mother has endometriosis.

Menopause.

In general, menopause does cure endometriosis, which is why a hysterectomy is performed. But a severe case of endometriosis can be reactivitated if you begin hormone replacement therapy or continue producing hormones after menopause, which is common. In fact, the oldest woman to be diagnosed with endometriosis was age 78. Some doctors suggest no replacement hormone be given for about three to nine months after menopause or a hysterectomy procedure. Menopause is discussed in more detail in chapter 13.

The Future of Endometriosis

The first case of endometriosis may have been documented in 1600 B.C., according to ancient Egyptian writings. However, endometriosis has been recognized as a real disease only in the 20th century. In the past, endometriosis either was considered rare or was simply undiagnosed; today, it's a major cause of painful periods and infertility in women.

Until recently, a large percentage of endo patients (one endometriosis clinic reports as many as 75%) were dismissed as neurotic or overly sensitive to pain. The pain breakdown goes something like this: 45% complain of painful periods (cramps, back pain); 37% complain of painful intercourse. At a recent conference on endometriosis, representatives of patient self-help groups from the United Kingdom and North America emphasized the frequent delays in diagnosis. A study revealed that 27% of endometriosis patients complained of symptoms *for six years* before a diagnosis was made. Diagnosis and education about endometriosis are improving, but the most important thing you can do if you have the disease is to educate yourself.

Adenomyosis: Internal Endometriosis

There is a sister condition to endometriosis known as *adenomyosis*, in which the endometrial tissue (the uterine lining, glands, and connective tissue) invades the deeper muscle layers of the uterus. Usually there's a barrier between the endometrium and the deeper layers of the uterine wall that acts as a defense against invasion from endometrial tissue. Women who develop adenomyosis don't seem to have this defense.

Unlike endometriosis, some researchers believe that adenomyosis may set in after pregnancy and delivery; women in their 40s and 50s who have given birth to at least one child are more likely to develop adenomyosis. Other researchers believe that, like endometriosis, genetics plays a role, and still others believe it may have to do with some sort of hormonal imbalance. The bottom line is that no one knows exactly what causes it, but treatments are available.

Looking at the Symptoms

About 40% of the time in cases of adenomyosis, women have no symptoms, but when they do, the symptoms are similar to endometriosis: painful and heavy periods and sometimes chronic pelvic pain. The more involved the uterine glands are, the heavier the flow; the deeper the penetration into the uterine wall, the greater the discomfort.

Diagnosis and Treatment

In the past, adenomyosis was diagnosed only by a pathologist, often after a hysterectomy was performed for another uterine problem. Adenomyosis is often present in conjunction with other uterine conditions such as fibroids (discussed in chapter 7). Therefore, to diagnose this condition accurately, your doctor must play detective. The diagnosis is difficult. It may be possible to detect adenomyosis with a magnetic resonance imaging (MRI) scan or a hysteroscopy (a telescope, similar to the laparoscope, placed through the cervix). However, an MRI is expensive, while a hysteroscope will at least rule out fibroids (discussed in Chapter 7) under the uterine lining.

Until recently, a hysterectomy was the suggested course of treatment for adenomyosis, but many doctors believe that adenomyosis can be treated the same way endometriosis is. Women have responded well to danazol, progesterone, or oral contraceptives. If conservative regimens fail, then unfortunately a hysterectomy is the only solution. Hysterectomies are discussed in chapter 7.

Zen and the Art of Menstrual-Cycle Maintenance

When you're menstruating regularly and your cycle and flow are normal for *you*, it's a sign that you're in good gynecological health. There are a number of good habits to get into—and out of—that will *keep* you healthy.

The Importance of Good Nutrition

Practice good nutrition and avoid excessive dieting. As mentioned earlier, when the body is malnourished, it stops ovulating as a protective mechanism. Any kind of obsession with your weight, continuous crash/fad dieting, or a starvation/purging habit is a sign that you have a problem with food. If you don't solve the problem, you may be a candidate for a serious eating disorder (such as anorexia or bulimia) that will wreak havoc on your entire menstrual/ovulation cycle. Don't be afraid to ask your family doctor to recommend a nutritionist or a *legitimate* weight clinic. (Usually, a good weight clinic program will point out that the *way* you eat is more of a problem than *what* you eat.) Studies have proven that most weight problems and eating disorders are rooted in a woman's perceptual distortions of what the female body looks like and what her relationship to food should be. A good primer for any woman obsessed with her weight is *The Beauty Myth,* written by former anorexic Naomi Wolf.

The Tampon Controversy

In the early 1980s, tampons were placed on the list of high-risk medical devices, along with intrauterine devices (IUDs) and heart pacemakers. This was in response to the outbreak of toxic shock syndrome (TSS) and its association with tampons. There is simply not enough information and education provided to women about the risks associated with tampons.

TSS is defined as a group of symptoms. It is actually caused by a bacteria already present in the vagina that adheres to the tampon. The bacteria then starts producing a toxin that attacks other parts of the body. The initial symptoms of TSS are fever, nausea, vomiting, diarrhea, sore throat, and dizziness. Other symptoms include a sunburnlike rash, peeling of the skin (especially on the hands and feet), and low blood pressure. All of these symptoms are vague and can be attributed to a host of other diseases. Women with TSS can easily be misdiagnosed, particularly if they have some but not all of the symptoms. Currently, the list of symptons is being revised.

Aside from TSS, there are other problems tampons can cause. Because tampons actively absorb menstrual blood and do not differentiate between blood and vaginal mucus, the skin that lines the vaginal walls dries up, which can lead to microulcerations and infection. Tampons should, therefore, never be used between periods, during pregnancy, or when you already have a vaginal infection.

Hygiene No-Nos

One family doctor told me that in order to practice gynecology in her office, she relies regularly on a small, surgical instrument designed to pull out old, long-forgotten tampons. Believe it or not, many women *forget* to remove their last tampon. Furthermore, many women with extremely heavy flows are in the habit of using *more* than one tampon at the same time. If you're among them, break the habit *now*. The second tampon can get pushed so far into your vagina that you can't retrieve it yourself. You should change your tampons every 4–6 hours. Official warnings on the box state that tampons left in for longer than 12–18 hours may put you at risk for toxic shock syndrome.

Another hygiene no-no is feminine deodorant products. Never use scented tampons or pads; they can cause irritations. Even if you've used deodorant tampons and have never had a problem with them, it's important to reduce the risk of irritations. Moreover, don't use any feminine deodorants to mask the menstrual odor. The odor is normal and natural, and deodorants can irritate your system. Don't douche—unless your doctor recommends it. Douching rids your vagina of friendly bacteria that are very important for maintaining its ecosystem. Douching is not recommended after menstruation. As long as you bathe regularly, your vagina and uterus are self-cleaning and will do everything that's necessary on their own. Finally, avoid perfumed and colored toilet paper. Again, the perfumes and dyes can irritate your vagina.

Oral Contraceptives and Your Menstrual Cycle

It's common for younger women in particular to be placed on oral contraceptives as a way of controlling severe PMS symptoms, irregular cycles, or dysmenorrhea. As long as you see a doctor regularly and don't have any adverse health problems that oral contraceptives can complicate (discussed in more detail in chapter 4), you can stay on them for a long time. Combination oral contraceptives (as opposed to progesterone-only pills) stop ovulation. Carefully controlled levels of synthetic progesterone, however, will cause you to shed the uterine lining once a month. As many of us know, when we're on oral contraceptives, periods are a dream come true: Cramps are relatively mild, flow is medium-to-light, and the period comes at around the same time each month. Many women are surprised to find that when they go *off* oral contraceptives, their menstrual problems return. If their cycles were irregular before the oral contraceptives, they may continue to be irregular after the pills are discontinued; if they suffered from painful periods before, they will probably have painful periods after; and so on. Oral contraceptives may be only a *temporary* solution for menstrual-cycle problems.

Some women do remain regular when they go off oral contraceptives. This is usually because when they initially went on them, they were younger and had less mature ovulation cycles. A woman's ovulation cycle does mature as she gets into her 20s and 30s, and the cycles may normalize. But as mentioned, the original cycle, however flawed, often returns. In addition, it can take up to six months for your ovulation cycle to kick in and return to normal. If you're planning to get pregnant, allow at least that much time. Doctors will tell you to wait until you have two natural periods before you try to conceive. Don't panic if you don't conceive after your third, fourth, or fifth cycle. We mistakenly believe that as soon as we go off oral contraceptives we'll get pregnant. This is simply not true. Couples having intercourse every other day can sometimes wait a year before conception actually takes place. (Fertility is discussed in chapter 12.)

Much of what has been discussed in this chapter falls into the gray area of gynecological care that was once historically undiagnosed. What was once considered "phantom pain" is now perhaps recognized as endometriosis; what was once dismissed as emotional overreaction is now seen as PMS. Finding and maintaining good gynecological health care and communicating with your doctor are vital to getting adequate care. In an age of rising costs and volatile standards, being proactive about your gynecological care is crucial.

CHAPTER 3

Finding a Plumber: A Woman's Guide to Gynecological Care

As a woman, the most important doctor-patient relationships you will have are those with your family doctor and gynecologist. Since most family physicians are qualified to practice basic gynecological care, which is what we usually require, you would think that gynecological care is split evenly between gynecologists and family physicians. It isn't. In fact, 70% of the women who regularly see a gynecologist have *no* other doctor. More gynecologists are acting as *primary care* (that is, overall care) physicians for women than are family physicians, which can lead to problems. The confusion lies in determining what constitutes primary care for a woman. The purpose of this chapter is to guide you through the maze of decisions you need to make as a medical consumer, and to help you maximize the use of both a gynecologist and a primary care physician. Also highlighted is the range of specialists most women are likely to encounter at some point in their lifetime.

Who Should Be Your Primary Care Physician?

Gynecologists are doctors who specialize in caring for a woman's reproductive organs (her vagina, uterus, cervix, fallopian tubes, and ovaries) as well as her breasts (they will do breast examinations and perform mammograms, but usually do not treat breast cancer). Some residency programs now include breast care, though. *Are these the only parts that require care?* Apparently 7 out of 10 women think so.

Many gynecologists serve as excellent primary care physicians. A 1985 study found that, with the exception of cholesterol screening, obstetrician-gynecologists (OB-Gyns) perform what are considered primary care services for women on a more routine basis than traditional primary care physicians. During a routine visit, OB-Gyns are much more likely to do breast, pelvic, and rectal exams, cervical cancer screenings (Pap smears), blood pressure checks, and urine testing than are general practitioners (an M.D. with four years of medical school and one year of internship), family practitioners (an M.D. with four years of medical school and up to three years of residency training in general/family medicine), or internists (an M.D. with four years of medical school and up to three years of residency training in nonsurgical treatment of several different illnesses). In a competitive industry, many gynecologists, as specialists, have been forced into a generalist role because of real financial pressure to keep women's primary care dollars in their pockets.

When you consider that a gynecologist has only *one year* of training in general medicine and *three years* of training in obstetrics and gynecology, is it wise to use a gynecologist for primary care? Meanwhile, a family practitioner or internist spends *three or more years* training to become a primary care doctor.

The Doctor Wars

As medical consumers, women are caught in an ongoing debate between gynecologists and family practitioners. On the one hand, many gynecologists argue that since they specialize in women's health, why does a woman need to go elsewhere? They are far more qualified to perform gynecological exams than are family practitioners who may have only minimal training in gynecology. The truth is that gynecologists specialize only in women's *reproductive* health. What if a patient has a heart condition, diabetes, high blood pressure, epilepsy, or thyroid disease? Is a gynecologist more qualified to handle all of these conditions when he or she is not trained to do so?

On the other hand, family practitioners feel they are more qualified to assess the bigger picture, juggle a cross section of different health concerns, refer patients to a variety of specialists when necessary (including a gynecologist), and provide basic gynecological care—the same way they provide care in other health areas. (After all, do you insist on seeing a cardiologist to get a routine cardiovascular checkup? Or an endocrinologist for a routine diabetes screening?)

The job of a family practitioner or internist is to act as your "general contractor," overseeing and managing your entire health structure and deciding when to call in the "experts." When it's time for a special job, they'll refer you to a gynecologist, nutritionist, endocrinologist, oncologist (cancer specialist), physical therapist, or whoever. A gynecologist is best utilized as a specialist, because that's what they've been trained to be.

As a sexually active woman, you need two physicians: a primary care physician in the form of a good family practitioner, general practitioner, or internist (see Plan A below), and a gynecologist. The gynecologist can be someone you've found on your own, or you can ask your family doctor to recommend one or two. Each time you see one doctor, make sure he or she sends a copy of all of his or her latest findings to the other.

If you are in a high-risk category for gynecological problems (you have a history of cancer, have been sexually abused, or are a DES daughter, see pg. 61), Plan B is more appropriate for you.

Plan A: Using Your Family Physician as a Basic Gynecologist

Using your family doctor for *basic* gynecological care is just fine if you're healthy and have never had any gynecological problems, such as cancer, positive Pap smears, or sexually transmitted diseases (STDs). But, if your primary care doctor doesn't do pelvic exams on most of his or her female patients, this is a sign that he or she isn't as qualified to manage your basic gynecological care as a primary care physician who does. When the service is offered, however, this can be an ideal option. Your family physician can perform routine Pap smears and pelvic exams, provide you with contraceptive options, and advise you on family planning (pelvic exams and Pap smears are discussed later in this chapter). All of these fall under primary care for a sexually active woman and are usually performed when you go for your annual checkup. You can also see your family doctor for garden-variety vaginal or vulvar irritations, yeast infections, and bladder infections.

During an annual checkup, your family doctor will also check your overall health: Your cholesterol, hemoglobin, and hormone levels will be screened, you'll provide a urine sample, and your cardiovascular health, reflexes, eyesight, and hearing will be checked. As with any serious problem, your family doctor will refer you to a gynecologist or a gynecologist with a *subspecialty* if he or she finds anything abnormal in your gynecological exam, such as a positive Pap test, a particularly nasty yeast infection, an unexplained vulvar irritation, pelvic pain, difficult periods or irregular cycles, problems with fertility, or irregular bleeding. The beauty of a family doctor is that he or she is trained to pinpoint the specialist you need. For a fertility problem, you would more likely be sent to a reproductive endocrinologist who specializes in hormones, or a gynecologist who subspecializes in reproductive endocrinology. If you had a positive Pap smear in Canada, you'd be referred to a gynecologic oncologist for a colposcopy. In the United States, you'd probably be sent to a normal gynecologist who does colposcopy.

In the United States, a family doctor will also refer you to an obstetrician when you're pregnant. Malpractice insurance goes up when doctors practice obstetrics. For this reason, to avoid the risk, as do many gynecologists, most American family doctors don't even attempt to practice obstetrics (even though they're qualified). Yet in Canada, family physicians will very often manage all aspects of a normal pregnancy and refer patients to obstetricians only when there's a problem. (Appropriate doctors during pregnancy are discussed in chapter 10.)

Let's say you have a more "colorful" gynecological medical history. As long as you've been treated successfully for your condition under the supervision of a gynecologist and have had three to six normal Pap tests and pelvic exams, you can resume basic gynecological care under your family physician. Make sure that your gynecologist sends your family doctor a complete record of your previous diagnoses, treatment, and current gynecological status.

Even though you're under the care of a family physician, you should shop for a gynecologist and "register" as a patient when you find a good one. That way, if there *is* a problem down the road, you'll already have a gynecologist in place. There's nothing worse than having a gynecological emergency and having to be treated by someone with whom you're unfamiliar.

The benefits of Plan A are as follows:

- *You have the benefit of two gynecological perspectives: those of your family doctor and your gynecologist.* In the event of a minor problem, if you're not satisfied with your family doctor's explanation or recommendation, you can go for a second opinion, or vice versa.

- *Your overall health will be better managed.* Because family doctors are trained longer in general medicine (with the exception of a general practitioner), you'll receive better primary care with a good family doctor.
- *Better access.* Family doctors are often more accessible than specialists. They're not as heavily booked, are usually free to take phone calls or book last-minute appointments, and can spend more time with you.
- *A more intimate relationship.* Family doctors are more aware of your family medical history because they often treat other members of your family.
- *A more balanced approach to health care.* Family doctors see the big picture and are less myopic about your health care. Say, for example, that a woman with high blood pressure has small fibroid tumors. A gynecologist may recommend a hysterectomy, while a family doctor may choose only to monitor the tumors, not wanting to worsen her blood pressure by subjecting her to major surgery that isn't yet necessary.

Plan B: Separating Gynecological Care from Primary Care

This involves paying separate but equal attention to both your family doctor and your gynecologist. Tell your family doctor that you have a gynecologist who manages *all* your gynecological care, and vice versa, but request that both doctors communicate with each other about your health and report their findings on a regular basis. Then, if there's a health risk your gynecologist isn't taking into consideration when he or she recommends a certain treatment, your family doctor can alert him or her.

Your gynecologist can also be helpful in primary care diagnoses. For instance, you see your family doctor about frequent, but not chronic abdominal pain and painful bowel movements. Your family doctor may want to send you to an internist (if he or she isn't one already) or may suspect a variety of problems, and order a battery of tests to find out what's wrong. Upon communicating with your gynecologist about your situation, your gynecologist suggests that the symptoms may indicate endometriosis, and may prompt your family doctor to ask more specific, conclusive questions: "Do your pains seem to coincide with your period?" instead of the standard "When do you have these pains?" You may not have noticed the pains are coinciding with your period. Your gynecologist's interactive relationship with your family doctor would save you the time and expense of a series of unnecessary tests, and your family doctor would send you to your gynecologist for confirmation. This is the plan to take if you have a history of sexual abuse, cancer, or other gynecological problems, or if you are a DES daughter.

The benefits of Plan B are as follows:

- *You create a partnership between your family doctor and your gynecologist, not a competition.* Since each doctor is doing what he or she was trained to do, they work together to give you the best care possible. By asking a gynecologist to provide primary care, you may inadvertently create competition between the gynecologist and your family doctor (if you have one) or suffer the consequences of an unbalanced approach to health care.
- *A system of checks and balances.* If you have a question about a recommended treatment you can follow up with either one and get a second opinion. Seek out the other's opinion to confirm or alleviate your suspicions.

Guidelines for Choosing a Family Doctor

If you have the luxury of choosing any doctor you wish, or if you are on an insurance plan that offers you a wide selection of doctors, here are some general guidelines. Traditionally, family doctors treat the entire family and therefore develop an intimacy with each particular family member and familiarity with their health problems. Today, however, the family doctor's role has changed significantly in that the doctor often has no connection with the health scenario in your family. If you're in this situation, make your doctor aware of not only your own history, but your family's medical history as well.

You can also encounter problems with a doctor who has in fact treated your whole family. Often the worst thing to do is to go to your mother's doctor after you're 18. The doctor may continue to treat you like a child and may discuss your health situation with your parent(s), bypassing you in the process. If you're between the ages of 20 and 35 and uncomfortable with a doctor you've seen since childhood, explain the reasons for your discomfort and ask him or her to recommend a separate family doctor. You can also ask your gynecologist or another specialist (an allergist, for example) to recommend a family doctor, or ask your friends and neighbors for some names.

Of course, if you *are* comfortable with the same doctor who treated your mother or father, you don't have to switch, but you should make a point of *evaluating* the doctor. You may even want to see a few other doctors just to get an idea of who's out there. If you're a woman between the ages of 39 and 55, you should also re-evaluate your situation. Menopause is a very sensitive time, and the worst thing is to have a doctor who is insensitive to you. What may have worked for you in your late 20s and early 30s may not work anymore. Forget about loyalty. If you are not comfortable with your doctor, you may avoid going to him and endanger your own health in the process.

Try not to take your doctor's word as gospel. The older you are, the more abused you can become: You're given less information, you're often not treated as equally as someone closer to the doctor's age, and if English is not your first language, you may be easily intimidated. No matter how old you are, if you don't speak English well, you're at an immediate disadvantage. It's important to find a doctor who speaks your language. If you can't find one who does, call an association or organization affiliated with your ethnic origin and ask them. Should you have a female doctor or a male doctor? That's up to you. The most important factor is whether you're comfortable with your doctor. Here is a quick checklist you can use to evaluate your current comfort level:

- *What does your doctor call you?* Your doctor should call you by your first name. It's more relaxing for both of you. Some doctors even tell you to call them by their first name.
- *Can you ask your doctor questions?* How open is he or she? If you can't question your doctor, that's a bad sign.
- *Where is your doctor located?* Is the location convenient, or does it take you over an hour to get to? Waiting to see the doctor is stressful enough, but if you're hiking across the country just to go to your doctor, consider the stress involved with your doctor appointments.
- *How do you reach your doctor after hours?* Can you just pick up the phone and call him or her any time to talk about a particular health situation? If you can't, is it because the doctor is truly busy or not accessible to patients after hours? Some doctors leave a number where they can be reached in the event of an emergency.
- *If he or she weren't your doctor, would you want him or her as a friend?* If you wouldn't be caught dead having a cup of coffee with your doctor, why would you allow him or her access to your vagina?
- *Does your doctor make house calls?* If he or she does, you probably have a gem on your hands.

When Do You Need a Gynecologist?

Healthy Women

You should have your first pelvic exam after you have sexual intercourse, either vaginally or anally. This is what your doctor means when he or she asks you if you are sexually active. Although you can be a virgin and still be sexually active if you engage in heavy petting, use lubricants, vibrators, dildos, and so forth, or engage in oral sex, technically you are not sexually active until you begin having intercourse.

If you are not sexually active by the age of 18, this is still a good time to have a pelvic exam. At this point, the pelvic exam would be an opportunity to discuss future sexual activity and address questions about safe sex and contraception. It is also an opportunity for your doctor to determine any potential problems at this point. Even if you're a virgin, a pelvic exam needn't be a painful ordeal with the appropriate instruments and a sympathetic examiner. Women who use tampons can be examined quite comfortably. The pelvic exam includes the Pap test, which was invented by Dr. George Papanicolaou to detect and help prevent cervical cancer. A sample of cells that line the cervix is taken and investigated for abnormalities. The vast majority of cervical cancer is associated with one strain of an STD called *human papillomavirus* (HPV), the virus that causes genital warts. HPV invades the cervix and causes the cells on the cervical lining to change; it is usually transmitted through sexual intercourse. Today, women become sexually active anytime from 12 years of age and up (sometimes even earlier if abuse is involved). Once you enter high school, a good family doctor will start to question you regularly about your sexual activity and based on your answers, may suggest a pelvic exam before you've had intercourse and before you reach 18. When you're 18, your doctor may suggest an annual pelvic exam despite your insistence that you're not sexually active and still a virgin. Regardless of whether you're sexually active or not, when it's time for your pelvic exam, you can choose to follow either Plan A or Plan B. Both plans are fine.

Women Under 18 and Children

If you're under 18 and are or have been sexually active, you'll need to have an annual pelvic exam, as discussed above. Sexual activity before 18 includes rape and sexual abuse of any kind. For example, if you were abused as a child and the abuse stopped when you reached puberty, you'll need to have a pelvic exam as soon as possible. If you're a mother of a two-year-old child who has been abused, that child will need to have a pelvic exam. Sexual abuse need not involve intercourse. The abuser may have inserted objects or his or her fingers into the vagina. If you were abused or began having sex at a particularly young age (before 14), then Plan B is a better route for you.

DES Daughters

Any woman born in the United States between 1941 and 1971 (and perhaps just before or after that) may be a DES daughter. During this period, five million pregnant women took the drug *DES* (*diethylstilbestrol,* a synthetic estrogen) to prevent miscarriage. Any daughter born to a mother who took DES runs a higher than normal risk for reproductive organ abnormalities, cervical and vaginal cell changes, and cancer. DES Action, a nonprofit consumer group, warns that DES daughters run the risk of receiving inappropriate medical treatment because some doctors shrug off DES concerns as a thing of the past. If you are a DES daughter, you'll need to have all of your gynecological needs handled by a gynecologist rather than a family doctor. You'll also need to have a special DES pelvic exam and Pap smear, where cells from all corners of your vaginal wall and cervix are annually investigated. You're definitely a Plan B patient.

The best way to find out whether you're a DES daughter is to ask your mother if she took any drugs while she was pregnant with you. If she did, ask her if she can remember the hospital you were born in. Contact the hospital and give them your mother's name and your date of birth. Request a list of all prenatal medicine on your mother's record. You may also be able to contact your mother's old pharmacy as well. Some keep records on file for years. Your mother may also be able to contact the obstetrician or doctor who delivered you, or if that doctor is retired or deceased, the physician who took over the practice. As a last resort, call your local medical association to find out where old records are sent. Unfortunately, sometimes these records just aren't locatable.

If your mother is no longer living, it may still be worth going through the above procedures just to be sure. If your mother can't remember whether she took anything, ask her if she had any problems during her pregnancy: bleeding, miscarriages, premature labor or delivery, or diabetes. If she did, you should investigate as outlined above.

DES was administered under a host of different labels. If you can find out the name of the drugs your mother took, contact DES Action at 510-465-4011 and ask them to check if any of the drugs you discovered match the drugs on their list. DES Action has a nationwide referral service of doctors who specialize in the treatment of DES-exposed women.

The DES exam includes:

- A Pap smear not only of the cervix, but four additional smears (called a four-quadrant smear) from the vaginal walls surrounding the cervix. These smears help to determine if a biopsy (tissue sample) needs to be taken to check for clear cell cancer.
- Careful palpation (feeling) of the vaginal walls for any lumps or thickening.
- Use of an iodine stain to check the vagina and cervix for adenosis tissue, a glandular tissue not normally found in the vagina that can harbor clear cell cancer. (Regular tissue stains brown; adenosis tissue doesn't.)
- A colposcopy, which is an examination that uses a magnifying instrument to examine the cervix and vagina more closely.

How to Find a Good Gynecologist

Generally, you can find a good gynecologist the same way you find a good hairstylist: ask your friends, neighbors, relatives, and so forth. You can also find a gynecologist through a family doctor. Or, if you have another specialist you respect, such as an endocrinologist, oncologist, surgeon, chiropractor, or dentist, ask for the name of either a good family doctor (since you need one anyway) or a good gynecologist. If this specialist is a woman, who is *her* gynecologist? If this specialist is a male, who is his *wife's* gynecologist.(I found my gynecologist through a thyroid surgeon, and my family doctor was recommended by my radiotherapist, who trained her!)

Do you have a particular condition, such as endometriosis, or do you fear infertility? Contact a self-help or nonprofit association/organization and ask *them* for names. Are you an immigrant? Perhaps you don't speak English very well? Contact your local ethnic association and ask if they have a list of doctors who speak your language.

When you do find a gynecologist you like, here are some questions you should ask when you go for your first visit:

1. *Are you board-certified?* This means that he or she has completed a residency training program that has met the standards set by ABOG.

There's a 1 in 2.5 chance that any gynecologist you see is not board-certified. To check a doctor's credentials, call the American Board of Medical Specialties at 1-800-776-CERT during business hours. They can tell you whether any doctor, regardless of specialty, is board-certified.

2. *Are you board-certified in any subspecialty?* Does your gynecologist handle gynecologic oncology, maternal and fetal care, reproduction and endocrinology? In the United States, most gynecologists manage some kind of gynecologic oncology and reproductive endocrinology. In Canada, you'd need a referral to a subspecialist. Try to find at least one that does gynecologic oncology. If you're sexually active, chances are you'll have at least *one* positive Pap experience in your lifetime. (Pap tests are discussed below.)
3. *Do you do obstetrics?* Not all gynecologists do. If you're planning to get pregnant, this might be a good idea. If you're finished with your family, or are living childfree, then your visits won't be interrupted by deliveries.
4. *What kind of hospital privileges do you have?* Full operating privileges are best.
5. *Do you share copies of medical records and test results with your patients at their request?* If he or she won't, that's a bad sign.
6. *Are you available for occasional phone calls?* Find out if the doctor is accessible or if you have to make an appointment just to ask him or her a question.
7. (If he's male) *Is a female assistant present in the room when you perform a pelvic exam?* If not, would you object if I brought along a friend or my spouse? If the male doctor performs "solo pelvics" only, that's a bad sign.
8. *What's your philosophy on hysterectomies?* Do you feel a woman's reproductive organs are worth preserving? You'd better find out so you can avoid becoming the next "unnecessary hysterectomy" statistic.
9. *How do you feel about hormone replacement therapy? Abortion? At what age do you recommend annual mammograms?* All of these questions are important issues. The response you get will tell you about the doctor's ethics and flexibility, as well as expose his or her level of skill, education, and awareness regarding women's health issues.

The Pelvic Exam

A pelvic exam is the most vulnerable procedure a woman may undergo. It's crucial that you know what to expect in this exam and who is qualified to perform it. I've included some excerpts from my own and other women's experiences just to give you some insight into how common mistreatment is. Only in the last five years or so have women been encouraged to report mistreatment from a gynecologist. This is partly because the boundaries of what constituted mistreatment were gray, and partly because women were ashamed of their experiences and made to feel somewhat responsible for them.

Who Should Perform It?

A family practitioner, internist, general practitioner, and, of course, any gynecologist is qualified to perform a pelvic exam. A medical student, intern, or resident should not be allowed to perform a pelvic exam unless a senior practitioner qualified to perform a pelvic exam is in the room or supervising.

You'd be surprised how many women allow *anyone* wearing a white coat access to her vagina—myself included. For example, after I had been admitted to a hospital for major surgery, a fourth-year male medical student entered the room to take my medical history. That's fine. He asked me what procedures I had in the past year in which I was put under a general anesthetic. It so happened that a few months earlier, I required a minor gynecological procedure under a general anesthetic. Trying to be a good patient, I disclosed to him that I had had this procedure. "What was it?" he asked. I told him. "Okay," he said, "lie down and take off your panties, please. I just want to have a look." Foolishly, and blindly trusting that this was standard procedure, I did as he asked. No female assistant was in the room, and this student was not even a licensed doctor yet—and certainly not qualified to be anywhere *near* my vagina without a senior practitioner present. The student never actually performed a "routine" pelvic exam with a speculum (see below), but he opened up the vaginal lips and took a look. This was, in fact, misconduct. At the time, in 1983, there weren't any strict rules in place about a female being present in the room. Even then, this form of misconduct was accepted. I myself didn't consider this misconduct until years later. For the record, a male doctor, regardless of his credentials, should *never* perform a pelvic exam without a female assistant or colleague in the room. It's foolish for both yourself and the doctor. If there isn't a female available, it's your right to refuse the procedure until suitable arrangements can be made. Don't let anyone tell you otherwise.

A female doctor, however, can perform the exam alone, with no one in the room except you and her. The reasons for this seemingly biased rule are obvious. To date, there have been no reports of female-to-female sexual abuse recorded during a pelvic exam. If you do happen to be a lesbian, and you know for a fact that your doctor is also a lesbian, you might inquire about requesting another female in the room during a pelvic exam. If you know for a fact that your male doctor is gay, you still need to have a female present in the room.

What to Expect

Before the actual pelvic exam begins, whoever is performing the exam may ask you some questions about your gynecological history: your family's history of breast cancer or cancer of the reproductive organs, details about your menstrual cycle, whether you're sexually active and have ever been pregnant, whether you use contraception, and whether you've ever had STDs, as well as questions about your general health. Sometimes they might (and should) ask you about your mental health history. They will probably do some routine things, such as taking your blood pressure, urine sample, weight, pulse, and so forth.

You'll then be asked to take off your panties and sometimes your bra (for a breast exam) and lie down on an examination table, placing your feet in two metal stirrups, which are semicircles that hold your feet in place. (You may want to urinate first. The exam sometimes can put pressure on your bladder and you'll feel like you need to "go.") The stirrups are there to support your feet. Some doctors have "stirrup mitts" that make the stirrups less cold and uncomfortable. Other doctors have cartoons on their ceilings as a pleasant distraction. A sheet covers you, and the doctor will lift the sheet and work under it. The sheet is provided for comfort and modesty purposes. Depending on where you are, a nurse practitioner may take your history and ask you to undress and have you wait for the doctor. If the doctor is male, the nurse will stay (or enter at this point) and perhaps even assist. If the doctor is female, the nurse will leave.

The doctor will first do a breast exam, checking your breasts and armpits for any lumps. Your breasts will be pressed and squeezed so the doctor can feel for anything unusual. The doctor will also squeeze your nipples to make sure there is no discharge. The doctor should also check your thyroid gland for any enlargement or nodules. The doctor will feel your abdomen, pressing down and feeling the size and consistency of your internal organs, spleen, and liver.

Then the actual pelvic exam begins. You'll be asked to slide down toward the stirrups until you're in a squatting position. The doctor should put on surgical gloves. The doctor will visually inspect your vulva, looking for irritation, herpes sores, genital warts—anything suspicious. The doctor will gently spread the folds of skin around your vagina.

Next, the doctor will insert a speculum, a metal or plastic device resembling a duckbill with a handle. It comes in four sizes, and the doctor will choose the right size for you. If you've never had intercourse, you'll need the smallest size. The device is opened up inside you so that the doctor can see your cervix and the inside of your vagina clearly. The speculum also allows the doctor to insert other instruments into your vagina without constantly touching the vaginal walls, which can irritate them. The doctor checks your cervix for redness, discharge, and rough spots, which could mean precancerous cell changes.(If you've never been sexually active, you may request that the doctor postpone this portion of the exam until you are, for the reasons discussed above.) Most doctors run warm water over the speculum to warm it, and lubricate it before inserting it. If your doctor doesn't, you might want to suggest it. Many doctors will also insert a lubricant into your vagina for comfort, but if a Pap smear is being done, no lubricants should be used because they can taint the test results.

The doctor will then do a Pap smear, which is discussed in detail below. The doctor will then take out the speculum and insert one or two gloved, lubricated fingers into the vagina until they are against the cervix. Then, with his or her other hand, the doctor will press on your abdomen, feeling the size and shape of your uterus and checking for masses that might be on your ovaries or fallopian tubes. Finally, the doctor may insert one gloved, lubricated finger into your rectum and one into your vagina. This makes it easier for him or her to feel your ovaries. It also allows the doctor to check for signs of endometriosis, abscesses, and tumors. The doctor should tell you what he or she is doing each step of the way, and what he or she is finding as he or she goes along. If everything is normal, you can get up and get dressed, and your doctor will tell you that you'll be notified about the Pap test results only if they're abnormal. (It's always a good idea to follow up. Call the office yourself in two weeks to make sure that the Pap smear is normal.) If there is a problem, the doctor will have you get dressed and will ask you into her/his office for a further discussion.

When You Suspect Misconduct

There are two kinds of misconduct: attitude misconduct and practice misconduct. Attitude misconduct includes uncalled-for remarks and rudeness, inappropriate jokes, or comments about your appearance ("Anyone ever tell you you're a beautiful woman?" or "You ought to do something about your facial hair!") or questions about your sexual habits that have *nothing* to do with your gynecological health. For example, asking you if you have orgasms, perform fellatio, or masturbate are inappropriate unless you have specifically requested advice on your sex life; asking you whether you have anal sex or practice contraception *is* relevant, however, and *does* have bearing on your gynecological health. If you're tense during the exam your doctor shouldn't yell at you or rudely command you to relax. A doctor who discloses to you details about his or her own personal life that make you uncomfortable, or a doctor who chats with the assistant present in the room during your exam and ignores *you*, is mistreating you.

Here's an example of misconduct from one of my mother's pelvic exams, circa 1975. After undressing and placing her feet in stirrups, her gynecologist entered the room, looked her over, and said: "Apparently, any problems you're experiencing down *there* haven't interfered with your appetite!" Even more shocking is the fact that my mother, an intelligent and sophisticated woman, thought that was *funny*.

If you suspect attitude misconduct, go back to the person who referred you and find out if there are similar complaints. If you were referred by a friend who's also a patient, ask her how the doctor behaves during your friend's pelvic exams. If you were referred by a doctor, recount the misconduct and see what he or she thinks. That way you can decipher whether the doctor's behavior is unusual in your case or whether you just clash. Usually, attitude misconduct doesn't cause any physical damage, but if you feel your misconduct has caused you to seek out therapy, you may have been damaged. Call the ABOG or the American College of Obstetricians and Gynecologists and ask to speak to someone in standards and practices. Report the mistreatment and find out if you have grounds for complaints and further action. In Canada, call the provincial College of Physicians and Surgeons and ask for the standards and practices department.

Practice misconduct includes doctors performing a pelvic exam when they're not qualified; male doctors performing a pelvic exam without the presence of a female assistant; any kind of inappropriate touching or fondling during the exam; not using surgical gloves; using the wrong-size speculum, which can tear your vagina or damage your vaginal walls; suggesting surgical procedures on the spot (I've just perfected a technique that enhances clitoral stimulation during sex. I can do it right now if you like!") ignoring a symptom that concerns you ("Painful cramps are normal. You're just oversensitive to pain," or "I can tell right now that this is not a cancerous lump. You're overreacting. Just leave it alone."); refusal to answer your questions; and ordering diagnostic tests without explaining the procedures to you.

Remember my mother's rude gynecologist? Guess who saw him for a yeast infection when she was 16? Since it was my first visit, the doctor, a man in his 60s, asked me some questions about my sexual activity:

"Are you a virgin?"

"Yes."

"DON'T *LIE* TO ME!"

"I'm not lying."

"What were you *doing* down there that makes you think you have a yeast infection?"

And so on. I was terrified, but at the time (1979) had no way of knowing that I was being mistreated. It got worse. The doctor believed I had actually lied about my virginity. He inserted an adult-size speculum into my vagina (of course, there was no female present in the room, either). My vaginal opening was so small at the time that I had difficulty using a tampon. I screamed in pain. The doctor took out the speculum and quickly inserted a child-size speculum. "Well, you certainly weren't lying about being a virgin, that's for sure!" In 1993 this doctor would have had his license revoked. And in retrospect, it's amazing I didn't require years of psychiatric treatment. But these examples of blatant practice misconduct constitute volumes of gynecological history. The experience recounted above isn't even unusual.

Practice misconduct is often a gray area. If you leave a gynecological appointment feeling uneasy and unsure why you're having a procedure, your gynecologist hasn't given you a satisfactory explanation. Or, if you leave the office with a bad taste in your mouth and are hesitant to return, something is wrong. Retrace the exam and try to figure out what made you so uncomfortable about the visit. Usually there's a reason for your uneasiness.

The Pap Test

The Pap smear determines only the condition of the cervix. It's done once a year because that creates a greater likelihood of picking up changes in the cervix. Cervical cancer can take up to 10 years to develop. So if you have a Pap test once a year and it does happen to come back positive (meaning only that something "fishy" was detected, not that you *have* cancer), you'll be treated for your condition before it has a chance to develop into cancer. A Pap smear can also pick up yeast and HPV, which causes genital warts. In fact, certain people can have HPV present without ever developing warts, and certain strains of HPV are more likely to cause cells lining the cervix to change. A Pap smear can also detect cell changes on the vaginal wall, which are signs of vaginal cancer.

To do a Pap smear, the doctor inserts an instrument that looks like a mascara brush and gently scrapes some cells off your cervix. The doctor will then smear the cells onto a glass slide and spray the slide with a fixative, a chemical that preserves the cells' state. The slide is then sent to a laboratory, where it will be examined under a microscope for signs of cancer, infection, and inflammation. Your doctor may also use a long Q-tip to do the Pap smear or a spatula-type instrument.

A Pap test is used only for determining cancer and should not be confused with a "wet prep" (called a swab in Canada), in which a long Q-tip is inserted and used to soak up discharge to diagnose for yeast, trichomoniasis, bacterial vaginosis (a.k.a. gardinerella), or other vaginal infections (see chapter 6). A separate swab is used to obtain cultures for chlamydia and gonorrhea. There's a newer test for chlamydia that requires a swabbing inside the cervical canal. When you see your doctor for any kind of irritation, infection, or discharge, this is when you'll be swabbed. In fact, the Pap test is not done (at least it shouldn't be) when there's an infection.

As discussed earlier, anyone who is sexually active needs a Pap test once a year. Women who are at higher risk of developing cervical abnormalities include: women who have had more than two partners in their lifetime (most of us!); women who had sexual intercourse before age 20; smokers; women with a history of genital warts; and women who are HIV positive (see chapter 5 for more details).

Getting Positive or Negative Results

If your Pap smear comes back *negative,* then it was normal or *clear.* If it comes back *positive,* it can mean a whole bunch of things. It may have picked up an infection, such as HPV, herpes, or yeast, which can cause inflammation of the cervix, known as *cervicitis.* In this case, your doctor will treat and repeat. First, he or she will treat the infection, then ask you to repeat the Pap smear to make sure the infection has cleared up. If it hasn't, you may be referred to a colposcopist (see below). Depending on where you live, there are two ways your Pap test results will be classified. In the United States, the most current system is called the Bethesda System. Prior to 1993, some regions in North America, as well as outside the continent, may still have been using the older, Papanicolaou classifications, indicated in the brackets below.

In the Bethesda System, your Pap smear is classified into various descriptions: "normal"; "atypical squamous cells or glandular cells of undetermined significance," which means that your Pap smear has picked up something unusual, but that nothing may be necessarily wrong; "low grade or high grade squamous intraepithelial lesion," which means that the cells are growing in an inappropriate manner (a.k.a. CIN 1—*cervical intraepithelial neoplasm* or *mild dysplasia,* CIN 2, or CIN 3—ranging from *moderate to severe dysplasia).* A Pap smear will also pick up *cervical carcinoma insitu,* a precancer, and *invasive cervical cancer,* which means that your cancer may be limited to the cervix, but may be in a more advanced stage.

Essentially, anything short of invasive cervical cancer is really akin to your dashboard "emergency indicator" light going on while you're driving; there's more than enough time to drive to a service station and fix the problem. Here, the indicator light goes on as a warning to get the problem diagnosed and looked after. When the Pap smear detects invasive cancer, this is more like blowing out a tire on the road; the problem *is* fixable, but it needs to be tended to immediately before you can drive any farther.

When the Pap smear picks up harmless, abnormal cells, called *benign atypia,* you'll need to repeat the test in six months' time. Benign atypia usually clears up on its own. If this is the case, you'll simply repeat the Pap in a year, as you normally would. If benign atypia persists, you'll be referred to a colposcopist.

Occasionally, with mild dysplasia and a clean Pap history, the family doctor or gynecologist may simply choose to repeat the test and see if it clears up on its own. If you have moderate to severe dysplasia, you'll be referred to a colposcopist for further investigation.

Colposcopy is the most common referral in gynecology. The incidence of positive Pap smears has skyrocketed in the last 10 years. Not only has sexual behavior changed, but more women are going for Paps. As a result, we're able to pick up more cervical abnormalities *because* of the Pap. Death from cervical cancer has dropped dramatically, however, since the test was introduced.

Colposcopy

If you've been referred to a colposcopist, chances are either you have HPV (condyloma) or you have dysplasia. Both of these conditions are precancerous and have been known to *develop* into cancer, but are not yet cancerous. In a colposcopy, an instrument is used that allows the cervix to be viewed microscopically. Before viewing, the cervix will be stained with vinegar. Most American gynecologists perform colposcopy, but in Canada those that do usually subspecialize in gynecologic oncology. Because of the frequency of colposcopy, most gynecologists and many family doctors are now upgrading their skills and training to perform it. Your colposcopist may at this point want to do a biopsy (described below). Depending on what he or she finds, you may require treatment for your condition in the form of loop electrocision procedure (LEEP) discussed below, laser therapy, cryosurgery, or a type of sloughing cream. For mild dysplasia, you may just be followed with a Pap smear and colposcopy. When you first meet your colposcopist, ask the following questions:

1. *What did my Pap smear show?* This will tell you whether you have an infection, CIN, dysplasia, and so forth. Then you'll be able to better gauge whether the treatment your doctor suggests is reasonable.
2. *Is it possible that the lab report was wrong?* A 1987 *Wall Street Journal* report found that a large majority of Pap smears were sent to cut-rate labs with overworked, underpaid technicians. A large percentage of Pap tests are currently inaccurate. You could wind up being treated for a condition that would have cleared up on its own, or worse, pass your Pap test when you should have failed. Ask your doctor if your Pap smear was analyzed by a lab that is certified by the American College of Pathologists or American Society of Cytologists. If the answer is no, request a second opinion from a lab that *is*. Then, if both reports come back the same, you can be sure you're being treated appropriately. Even a properly obtained and properly inter-

preted Pap smear can be falsely positive or falsely negative. A false positive results because the problem may resolve between the time you have the Pap and the time you see the colposcopist. The worst problem with a false positive is the anxiety and expense. The danger with a false negative smear is that a significant problem may not be diagnosed and treated. False negatives can result if the abnormality is too high in the cervix for the Pap smear to reach it or if it's not shedding abnormal cells for some reason. Because of the possibility of a false negative, it's best to have regular Pap smears performed. It's unlikely that you'll have two false negatives in a row.

Biopsy

Once you're comfortable that your Pap smear was analyzed correctly, your colposcopist will most likely do a cervical biopsy. This means that he or she will remove bits of tissue from the cervix, using a colposcope. This procedure can take anywhere from 5 to 20 minutes. It is relatively painless. The tissue samples look like pieces of grain or rice and are obtained with an instrument that looks like a hole puncher. At this point, the colposcopist will also scrape cells from the cervical canal, and send them to a pathologist for examination. It is possible to have a negative biopsy with a positive Pap smear. This means that your condition may have cleared up on its own or that your Pap smear is inconclusive. You may not require any further treatment and be asked to repeat your Pap test again in about three months to see if the condition either has cleared up or remains clear. This negative biopsy/positive Pap smear combination is rare, but it does happen. You will most likely have a positive biopsy and will need treatment.

Treatment

If your biopsy comes back positive, it simply means that you do have cell changes on your cervix. It does *not* mean you have cancer. There are three kinds of treatment available for cell abnormalities on the cervix: cryosurgery, laser surgery, and sloughing cream. In cryosurgery, the lesions or cells on the surface of the cervix are destroyed by freezing via nitrogen gas. With laser surgery, the lesions are vaporized with a carbon dioxide laser. With either procedure you may have bleeding and cramping afterward. If you're told that the procedure is painless, it's not true.

If you take a nonsteroidal painkiller prior to the procedure, it really helps. Another treatment option is an external sloughing cream called *5-fluorouracil* (5-FU, or Efudex) that has been used in the past for skin cancers, and essentially gives your cervix a "facial." You insert the sloughing cream with an applicator, and the surface cells will slough off your cervix. The cream may cause a burning sensation on the outer portions of your vagina or vulva. This can be easily prevented by coating your vulva and outer lips with Penaton cream, a thick cream used for diaper rash.

Laser surgery is the third option. Here, your cells are removed with a laser. A newer procedure, known as loop electrocision procedure (LEEP), involves a wire that cuts through the cervix easily, producing a far lower infection rate and superior healing. The benefit of laser surgery is that you may need only one treatment; 95% of the time cryosurgery requires only one treatment. If you choose to use the sloughing cream, you can apply it yourself at home, and you'll need to see the doctor only for Pap tests. Treatment for cancer of the cervix is discussed in chapter 9, but most times you're referred to a colposcopist for a precancerous condition. After a suitable number of clear Pap smears and normal pelvic exams (anywhere from 3 to 6), whoever is performing the colposcopy will decide when to send you back to the doctor who is handling your basic gynecological care.

How to Use a Primary Care Physician

As you may have guessed by now, I'm a big fan of family physicians. There's a right way and a wrong way to use them, however. Regardless of whether your primary care physician is a family practitioner, a general practitioner, a gynecologist, or an internist, that doctor *is* your family doctor. Since your family doctor is often the first doctor you'll see about a gynecological problem, it's crucial that you understand the role a family doctor plays in today's health care system. Whenever you're not well, it's your family doctor who initiates the diagnostic process, which may include referrals to a specialist. Because medicine *is* a business, doctors are very concerned about costs, so they try not to order too many tests or "unnecessary" procedures. This can leave you misdiagnosed.

As a patient, you have to be responsible for making sure your doctor is acting in your best interests. To do this, you have to assert your rights and act responsibly. For example, if you keep certain information about your medical history hidden from your doctor, you can't expect your doctor to make an accurate diagnosis. Similarly, if you don't ask questions about your health, you can't expect your doctor to read your mind and give you all the answers.

The Wrong Way

Here's a classic example of how a misdiagnosis occurs. You are a single, 30-year-old woman with classic endometriosis symptoms but don't know it. In this case, your endometrial tissue growths are small and cannot be felt externally by the doctor. An accurate reporting of symptoms (that is, pains coinciding with periods) and a laparoscopy would easily confirm the diagnosis. You've had painful bowel movements every so often, and regular pains in your "stomach" (actually, they're in your lower abdomen, where your ovaries are located, but you're unaware of this). The pains are frequent but sporadic—you never know when they'll strike. You think you might have an ulcer.

Concerned, you decide to set up an appointment with your family doctor. You call the office and are asked by the receptionist what the nature of your visit is. You're embarrassed about your symptoms and simply say that it's "just a checkup." The receptionist is asking you about the nature of your visit so that he or she will know *how much time you'll need* with the doctor. By not being up front, you've just cut your appointment time in half without knowing it. Routine checkups usually require about 15 minutes.

On the day of your appointment, you arrive to discover that the doctor's office is packed. She's overbooked again. When she's finally ready, you go into the examination room.

DOCTOR: *And how are we this morning?*
(Translation: The doctor wants to know if you're there for a particular problem.)
PATIENT: *I've been finding lately that I have these pains.*

DOCTOR: *Where do you feel the pain?*
(Translation: I probably need more time with you, but it's too late now. I hope you'll be specific.)
PATIENT: *In my stomach.*

DOCTOR: *I see. How frequent are these pains?*
(Translation: You're being too vague.)
PATIENT: *Well, I don't get them all the time, just sometimes.*
(Translation: Just often enough to notice. I haven't been keeping track.)

DOCTOR: *Do the pains coincide with a particular food? Do you get it after you eat something?*
(Translation: I'm going to take a wild stab here and investigate gastrointestinal disorders, such as ulcers, or food allergies, such as lactose intolerance.)
PATIENT: *I'm not sure.*
(Translation: I haven't been keeping track.)

DOCTOR: *I see from your chart that you just had a physical last month. You didn't complain about these pains then, did you?*
(Translation: Obviously this pain is recent, not chronic.)
PATIENT: *No, I guess I didn't.*
(Translation: I *did* have the pain, but I didn't bother mentioning it because I thought it would go away. I didn't want to pay for any extra tests.)

DOCTOR: *Are your periods regular?*
(Translation: Are the pains connected to your period?)
PATIENT: *Yes.*
(Translation: I haven't a clue. My periods are so irregular I've lost track. But how it would look to tell the doctor I can't remember when I last had a period?)

DOCTOR: *Painful urination or bowel movements?*
(Translation: Nope. No connection to her period. Let's try again.)
PATIENT: *Sometimes my bowel movements are painful, come to think of it.*
(Translation: I should have told her this earlier. Now I look like a complete airhead!)

DOCTOR: *When do you get painful bowel movements? Do they seem to coincide with your stomach pain?*
(Translation: Give me something to work with here. Your symptoms are still too general.)

As the doctor questions you, she feels and presses all

around your stomach to see if anything feels enlarged or if the pain comes back. It doesn't.

PATIENT: *I don't know . . . Wait . . . no. I don't think they do.*

(Translation: I never thought about a connection. I don't want to waste her time. I'll just say no.)

DOCTOR: *Have you been under any stress lately? Problems at work or at home?*

(Translation: This could be stress-related. Gas, stomach acid, and so on.)

PATIENT: *No. Everything's fine.*

(Translation: It's not just stress!)

DOCTOR: *OK. I think I've got enough information. I would like to order some tests to get to the bottom of this. I'm going to schedule an ultrasound, and I want you to give me a stool sample. If nothing shows up, we'll just sit tight and wait until the pains come back. As soon as they do, give me a call, and we'll take a look then.*

(Translation: You're giving me zero to work with. I'll make sure you don't have an ulcer and that your stools are clear. Next time, come back when the pain is actually there, and maybe I can find something.)

The problem here is that both your time and the doctor's time have been wasted. You gave the doctor too little information to work with, and as a result, the doctor was only able to eliminate the obvious problems, not connecting pain to your menstrual cycle. In addition, the ultrasound she ordered won't show any small endometrial tissue implants. Ultrasound tests aren't very good tools for diagnosing endometriosis, unless the disease is already quite advanced.

You clearly were not very aware of your own body and weren't paying enough attention to other clues that would have given the doctor more to work with. Not connecting the pains to your period was a key missing link. Because you hadn't kept track of *when* your pain occurred, you are uncertain about connecting the symptoms. Since your periods are irregular, the pain may not come back for weeks, and when it does, by the time you call the doctor and make an appointment again, the pain will have subsided as your period ends. You will probably be continually dismissed or sent for the wrong tests until your next pelvic exam, which may or may not turn up something. The endometriosis may worsen, and infertility could set in. You may not notice the infertility until it's too late.

The Right Way

Whenever you notice *any* kind of pain or general symptom, the best thing you can do is chart your symptoms as they correspond to your menstrual cycle. Then, you can immediately link certain pains or symptoms to certain times in your cycle, or conclude that the symptoms *don't* correspond to your cycle. This will prevent your doctor from diagnosing in the wrong direction. Do a mental check of other things you've noticed so that you can give your doctor more than just one general symptom to work with. Try to answer at least some of the following questions:

Q. Am I looking different than usual? How?
A. I seem to look more bloated.

Q. Has my morning and evening bathroom routine (e.g., washing up and so forth) changed at all? Am I going through certain products faster than usual?
A. I seem to be using more pads than usual (maybe that's because your periods are heavier than usual), and I seem to be using more Tylenol (you're using more painkillers).

Q. Am I going to the bathroom more or less often than usual? If so, when?
A. I seem to be constipated around my periods, and then have pain when I try to go.

Q. Am I eating differently than usual to cause this, or trying to eat differently to remedy this situation?
A. I do eat All-Bran when I'm constipated, but the pain is still there. (So, despite your efforts to correct your diet, the pain still persists.)

Q. Am I feeling different than usual?
A. I'm feeling more bloated.

Q. Am I dressing differently than usual?
A. I always wear an elasticized waist now. (Perhaps you've gained more weight or experience discomfort when you wear tighter, more restricting clothing.)

Q. Did my grandmother, mother, or father suffer from any kind of condition or ailment when she or he was around my age?

A. My mother had difficulty getting pregnant after I was born. That's why I'm an only child. My mother is also an only child. I wonder if her mother had trouble getting pregnant, too?

Q. Have you been under any unusual stress lately?
A. No. (Now you can rule out stress-related symptoms.)

When you do it this way, you've taken a lot of the routine guesswork out of your doctor visit and can help the doctor get to bottom of your symptoms faster. Let's replay that earlier visit:

DOCTOR: *How are you this morning?*

Go for it! Don't hold back. Give her as much information as you possibly can. Symptoms run in groups, and you want to get the doctor thinking about things that go together.

PATIENT: *I'm actually not that great. I haven't noticed any change in my daily routine, and I'm not under more stress, but I'm finding that I seem to have pains in my stomach and painful bowel movements with my periods. My flow is also a lot heavier, and I seem to be more bloated before my periods than I usually am. I also get more constipated around my periods. At first I thought that the pain was just drier stools, but even when I'm on a high-fiber diet the pain is still there during periods. I don't know if* this *means anything, but I do know my mother and grandmother had difficulty getting pregnant around my age. Do you think there's any connection?*

DOCTOR: *You say the pains are in your stomach, or are they a little lower, just above your hips?*

(Translation: She may be confusing her stomach with her entire pelvic region. I'd better make sure.)

PATIENT: *The pains are just above my hips. Isn't that my stomach?*

DOCTOR: *Actually, that's where your ovaries and uterus sit. Because you're getting these pains with your periods, I don't think they have anything to do with stomach problems; I think they're originating in your uterus. I'm going to schedule an appointment with your gynecologist. Let's see what he can turn up before I go any further.*

Wonderful. You haven't hit the nail on the head exactly, but this way the doctor is a lot "warmer" than in the first scenario and has determined the source of your problem. These kinds of symptoms still could involve some guesswork, but because you revealed a little bit about your family medical history in conjunction with your own symptoms, the doctor has some idea of the kinds of conditions you may be prone to. Remember, endometriosis does run in families, and if you recall a long line of only children, it's a sign that infertility may run in your family.

From this point on, the doctor will probably ask more specific questions about your condition to try to get an even clearer picture. Every time you see him or her write something down on your chart, ask about it. "What are you writing on my chart? Why is this or that significant?" In other words, don't be afraid to challenge the doctor. Ask questions. If you don't understand something, keep asking until you do.

DOCTOR: *Are you currently sexually active?*
(Translation: How fertile are you?)
PATIENT: *Yes.*

DOCTOR: *Are you using any contraception?*
PATIENT: *I've been in a monogamous relationship for the past two years, so we're just using foam.*
(Translation: I don't know why they say foam isn't enough on its own. It works great for me.)

DOCTOR: *No condoms or diaphragms?*
(Translation: Foam isn't very effective. I'm concerned that you may not be *able* to conceive.)
PATIENT: *No. The foam seems to be very effective.*

DOCTOR: *How often are you having sex?*
(Translation: Is it just blind luck that you haven't gotten pregnant?)
PATIENT: *A few times a week. What are you writing on my chart?*

DOCTOR: *I'm just noting that despite inadequate contraception, conception* hasn't *occurred.*
PATIENT: *Well doesn't the fact that I haven't gotten pregnant mean that the foam is working?*

DOCTOR: *No. It simply means that you're not getting pregnant.*

PATIENT: *You mean you think I* can't *get pregnant?*

Depending on your doctor, he or she might try to end your line of questioning to avoid you from panicking or jumping to conclusions, or he or she may have a time constraint. But don't stop. Remind the doctor who's in charge of your body. If things get really bad, ask him or her for some literature on the subject or a number you can call for more information.

DOCTOR: *Look, there's nothing to worry about yet. I'm just making some routine observations. I want to wait and see what the gynecologist says before I discuss anything further.*

PATIENT: *Can I make an appointment with you next week to discuss my symptoms in more detail? Or do you have any literature on these symptoms I can read in the meantime?*

DOCTOR: *Let's schedule an appointment for next week. By that time I'll have set up an appointment with your gynecologist, and we can discuss the kinds of tests you'll undergo. You can ask me anything you want then.*

Good. Now you're being assertive as well as sensitive to the doctor's schedule. Scheduling a separate appointment for questions is an excellent way to gain a better understanding of your health problem and a smart way to use your doctor's time. Asking for literature indicates to the doctor that you're willing to educate yourself and participate in decisions. Because the family doctor only *suspects* endometriosis, he or she may not want to alarm you. In this case, a question-and-answer period is a good idea. You can go home and write down your questions and concerns logically. If you have a doctor who is unwilling to answer your questions, you need to address the problem.

The Patient's Bill of Rights

In the past, doctors were expected to be godlike creatures, and patients were expected to play passive roles. This kind of doctor-patient relationship doesn't exist anymore. We are now consumers of health care. We've gone from patient to *im*patient. We want results; we want value for our money. Whether we live in the United States or Canada, the patient is the customer, the one who ultimately pays the doctor's salary. (Canadians pay for health care with their taxes.) As a result, the doctor-patient relationship is now a two-way street, not unlike a marriage. Here's what you have the right to expect from a doctor:

- *As much information as you want.* You have every right to know your diagnosis, prognosis (the doctor's estimate of when you'll get better), alternate forms of treatment, and your doctor's recommendations and the basis of those recommendations (research studies, hunch, and so forth).
- *Time to address questions and concerns.* If your doctor doesn't have time to answer questions, you should be able to call him or her or make another appointment that serves as a question-and-answer period.
- *Reasonable access.* You and your doctor must decide together what "reasonable" means. Do you need weekly, quarterly, or annual appointments? Or do you just want to see the doctor whenever you feel like it? How much advance booking time do you need to get an appointment?
- *Participation in the decision-making process.* To do this, you'll have to ask questions and be willing to educate yourself about your illness.
- *Adequate emergency care and the name of your doctor's substitute.* Who do you see in case of emergency, and when your doctor is sick or on vacation? Is there a substitute doctor? Find out in case you need to see the substitute some day.
- *Knowing who has access to your health records.* How confidential are your health records? Can your doctor release them to just anyone—your employer, insurance companies, government authorities? What are your doctor's legal obligations with respect to health records, and what are yours?
- *Knowing what it costs.* If you live in the United States, you have the right to know what your bill is in advance. Get an estimate and have the doctor break down each charge so you know exactly what you're paying for and what your insurance plan is covering. If you live in Canada, make sure all appointments, tests, and procedures are covered by your province before you consent to anything.
- *Be seen on time.* If you're on time for an appointment, your doctor should be as well. Do you generally have to wait more than 30 minutes in the reception area before your doctor will see you?
- *The opportunity to change doctors.* Yes, you can fire your doctor. If you're unhappy with your current doctor or simply need a change, you have every right to switch. Make sure you arrange for your records to be transferred!

- *A second opinion, or a consult with a specialist.* If your doctor can't make an adequate diagnosis, you can insist on a referral to either another doctor or a specialist.

The Doctor's Bill of Rights

Remember, it's a two-way street. Your doctor has an unwritten bill of rights, too. Just as you're entitled to certain information and courtesies, so is your doctor. Here's what your doctor has the right to expect from you:

- *Full disclosure.* Doctors aren't telepathic. If you're hiding information (certain family or medical history, prescriptions, addictions, allergies, eating disorders, specific symptoms), it's unfair to expect an accurate diagnosis. What if your doctor prescribes a drug that you're allergic to, for example, or one that conflicts with your other medication?
- *Common courtesy.* Treat your doctor like a business associate. If you make an appointment, show up; if you need to cancel, give 24 hours' notice.
- *Advance planning.* Plan your visit in advance and think carefully about your symptoms. Don't go to your doctor with a vague complaint like "I'm not feeling well," and expect a full diagnosis. When you make an appointment, tell the receptionist how much time you think you'll need for a full examination, and write down your symptoms; give the doctor something to work with.
- *Questions and interruptions.* If you don't understand something, ask. Interrupt the doctor if necessary, and ask for simpler explanations of what's wrong. If you don't do this, you can't blame your doctor for not giving you enough information.
- *Follow advice and follow through.* Take medication as directed and follow advice. That's what you're paying the doctor for. If you're experiencing side effects to medication or have a problem with his or her advice, or if your condition has worsened as a result of the doctor's advice, let the doctor know. Full disclosure strikes again.
- *No harassment.* If you have a problem, go through reasonable channels; dial the after-hours emergency number the doctor leaves with the answering service, or call your doctor's office during business hours. Don't continuously call the doctor at home at 4 o'clock in the morning, and

don't call the office 10 times a day with every little ache and pain.
- *Enough time to make a diagnosis.* Diagnoses don't happen overnight. Allow the doctor enough time to examine you and run the necessary tests. Don't expect miracles in 15 minutes. This might mean that you need to wait longer for an appointment so your doctor can schedule enough time to fully examine you.
- *Room for disagreement.* What you think is in your best interests may not be what your doctor thinks is best. Allow for a difference of opinion and give your doctor a chance to explain his or her side. Don't just leave in a huff and threaten to sue. Maybe your doctor is right.
- *Professional conduct.* Don't request unusual favors that compromise your doctor's moral beliefs, and don't ask your doctor to do something illegal (such as writing bogus notes to your employer so you can claim disability pay).

Incidentally, if even a few of these "rights" are abused, your doctor has the right to resign as your physician and request that you seek care elsewhere.

When to Get a Second Opinion

Getting a second opinion means that you see two separate doctors about the same set of symptoms. The doctors can be in the same field or specialize in different areas. This can happen at either the diagnostic or treatment stage of an illness. Second opinions particularly come into play when your problem is gynecological. Often, your doctor will want you to see one of his or her associates or a specialist to confirm a diagnosis or a particular treatment approach; this is known as a referral or a consult. Usually, if a family practitioner finds something suspicious in a pelvic exam or wants to investigate symptoms of an irregular menstrual cycle, you'll be referred to a gynecologist (one of your own choosing) or someone your family doctor trusts. Sometimes it is *you* who requests a referral to another specialist to seek an alternate diagnosis or approach to treatment. In the United States, many insurance companies require second opinions before they'll cover a procedure.

When it comes to gynecology, second opinions can be tricky. First, doctors weigh a variety of factors in determining the best treatment. Take for example, a 38-year-old woman with four children, who has symptomatic fibroid tumors. She may be treated differently by two gynecologists. One may recommend a "watch and wait" plan to see if the fibroids get worse with time. He or she may feel this is preferable to subjecting this woman to a hysterectomy, even though she already has four children. The other gynecologist may feel that a hysterectomy will correct the problem faster, and delaying the operation is simply prolonging the woman's suffering. In both cases, the suggested course of treatment may be correct, even though they're completely different plans of action for the same problem.

A second opinion is a good idea if you have any reservations about a particular course of treatment.

General Guidelines for Seeking a Second Opinion

It's difficult to know whether you're justified in getting a second opinion. Just because you don't like the sound of your diagnosis doesn't mean you *require* another opinion. Let's say your doctor suspects you have endometriosis and wants to perform a laparoscopy to confirm his or her suspicions. You might not like the sound of this and decide to see a holistic doctor or a herbalist instead. The holistic doctor may tell you that you're under stress and need to rest and take various herbal vitamin pills. This is a much more soothing diagnosis, but the first doctor is the one who is right.

The following guidelines should help you decide whether a second opinion is warranted. If you answer yes to even one of the questions below, you're probably justified in seeking a second opinion.

1. *Is the diagnosis uncertain?* If your doctor can't find out what's wrong or isn't sure whether he or she is correct, you have every right to go elsewhere.
2. *Is the diagnosis life-threatening?* In this case, hearing the same news from someone else may help you better cope with your illness, or come to terms with the diagnosis. Diagnoses like cancer, however, usually won't change; the diagnosis is based on carefully analyzed test results, not just symptoms.
3. *Is the treatment controversial, experimental, or risky?* You might not question the diagnosis, but you might have problems with the recommended treatment. For example, if you're not comfortable with surgery, perhaps another doctor can recommend a different approach, such as hormonal therapy.
4. *Is the treatment not working?* If you're not getting better, maybe the wrong diagnosis was made, or the treatment recommended is just

not for you. Hormone therapy often doesn't work, and surgery might be the best approach after all. Seeking a second opinion may help to clear up the problem.

5. *Are risky tests or procedures being recommended?* If you don't like the sound of laparoscopy, hearing it from another doctor might make you accept the procedure more readily. Or, you may find out that a laparoscopy is premature and isn't necessary after all. Find out if there are alternate procedures that can confirm the same results.
6. *Do you want another approach?* An 80-year-old woman with heart disease and high blood pressure might be diagnosed with advanced breast cancer. She'll probably die from heart disease or a stroke before she dies from breast cancer, which tends to grow slowly in the elderly. As a result, her doctor may decide that she's too frail for surgery, chemotherapy, or radiotherapy, and opt to leave her alone. The woman's children may find this approach unacceptable and demand that her breast cancer be treated.
7. *Is the doctor competent?* When I asked my gynecologist if radioactive iodine (used for treating various thyroid disorders) would conflict with oral contraceptives, his response was, "What's radioactive iodine?" I left and never went back. Basically, if your doctor doesn't seem to know much about other health problems you have and doesn't bother to find out, find another doctor! Or, if you only suspect your doctor is deceiving you, find another doctor either to reaffirm your faith in him or her or to confirm your original suspicions.

Gynecological Guidelines for Second Opinions

We all know that hysterectomies are performed too often, and that other gynecological treatments carry risks. Even if you trust your doctor implicitly, there are some "red flag" gynecological conditions and procedures that are always controversial. Any time you're faced with making a decision about the following issues, you'll need a second opinion, and perhaps a third opinion as well.

- *Hysterectomy for* any *reason.* Make sure you really need a hysterectomy. Be wary of any doctor who recommends it for fibroid tumors, as a means of permanent sterilization, to prevent cancer, for cervicitis (inflammation of the cervix), for mildly abnormal patterns of uterine bleeding, for most cases of menstrual pain or PMS, or for abortion during the first and second trimesters. (See chapter 7 for more details.)

- *Ovary removal for any reason except ovarian cancer.* Just because you're having a hysterectomy doesn't mean your ovaries need to come out. They can be preserved, which can spare you the ordeal of hormone replacement therapy. Check it out.
- *Dilation and curettage (D & C) for any reason.* A D & C (discussed in chapter 7) is the third most common operation in the United States. It may not be necessary, particularly as a diagnostic tool. Ask about the possibility of having an endometrial biopsy instead.
- *Cautery (heat) or cryosurgery (freezing) for cervical abnormalities (found in a Pap smear.)* If you skipped the Pap section, go back and read it. You have options when your Pap test is positive.
- *Preventive or "prophylactic" surgery.* Sometimes, in families with a long history of breast or ovarian cancer, doctors may suggest removing breasts and ovaries before any evidence of cancer is present. Reconsider this if it's suggested.
- *Surgery for symptomless fibroid tumors.* If your fibroids aren't bothering you, you may not need surgery, or any treatment, for that matter. See chapter 7 for details.
- *Radiation therapy for any kind of pelvic cancer.* Even though you may need it, there are risks involved. Make sure you're aware of them.
- *Mastectomy.* Often, a lumpectomy is all that's necessary for early breast cancer. See chapters 8 and 9 for more details.
- *Radical mastectomy for breast cancer.* It's rare when you need this procedure, which is mutilating to say the least. Again, be sure that it's necessary. See chapter 9 for more details.

How to Use a Specialist

Specialists can be a different breed from family physicians. They're more academic: They may teach or run residency programs, they're involved with research, they frequently lecture at various academic centers, they regularly publish papers, articles, and books in their field, and they're recognized in their field. Specialists train longer than family doctors, make more money, and charge more for their services. As a result, many specialists are more egotistical, colder in terms of bedside manner, harder to get in touch with (they're usually booked months in advance), and, because they're pressed for time, impatient. Certainly there are many specialists who are very caring and do not fit this profile, but don't be surprised when you find one that does.

In addition, you usually don't have the luxury of shopping for a specialist the way you do for a family doctor or gynecologist (who is also a specialist but is seen more frequently and hence becomes part of our primary care "family"), because you're only referred to one when you need one. At that point, your main concern is getting better as soon as possible, and "getting in" to see another specialist can take months—time you really can't afford when you're ill. Again, you have rights, and specialists, like any other doctor, have their rights as well. Because their time is valuable (not to mention expensive), here are some guidelines that will help you make maximum use of your specialist:

1. *Tape record your visit.* Specialists often say a lot in a small amount of time. When you're upset or overwhelmed by all of the information being hurled at you, you often don't hear what the specialist is saying. Tape recording the visit is helpful because you can replay the information when you're more relaxed and can better understand what you've been told.
2. *Take a list of questions with you, and tape record the answers.* When you have a lot of questions, make a list. The specialist has an obligation to answer all of your questions, and if he or she doesn't have time, there are options. Give him or her your list and ask if he or she can address them in your next appointment. If that's not possible, agree on a time when the specialist can call you at home and address the questions. As a final resort, ask if there is a resident studying with the specialist with whom you can arrange a question-and-answer session. (Usually any resident—a "specialist in training"—can answer your questions.)
3. *Request literature or videos on your illness from the specialist, or the number of an organization you can call for more information.*
4. *If it's relevant, ask the specialist to draw you a diagram of your illness.*

A Map to the Specialists

In her lifetime, a woman will probably deal with at least three separate doctors when it comes to her gynecological health. The first is usually a family doctor or gynecologist, the one who will initiate the referral or consult process in case of a more serious illness. The following is a map to some of the specialists you may encounter, along with a brief description of when you'll be referred to each one.

- *Gynecologic oncologist:* This is a cancer specialist you might be referred to in the event that your Pap smear is abnormal and you require colposcopy. (Doctors who perform colposcopy are sometimes called colposcopists.) You'll also be referred to an oncologist for any kind of suspicious lump or tumor that requires further investigation. If you do require treatment for any kind of cancer, often you'll see an oncologist for the duration of your treatment, in conjunction with your gynecologist or family doctor.
- *Endocrinologist:* This is a hormone specialist or, more precisely, a doctor who specializes in the endocrine system. Since so many gynecological problems involve hormonal therapy or revolve around hormone deficiencies, an endocrinologist will understand all of the complexities involved. Seeing an endocrinologist for infertility problems is particularly common. In this case, you may see a reproductive endocrinologist.
- *Maternal and fetal medicine specialist:* This is an OB-Gyn who has been trained to handle high-risk pregnancies, multiple births, or problem pregnancies. He or she is also an expert in amniocentesis.
- *Urologist:* A urologist specializes in bladder function. Bladder infections are extremely common, and you may be sent to a urologist for treatment.
- *Radiotherapist:* If you have cancer and need external radiation therapy, your oncologist, gynecologist, or family doctor (whoever is managing your treatment) will send you to a radiotherapist (a doctor who specializes in external radiation therapy), who will manage the radiation portion of your treatment.
- *Gerontologist:* This is a doctor who specializes in diseases of the elderly. If you have an older parent who has multiple health problems, or if you are over 65 and juggling a variety of medications and illnesses, a gerontologist may be called in as a consultant. Sometimes it is the gerontologist who calls in another specialist.
- *Andrologist:* A doctor who specializes in male reproduction. If you're struggling with infertility or other problems that involve your partner, you may see an andrologist together.
- *Psychiatrist:* When your family doctor tells you your PMS symptoms are either stress-related or just your imagination, you could be sent to a psychiatrist.

Obviously, you need to know a lot when it comes to choosing the right combination of doctors, and making sure that you're receiving the best health care possible. There are a number of areas, however, where you can make your *own decisions*. Knowing how to prevent disease and infection is one thing, but making *informed decisions* about family planning is another. In either case, it's a matter of life and death.

CHAPTER 4

Safe Sex and Contraception

In 1980, *safe sex* meant not having intercourse in a moving vehicle; in other words, there was no such thing. Contraception was used to prevent pregnancy, period. Although sexually transmitted diseases (STDs) such as traditional venereal diseases and herpes were in fact widespread, they were not talked about openly. Heterosexuals and homosexuals were all "Looking for Mr. Goodbar." Monogamy was frowned upon, perceived as a 1950s' mentality in an era that celebrated personal expression and sexual freedom.

The first cases of AIDS popped up in New York City in 1981. Several gay males were suddenly struck with a bizarre kind of cancer that baffled the medical community. Otherwise healthy young men were being diagnosed with Kaposi's sarcoma (a rare skin cancer where large dark spots develop all over the body) and *Pneumocystis carinii* pneumonia. In the past, both diseases had been diagnosed only in patients who had no immune system or who were elderly. This new disease began spreading like wildfire amongst the gay population. The gay community was horrified; gay activists demanded government action. The medical community was stumped and had little funding with which to research this new disease. It would take two years before this new "homosexual plague" was even linked to sexual activity. By then, thousands of gay men were already dead.

Finally, the disease was given a name, acquired immunodeficiency syndrome (AIDS), and it was found to be caused by the human immunodeficiency virus (HIV). HIV, we were told, was a sexually transmitted virus. But when the virus started turning up in intravenous (IV) drug users, it was discovered that the infection was transmitted through the exchange of all bodily fluids, principally blood, semen, and vaginal secretions. Once HIV enters our bloodstreams (through transfusions of blood and blood products; needle sharing among IV drug users; exposure to needle sticks, open wounds, or mucous membranes; injections with contaminated needles; or transmission of bodily fluids), *anyone*, we were informed, could get AIDS.

But because AIDS *appeared* to be affecting only gay males, most single, sexually active heterosexuals were oblivious to it, even as late as 1985. That year, the virus finally hit the rich and famous when actor Rock Hudson died from it. Of course, by then the virus had also gotten into the Red Cross blood supply. The next group to be heavily hit by the virus would be anyone requiring transfusions or blood product for other conditions, such as hemophilia (a hereditary disease in which the blood doesn't clot). The virus traveled into the heterosexual world, affecting women, children (who were either infected in the womb or through transfusion), and heterosexual males. It also found its way into the heterosexual domain through sexual contact between heterosexuals and bisexuals, and between heterosexuals and IV drug users. The age of AIDS was born, changing the social fabric of our society forever. If you are a sexually active woman, and even if you're monogamous, *having sex can kill you.*

The Difference Between Contraception and Safe Sex

Contraception methods are discussed later in this chapter. All of these methods are perfectly effective for preventing pregnancy. However, none of them is effective for preventing an STD, whether it's the human papillomavirus (HPV), which can lead to cervical cancer, herpes, or HIV. Therefore, before we can even discuss contraception in any form, it's crucial first to explain what safe sex is, and what it means to your reproductive health.

Safe Sex and the AIDS Myth

Safe sex is not a medical device or a new product. It is an umbrella term that refers to sensible sexual behavior that reduces one's risk of contracting an STD. (*Smart sex* may be a more accurate term.) Many women think that safe sex means simply using a condom during intercourse. This is not true. Safe sex refers to an entire array of sensible, health-conscious practices that *include, but are not limited to, using condoms.* These practices are outlined further below.

The irony is that with the exception of AIDS, STDs have been around since the time of primal man. The term *sexually transmitted disease* is relatively new and has gradually replaced the term *venereal disease.* This shift in terminology reflects both an expanded awareness of infectious diseases transmitted through sexual contact, as well as an expanded array of diseases. Each era has always had a name for STDs. In the early 20th century, STDs were known as "the Clap," which was slang for gonorrhea, and syphilis was known as "bad blood"; in the '60s and '70s, STDs were known as VD, short for venereal disease. VD originally encompassed five traditional infections: *gonorrhea, syphilis, herpes (cancroid), lymphogranuloma venereum,* and *granuloma inguinale.* The term *STD* includes more than 20 organisms and syndromes, including HIV. Even before AIDS, STDs were rampant, occurring at epidemic rates. VD was once considered the most dreaded curse one could get, until AIDS made other VD seem mild in comparison. Here's an excerpt from a 1979 edition of *Our Bodies, Ourselves* on VD:

> There is at present a venereal disease (VD) epidemic so widespread that the incidence of the most common of these diseases is second only to the common cold.... We want to talk about more than just the bare facts that most public sources of information give. We want to help people to confront their problems in facing what VD is and in dealing with it. Therefore, we must explore why VD is still difficult to face and talk about. (p. 167)

In 1977, approximately 2 million cases of gonorrhea were reported in the United States *alone.* And yet most of us are led to believe that practicing safe sex is solely for the purpose of preventing the spread of HIV and AIDS. This is a myth. In fact, had safe sex been practiced decades ago, all *kinds* of diseases and deaths would have been prevented. It was only because of the introduction of antibiotics that gonorrhea and syphillis became treatable. What happened to people who contracted VD in the 1800s and early 20th century? A lot of them died, unfortunately. And what about all of the deaths that resulted from cervical cancer, uterine cancer, and other cancers of the reproductive organs? Many of these cancers could have been prevented through the practice of safe sex.

It is an absolute fallacy to assume that there wasn't a need *to practice safe sex prior to AIDS.* Safe-sex methods, as you'll see later in this chapter, are not at all revolutionary or new. Yet the practice has taken on new meaning since AIDS and has arisen out of our own fear of the disease. Why are we more terrified of AIDS than of any other STD? The answer, of course, is that there is no cure for AIDS. Had there been, safe sex may never have come into being.

High-Risk Behaviors

High-risk behavior refers to certain activities that place you more at risk of infection and disease than other activities. High-risk behavior is "remedied" through safe sex. Some of these behaviors are highlighted below.

Sexual Promiscuity

A person who is sexually promiscuous has sex with a large variety of partners within a relatively short time span. Promiscuity is high-risk behavior. However, it is our *interpretation* of promiscuity that has undergone the most radical change since the introduction of AIDS.

In 1976, for example, if you were a single woman in your late 20s, it would not have been uncommon for you to have had five or six one-night stands in the course of a summer, without the use of condoms or even adequate birth control. But if you were a *gay male* in your late 20s in 1976, it would not have been unusual to have had a one-night stand *every* night during that same summer.

Today, a person is considered promiscuous if he or she has five or six heterosexual or homosexual partners within a *one-year* span.

Why is promiscuity considered high risk? Basically, the more people you sleep with, the more chances you have of contracting a virus or infection. Every time you sleep with someone, you're sleeping with every person he or she ever slept with. Until AIDS, the risk of contracting VD or other STDs was not enough to scare people out of promiscuous behavior, because the dangers were not perceived as imminent. Antibiotics provided a cure for any deadly forms of VD. Herpes, although not curable, was not deadly, just miserable to have. Finally, not much was known then about other STDs; today, they are known to cause cervical cancer and other pelvic diseases and infections.

The safe-sex remedy for promiscuity.

As a single woman in the 1990s, being promiscuous is very dangerous. You risk not only HIV infection but all kinds of STDs (see chapter 6), which can lead to cancer of your reproductive organs and/or infertility. There are eight safe-sex rules you must adopt to "remedy" promiscuous behavior.

1. *Abstinence.* Never sleep with someone you don't know. You don't have to marry the guy, but abstain from intercourse until the relationship is serious and you know him better.
2. *Ask the difficult questions.* Get to know your partner *well.* Ask him about his sexual history (how many girlfriends he has had, how many one-night stands, how many long-term monogamous relationships, and so forth). Ask him if he is bisexual or if he has ever had any homosexual relationships. Ask him if he has ever had anal sex. Ask him if he is an intravenous drug user or has ever used drugs intravenously. Ask him if he has had any major surgery in the last 10 years (or prior to 1985, when the blood supply was finally screened for HIV). This will tell you whether he was at risk for HIV infection through a blood transfusion. Find out if he is a hemophiliac or has ever had sex with a hemophiliac. Ask him if he has ever had sex without a condom and what the circumstances were (a long-term relationship, for example, or perhaps he doesn't believe in wearing condoms). Finally, ask him if he has been tested for HIV. If he says he was and is HIV negative, demand to see proof; if he has never been tested, request that he *get* tested, and you should volunteer to take the test as well.
3. *Never have sex without using both a* latex *condom and spermicide, unless you and your partner are monogamous* and *have both tested negative for HIV infection.* Don't fall for lines like "All of my relationships have been monogamous," or "I don't fool around." Be sure. Unless you've been with the same person for more than two years, know for a fact that he's *never* strayed, and know for a fact that he *is* HIV negative, don't have sex without a latex condom and spermicide. It is believed that spermicide helps kill the HIV virus. How to use a condom (with spermicide) is discussed later in this chapter.
4. *Never perform oral sex on an "uncondomed" penis unless you and your partner are monogamous* and *have both tested negative for HIV infection.* HIV is transferred through semen. You don't want to swallow it.
5. *Carry latex condoms and spermicide with you at all times.* Whether you frequent singles' events or not. You never know when you *yourself*

will give in to your own urges without asking the right questions of your partner. If you weaken, at least you'll have a condom handy that you can insist he wears.

6. *Abstain from all sexual contact when you have your period.* That semen-to-blood contact is a real killer. Even if you're using condoms, you don't want to risk double trouble. What if the condom breaks or falls off? HIV infection is more potently transferred to the male through menstrual blood, and if you're bleeding, HIV-infected semen is more easily transferred to *you!* It's also important to prevent your partner from performing oral sex on you during your period for the same reasons, even though HIV technically is not transmitted through saliva.
7. *Abstain from all sexual activity when you have a vaginal infection of any kind.* Vaginal discharge can be more infectious to the male during this time; HIV is more easily transferred to you through this kind of vaginal discharge.
8. *Never have sex before you're ready.* Whether you're still a virgin or are simply unsure whether you *want* to sleep with someone, err on the side of health. If you're not comfortable, don't do it. If your partner doesn't understand, that's all the more reason *not* to sleep with him.

Anal Sex

Anal sex is *extremely* high-risk sexual behavior and is absolutely not restricted to homosexual activity. A Canadian journalist reported that anal sex is to couples in the 1990s what oral sex was to couples in the 1970s and 1980s. For heterosexuals, anal sex is the last taboo in heterosexual activity that hasn't been explored.

Public health professionals warn that for a heterosexual couple, the risks associated with anal intercourse *may* outweigh the pleasures. First, penetration causes tearing of rectal tissue and bleeding. ***This is why HIV can be so easily transmitted during unprotected anal sex. It provides direct semen-to-blood contact.*** Worse, the tears in your rectum are aggravated by bowel movements. This can mean permanent damage to your bowels and rectal tissue, and pain and bleeding when you have a bowel movement. During unprotected anal sex, a male can get feces on his penis, and then transfer fecal material into the vagina. This can introduce a whole gamut of nasty bacteria into your vagina. The bottom line is that women's rectums are not meant for penises. Although many women enjoy anal sex and need no convincing by their partners, some women *are* coerced by their partners. If you don't want to do it and your partner is pressuring you to "experiment," find another partner!

It's important to make a distinction between heterosexual anal intercourse and homosexual anal intercourse. For homosexual males, anal intercourse is the only form of sexual intercourse available to them. Unfortunately, it is this one, single, high-risk activity that is responsible for the AIDS lie: *Only gay men can get AIDS.* Infectious disease specialists speculate that HIV, an active virus in the Third World (and discussed more thoroughly in chapter 5), was by *chance* contracted and brought over to North America by a gay male, who then spread the virus to the gay community through anal sex. Again, because anal sex causes bleeding and open tears in the rectum, the seepage of semen into these open tears and the seepage of blood into the male's urethra create a particularly fertile breeding ground for HIV. To aggravate matters, promiscuity was typical homosexual behavior at the time of this probable "first contact."

General oral-anal contact is also not a safe activity. If a tongue comes in contact with an open rectal sore or tear, HIV infection can follow.

Safer anal sex. If you must have anal sex, here are the rules:

1. *Use two condoms and plenty of the proper lubricant.* The lubricant will moisten the orifice and help prevent the tearing of rectal tissue. Two condoms are necessary in case one condom breaks.
2. *Never use Vaseline or petroleum jelly as a sexual lubricant.* It can erode the condom and cause it to break, and it does not dissolve inside the rectum (or the vagina, for that matter). Use a proper sexual lubricant, such as K-Y Jelly.
3. *After anal intercourse, make sure your partner carefully washes and dries his penis, carefully washes and dries his hands, and puts on a fresh condom before continuing.* You want to make sure that no fecal material is transferred into your vagina, and that no blood from your rectal tears gets inside your vagina.
4. *After anal intercourse, reapply lubricant into your rectum to help soothe any irritation that results.*
5. *If you're engaging in regular anal intercourse, make sure you have a full pelvic exam twice a year, and ask for a rectal exam as well.* If anal sex is only a one-time occurrence for you, go for a pelvic exam as soon as you can after the experience. Report any bleeding, pains, or difficult bowel movements you may have after the incident.

6. *If you're having anal intercourse, make sure you inform your doctor.* Anal intercourse may affect the results of your pelvic exam. It's important that your doctor knows you're engaging in it so he or she can accurately analyze the results of your pelvic exam, and further advise you on safer sex practices.

Drug Use

Narcotic drug use has *always* been high-risk behavior, but with the advent of AIDS, narcotic drugs used intravenously are especially deadly. Although taking narcotics intravenously has *always* been unhealthy, and sharing dirty needles carries all kinds of germs and infections—including hepatitis B—until AIDS, the obvious risks associated with this kind of behavior have largely been ignored by drug abusers. Another problem with IV drug use is that when you're high, you'll be more careless about safe sex than you would when you're cognitive. In addition, drugs are often paid for in sexual "currency."

Safe-sex rules for IV drug users and abusers.

Even though drug use and abuse are not "sexual" per se, safe-sex practices need to be adopted here as well. Obviously, the first rule is that unless you *need* to use an IV drug for health reasons (such as diabetes or hemophilia) *don't use them.* Failing that, here are some safe-sex guidelines to live by:

1. *Always use clean needles; never share your needles, and never use someone else's needles.* There are needle-exchange programs set up all over the continent. Ask your doctor about where you can go to make sure you're getting clean needles.
2. *If you're taking drugs intravenously for legitimate health reasons, make sure you have regular checkups with your family doctor, and make sure you're using a screened blood product.* Don't use any product unless you know for a fact it's been screened for HIV infection.
3. *As a rule, get an AIDS test done once a year (or ask your doctor to recommend reasonable time intervals) to make sure you haven't been infected.* HIV can remain dormant for several years before it becomes active. Just because you've had one negative AIDS test doesn't mean you weren't infected with HIV. As an IV drug user, you are in the highest risk category for developing AIDS. So keep getting tested until you're absolutely sure.
4. *Avoid having sex with an IV drug user; if you must, use two condoms and*

plenty of spermicide. If *you* are the drug user, always disclose your drug use to your partner, and if you can't abstain from sex, insist on two spermicidal condoms.

Practicing Safer Sex During Normal Sexual Activity

Common sexual activities include vaginal intercourse, oral sex (fellatio and cunnilingus), deep kissing (French or wet kissing), mutual masturbation (or petting), masturbation, hugging, body rubbing, and massage. Sex toys (dildos, vibrators, flavored gels) are also part of normal sexual activity. To avoid the spread of STDs, the following are the new rules for normal sexual activity:

1. *Abstain from intercourse whenever possible, and substitute safer sexual foreplay activities, such as petting.*
2. *Use a latex condom with spermicide every time you have intercourse, and a spermicidal latex condom every time you perform fellatio. Ask your partner to use some sort of barrier, such as plastic wrap, every time he or she performs oral sex on you.* No more swallowing, and no cunnilingus during your period or when you have a vaginal infection.
3. *Deep kiss with caution.* So far, HIV infection has not been transferred through saliva, but deep kissing is classified as only possibly safe. That's why it's important to know your partner's sexual history before you plan to share mucus with him (as gross as it sounds). You might want to consider using a dental dam (a sheet of latex that you put over your mouth) for this as well.
4. *Do not share sex toys.* Sharing sex toys is no longer safe. Bacteria and germs are too easily transferred between them. However, if you are the sole user of certain devices, such as vibrators, it's fine to carry on as long as you keep your device in a private place and wash the device with soap and warm water before and after use. (Keep in mind though, that a sibling or roommate could borrow this device, share it with his or her lover, and return it without your knowledge.)
5. *All non-mucus-sharing activities are safe.* Hugging, fondling, and so forth are all fine. As much as possible, try to abstain from intercourse and oral sex, and suggest mutual masturbation instead. Just

make sure both you and your partner wash your hands before inserting fingers into your vagina.
6. *Don't share your toothbrush, douching equipment, or vaginal applicators with anyone.*

When Is Unprotected Sex Safe?

Presuming no other high-risk factors, if both you and your partner have been tested for HIV infection, are both negative, and are practicing mutual monogamy, then it is safe to resume normal sexual activity without condoms or other latex barriers, such as dental dams. However, if you're not planning to get pregnant, you'll need to use effective contraception anyway (discussed later in this chapter).

If you and your partner are mutually monogamous and have been together since *before* 1977, you don't have to be tested for HIV infection, and can engage in normal sexual activity without condoms. (The year 1977 is considered to mark the beginning of the HIV epidemic in the United States.)

The problem, of course, is that partners *lie* about monogamy and may stray without your knowledge, or vice versa. It's common for unfaithful spouses to infect their monogamous partners. If you don't trust your partner, don't have sex without using condoms. Use safe sex to "test" the boundaries of your relationship by getting to know each other better and uncovering common values, history, and so on. The outcome may prove beneficial for both of you. Seeking counseling may also be an option if you're not sure what to do.

Have You Been Exposed to HIV?

If you've had oral sex or vaginal or anal intercourse without using condoms—with more than one partner since 1977, you are *technically* at risk for having been exposed to HIV. This is a terrifying reality for a large percentage of the population. But it's important not to panic. Your answers to the 10 questions below will narrow down the possibility of HIV exposure.

1. Since 1977, have you (or any of your partners) had sex with:
   - a homosexual man
   - a bisexual man
   - a prostitute (male or female)
   - anyone from central, eastern, or southern Africa, or some Caribbean countries
   - anyone believed or known to be HIV positive
   - anyone who has ever been in jail (forced anal sex and IV drug use is common in prison)
2. Have you (or any of your partners) had five or more sexual partners in any year since 1977?
3. Have you (or any of your partners) ever had an STD such as gonorrhea, syphilis, herpes, or genital warts?
4. Since 1977, have you (or any of your partners) had sex without latex condoms (except for long-term, mutually monogamous relationships)?
5. Have you (or any of your partners) used needle drugs and shared injection equipment since 1977?
6. Have you (or any of your partners) ever blacked out from using alcohol or drugs, especially during sex since 1977?
7. Have you (or any of your partners) had any transfusions of blood or blood components between 1977 and 1985? (If you've had any major surgery between 1977 and 1985, or if you've been under a general anesthetic in that time span, find out if you were given any kind of transfusion.)
8. Are you a hemophiliac? Have you had sex with a hemophiliac since 1977?
9. Have you (or any of your partners) received donor semen, donor eggs, transplanted organs, or transplanted tissue since 1977?
10. Have you (or any of your partners) ever been exposed to blood in your work setting?

If you've answered *yes* to any of these questions, you should be tested for HIV exposure, even if you are as healthy as can be. Getting an AIDS test and interpreting what the results actually mean are discussed in detail in chapter 5. Moreover, if you're planning to have a family or are already pregnant and have answered *yes* to any of these questions, you'll need to ask your obstetrician whether an AIDS test is warranted. Knowing your HIV status is not only for your own protection, but for everyone else's as well.

If You Suspect Your Partner Is HIV Positive

HIV can remain dormant in an infected person for up to 10 years or more before any symptoms manifest. There are a number of symptoms you can look out for: weight loss, loss of appetite, fever, sweats or night sweats, skin rashes or pigmented lesions, general dryness of the skin, enlarged lymph nodes below the ear and around the neck, headaches, persistent cold symptoms, whitish or painful lesions around or inside the mouth, persistent cough or shortness of breath, abdominal pain, diarrhea, depression or severe mood changes, cognitive difficulties, bowel or bladder dysfunction (bed wetting), general muscle weakness, persistent oral yeast infections, persistent or chronic vaginal yeast infections in women for more than a year, and sores around the genitals, such as herpes, which fail to heal within a reasonable time.

All About Condoms

Mechanical barriers that cover the penis have been used for centuries for protection against both pregnancy and infection, for decoration, and occasionally to produce penile or vaginal stimulation. Such practices can be traced to 1350 B.C., when Egyptian men wore decorative sheaths over their penises. The Italian anatomist Fallopius described the use of linen sheaths in 1564. Protective devices from animal intestines soon followed. It was not until the 18th century, however, that penile sheaths were given the name *condoms* and became popular forms of "protection from venereal disease and numerous bastard offspring." Casanova (1725–1798) was among the first to popularize the condom as a contraceptive, but he was also aware of the protective effect of condoms against sexually transmitted infections as well. When rubber latex was invented in the 1840s, condoms became mass produced and were coined "rubbers."

Ironically, the early condoms were sold primarily as prophylactics, in other words, as devices to protect against disease. They were available in brothels as well as drugstores, where they were known in slang terms as *French letters* or *capotes.* They were also sold in barber shops and other places men frequented. But the quality latex condoms sold today would not became available for several more decades.

Choosing and Using a Condom

Millions of couples are currently using condoms for protection against STDs and as a contraceptive. They are also the second most widely used reversible contraceptive in the United States after oral contraception. Condoms are available in all drugstores, and you don't need a prescription. There are dozens of brands and colors to choose from. Some are ribbed (enhancing stimulation for the woman), some aren't; some are lubricated, some aren't; some have built-in spermicide, some don't. Basically, as long as the box says "latex," and you check the expiration date on the box, your choice is fine.

All condoms originally came in one size, and the assumption of one-size-fits-all was challenged only when the United States began exporting condoms to Asian countries and found that they were too large for many Asian men (not to mention Asian-American men). Most large international manufacturers now produce two basic sizes, Class I and Class II. In the United States, some manufacturers offer the smaller-size condoms, promoting them as fitting "snugger for extra sensitivity" rather than indicating they are for men with smaller penises. The latest *Consumer Reports* study on condoms found that its readers preferred lubricated latex condoms with a reservoir tip (which comes in handy, as you'll read below). One study tracked 245 couples in which one partner was HIV positive and the other was not. Out of 123 of those couples who used condoms correctly and consistently, none of the healthy partners became infected, but out of the 122 couples who used condoms occasionally or did not use the condom correctly, 12 of the healthy partners became infected. Does this mean that religious use of condoms will prevent HIV infection? Not according to a similar Italian study. Here, out of 171 couples who used condoms correctly and consistently, 3 healthy partners became infected. As for the remaining 134 couples who were inconsistent condom users, 16 healthy partners became infected.

If you've never used a condom before, it does take some practice. The most fumbling comes from putting it on the wrong way, with the lubricated side touching the penis instead of the other way around. You might want to practice first on a shampoo bottle. (Don't use the practice condom for sex. Throw it out.) Following are tips on using a condom:

1. Make sure you keep a supply of condoms in your purse and near your bed (nightstand, decorative box beside your futon, under the

bed in a shoebox). The oldest excuse partners use for having unprotected sex is not wanting to get out of bed to get the condoms. This ensures that you don't have to!

2. As soon as the penis is erect, open the condom package carefully to avoid tearing the condom. Put the condom on before you insert the penis into the vagina. Either partner can put the condom on. If you're having anal sex, put on two condoms.
3. Wait until the vagina is lubricated. A dry vagina can cause the condom to fall off or break.
4. Pinch the air from the tip of the condom to leave space for the semen. Air left in the condom will cause it to burst. Unroll it, lubricated side away from the penis, right down to the base of the erect penis.
5. Avoid Vaseline and oil-based lubricant products, such as Crisco (which apparently is popular). Use a water-based lubricant such as K-Y Jelly or Lubafax to prevent the condom from deteriorating. For additional protection, use a spermicide containing nonoxynol-9, a spermicidal condom, or Delfen (a spermicidal foam).
6. After your partner ejaculates, pull out the penis while it is still hard, holding the base of the condom firmly.
7. Remove the condom, being careful not to spill any semen.
8. Then check the condom for any tears. If it has torn or has come off inside the vagina, insert contraceptive foam or gel immediately. (Always keep contraceptive foam or gel on hand for this reason.)
9. Throw the condom away. Use it only once.
10. Don't store condoms anywhere near extreme temperatures; cars and wallets are bad places.

Condoms and women

Right now, a latex condom is the best protection women have against STDs and AIDS. But aside from HIV and AIDS, STDs such as gonorrhea and chlamydia are biologically *sexist* illnesses; they do more damage to a woman's reproductive organs than to a man's (this is discussed further in chapter 6). So even if AIDS did not exist, you still stand to lose a lot with traditional VD.

Women are more at risk for STDs than are men. Statistically, infected men give STDs to two out of three female partners, compared to women giving STDs to one out of three partners. In addition to HIV and AIDS, condoms will help protect you against unwanted pregnancy, vaginitis, pelvic inflammatory disease (PID), tubal infertility, genital cancer, and infections that can harm your baby if you already *are* pregnant.

It is your right to insist that your partner wear condoms; if he doesn't, you should abstain from having sex with him. Always have them handy. Don't rely on your partner to purchase them. It's also important to anticipate reluctance on his part. Have some quick answers ready so you won't be searching for the right thing to say on the spot. Even if your partner insists he's clean or disease-free, tell him that *you* may not be, that you may have an STD and not know it.

The Female Condom

There is such a device as the female condom, which passed FDA approval in May, 1993. The female condom (called the Reality Female Condom) is a variation of the male condom, but instead of fitting over the penis, it lines the inside of the vagina. The disposable condom is made of polyurethane, which is thin but strong (40% stronger than the latex used in male condoms). It's also very resistant to rips and tears during use. Its design consists of a soft sheath that is open on one end and closed at the other. It has two soft flexible rings. The ring inside the closed end is used to insert the device and to hold it in place over the cervix. The other ring forms the open edge and remains outside the vagina after insertion. So in addition to lining the inside of the vagina, this condom covers your labia and the base of your partner's penis during intercourse, reducing skin-to-skin contact.

The female condom was originally invented in 1985 by a Danish husband and wife team (he is a gynecologist; she is a nurse), Erik and Bente Gregerson. Polyurethane was chosen as a material not only because of its strength and skin-like fit, but because it is also resistant to oils, which means it isn't damaged (unlike latex male condoms) by oil-based lubricants, such as petroleum jelly, for example. It is also suitable for women allergic to latex, and is less likely to cause vaginal infections. Polyurethane also transmits heat between partners, which gives the material a more sensitive and "natural" feel. It may also allow more spontaneity since it can be inserted before sex, like a diaphragm. However, you don't need a plastic inserter to fit it, nor do you need a prescription or a fitting for one, and it's available over-the-counter at all drugstores. Like a male condom, it is intended for one-time use only.

This new product is designed as both a safer-sex tool as well as a contraceptive. Findings of a six month study conducted by Family Health International and the Contraceptive Research and Development Program (CONRAD) were published in the December 1994 issue of the *American Journal of Public Health.* CONRAD concluded that the condom was as effective in preventing pregnancy as other barrier methods (discussed on pages 98-102), but had the added advantage of protecting women from STDs. In other words, among the 262 women who took part in the study and used the condom correctly and consistently every time they had sex, the failure rate was 2.6%. Of those who didn't use the condom correctly, the failure rate was 12.4%—roughly the same failure rate cited for the diaphragm and cervical cap (see further on).

And what do female condom users have to say? Eighty percent of the women from the CONRAD study said they liked using it, and two-thirds of women in a New York City acceptability study said they liked it, too. Meanwhile, 73% of the New York City study participants said they preferred the female condom to the male condom. (These findings were presented in November, 1994 to the annual meeting of the American Public Health Association in Washington, D.C.) Interestingly, some women reported that the female condom sexually stimulated the clitoris during use, providing more orgasmic delights.

The female condom is manufactured by Chartex International in London, England, and is distributed in the United States by the Female Health Company, a division of Wisconsin Pharmacal Company, which developed the device. It is also sold in 13 other countries (not yet in Canada), where it is called *femidom®* or *femy.* The female condom was endorsed by the FDA's obstetric and gynecology panel, as well as the U.S. Centers for Disease Control and Prevention. The price per condom in the U.S. is about $3.

Although there are several forms of contraception already available to women, it's important for women to be able to protect themselves from STDs during intercourse without having to rely on male compliance. The female condom is an ideal option if you're looking for both a prophylactic and a barrier method. However, as with any condom, it is critical that you use it consistently and correctly every time you have intercourse in order for it to work. It should never be used when your male partner is wearing a condom; neither will work properly because of the friction this "condom combo" will generate. If your doctor advises you to use the female condom in conjunction with a male condom, show him or her this passage!

At this stage, critics of the female condom feel that any ineffectiveness reported is due to human error—couples not using the product properly. So here are the rules—compiled from the Reality instruction pamphlets:

1. Never use the female condom if your partner is wearing his own.
2. Use more lubricant if: the condom rides the penis; the outer ring is pushed inside; it is noisy during sex; you feel it's slipped out of place; or it comes out of the vagina during use.
3. Remove the female condom if: it rips or tears during insertion or use; the outer ring is pushed inside the pouch; it bunches up inside the vagina; or you have sex again.

Finally, please call the manufacturer's toll-free line for more information on the female condom. The number is 1-800-274-6601. (Also listed in Appendix A.)

Preventing Pregnancy

The primary purpose of contraception is not to protect you against STDs, but to prevent pregnancy. The last few years have been particularly revolutionary in contraceptive technology. Before 1960 there were no hormonal methods of contraception, and intrauterine devices (IUDs) were just becoming available. Women relied on coitus interruptus (pulling out), diaphragms (available only to *married* women), condoms, or the rhythm/calendar method. You must know the old joke: *What do you call a man who uses the rhythm method? Daddy!*

When oral contraceptives (OCs)—the Pill—were introduced in the 1960s, contraceptive technology evolved around refining OCs. Women not taking OCs had to rely on fairly ancient but reliable barrier methods, such as foam, diaphragms, and IUDs. By the early to mid-1980s, more barrier methods became available to North American women, methods that had been popular in Europe for decades. These included the cervical cap and the vaginal sponge. But by the late 1980s, there was a comparative explosion in new contraceptive products that are now FDA approved and readily available to American women (Canadian women are still awaiting approval on some of these methods). The products include subdermal implants (Norplant), contraceptive injections (Depo-Provera), the abortion pill (not yet available in North America), and the female condom (discussed above). There are now probably as many estrogen/progesterone combination OCs as there are cough medicines. (In the late 1980s, the mini-Pill came out, which is a progesterone-only OC. It was developed because many women suffer side effects of estrogen, discussed below.) Several male oral contraceptive products are also being developed and may be ready for use by the late 1990s or early 2000s.

Why this sudden explosion in contraception? AIDs is one reason, but as consumers, women are demanding more innovative products and better value. It is this push for value that is helping to drive the pharmaceutical industry. Whether or not these new contraceptive products are currently safer than traditional methods, they will nevertheless *become* safer because their very invention will force *quality and safety through competition.* The bottom line is that with more choices, women will be able to find the right contraceptive for their individual needs, and hence take fewer risks.

The New Kid on the Block: Norplant

Norplant is a *subdermal* implant, which means that it's inserted underneath the skin. The Norplant contraceptive was approved by the FDA in December 1990, and has been on the market since February 1991. It consists of six silicone-rubber, matchstick-size capsules that release a synthetic progestin hormone, long used in oral contraceptives, into the bloodstream. The hormone prevents ovulation and also causes the mucus of the cervix to thicken, making it more difficult for sperm to reach the egg. In addition, the lining of the uterus becomes thinner, making it less receptive to an egg's implanting in it.

Norplant should be inserted either during your period or no later than the seventh day of your menstrual cycle. The reason for this is to prevent inserting it during a possible pregnancy. It absolutely should not be inserted if you either are or suspect you're pregnant. Norplant can also be inserted immediately after an abortion or miscarriage, or six weeks after delivery, and it does not interfere with breastfeeding. Norplant is effective within 24 hours after insertion, and one insertion works for five years.

The insertion process is fairly simple. First, you'll be given a local anesthetic. Your doctor will then make a tiny incision. Using a special instrument called a *torcar,* your doctor will place six capsules, one at a time, in a fan shape just under the skin of your upper arm. The incision is then covered with protective gauze and a small adhesive bandage. Stitches are not required. The bandage should be left on for three days and kept dry. When the anesthetic wears off, there will be some tenderness or itching and even some discoloration, bruising, and swelling. This is normal. If it doesn't clear up, it may mean you have developed an infection, and you'll need to see your doctor. (Infection is pretty rare, however.) You can't see the capsules once they're in place unless you're very thin or muscular, and even then, the capsules look like protruding veins. The inserts have also been known to come out, which can happen only if they're not inserted properly. (Again, this is rare.) The insertion process takes between 15 to 20 minutes. The upper arm was chosen as a site because it's not a noticeable part of your body. Unlike breast implants, these inserts do not move around. They're made from the same material as heart valves and other surgical devices—material used in surgery since the 1950s. The implants can be taken out *at any time,* and the removal process is the reverse of the insertion process. However, removal takes longer because scar tissue can form on the implants. If it's really difficult, you'll need to to go home and come back to the doctor to complete the removal process.

Each Norplant capsule is about one-tenth of an inch in diameter, and just under one and a half inches long. It holds 36 milligrams of the synthetic progestin *levonorgestrel* in the form of powdered crystals. The tubes are made of silastic, a silicone material. The hormone seeps through the permeable tubes into the bloodstream, initially at a rate of about 85 micrograms a day. The amount declines gradually to about 50 micrograms by 9 months, 35 by 18 months, and about 30 micrograms at the end of five years. In comparison, oral contraceptives that contain progestin release about 50–150 micrograms of progestin a day, *plus* estrogen. The progestin-only pill, or mini-Pill releases about 75 micrograms of levonorgestrel a day. When the capsules are removed, fertility is restored 5–14 days later. Twenty percent of Norplant users got pregnant within the first month of removal; 49% got pregnant within four months of removal; 73% got pregnant within six months of removal, and 86% got pregnant within one year of removal. No side effects have been reported in children conceived after Norplant removal. (Keep in mind that the product is still too new for enough data to be compiled.)

Interestingly, Norplant has been marketed in other countries for several years. More than half a million women in 46 countries have used Norplant since it was first approved in Finland in 1983. It now has regulatory approval in 17 other countries, including Sweden, Indonesia, the Dominican Republic, Thailand, China, Peru, and the United States. In fact, the first subdermal implants were tested in 1968, and what was to be called Norplant was developed in 1974.

How Effective is Norplant?

Very. With the exception of male sterilization, *Norplant is comparable to tubal ligation.* Pregnancy rates, however, were slightly higher in women weighing over 153 pounds (who probably needed a higher dose). Among 100 women of all weights using the implant for five years, four will become pregnant on Norplant. That compares to 15 out of 100 women becoming pregnant on OCs. The main reason why Norplant is so effective is that it doesn't depend on patient compliance: there are no pills to forget, no human error involved. It's also important to remember that Norplant does not protect women against STDs. Used with a latex condom, however, it is an excellent contraceptive/prophylactic system.

What are the Side Effects?

The most common side effect is menstrual cycle irregularity and irregular bleeding. The bleeding irregularities result from the *continuous* hormone release and the thinning of the endometrium. Basically, there's no thickened lining to be shed. With OCs, estrogen and progestin are taken for three weeks and withdrawn for one week, causing *regular* bleeding. Over a five-year period of use, about 45% of Norplant users will have irregular periods, and another 45% will have normal periods. The remaining 10% will have long periods of time (3–4 months) with no bleeding. Usually, the number of days of menstruation increase, while the flow decreases. In the first year, about 70% of users will experience changes in their menstrual cycle. Studies show that Norplant causes irregular periods in the first year, with regular periods developing over the next four years. Twenty-five percent of users will have no periods at all for the first 90 days. If you decide to use or are already using Norplant, chart your periods. If you go longer than six months without any bleeding, see your doctor or gynecologist and find out whether you should continue to use Norplant. Often, you need to wait out the first year before your cycle gets more regular.

Other side effects are headaches, nervousness, depression, nausea, dizziness, skin rash, acne, change of appetite, breast tenderness, weight gain, ovarian cysts, and excessive growth of body or facial hair. Breast discharge, vaginal discharge, inflammation of the cervix, abdominal discomfort, and muscle and skeletal pain have also been reported. Note, however, that many of these latter side effects are also common complaints in general, and have not yet been linked specifically to Norplant, as irregular bleeding has. If you do happen to suffer side effects other than irregular bleeding, they will most likely be weight gain, headaches, acne, depression, excessive hair growth, occasional itching at the site of the implants, and possibly a benign ovarian cyst.

Don't let this discourage you from using it. The major reason why women discontinue Norplant is because of irregular bleeding. The statistical breakdown of why women stop Norplant goes like this: 9% stop because of irregular bleeding; 5% stop because of other symptoms, such as dizziness or headaches; and 5% stop because they want to conceive. Most countries report a very high continuation rate after one year (80–98%) and more than 40% continuation after five years (meaning they've had it reinserted.) Meanwhile, 50% of the women who stop using OCs do so after one year.

Are You a Norplant Candidate?

You should definitely avoid Norplant if you're pregnant or have acute liver disease or liver tumors (benign or malignant), unexplained vaginal bleeding, breast cancer, or blood clots in the legs, lungs, or eyes. If you become pregnant while Norplant is in, have it removed as soon as possible. You should also avoid Norplant if you

- are happy with your current form of contraception;
- cannot afford the upfront cost of Norplant (see below);
- cannot tolerate irregular menstrual bleeding; and
- don't want to visit a doctor to control your own contraception.

Norplant is perfect for women who want a highly effective, low-dose hormonal contraceptive. It's also ideal if you want long-term contraception after having a family but don't want sterilization. If you don't do well on OCs with estrogen, Norplant might also be an alternative. Norplant is also safe for smokers, older women, women with high blood pressure, and women who are breastfeeding. In the United States, a single Norplant system of six capsules, lasting for five years, costs about $350, plus the fees for insertion and removal, which vary depending on your doctor (the average is $150 for insertion and $100 for removal). The average cost for pharmacy-dispensed OCs for five years is about $1000. Unless you're on Norplant for at least three years, it may not be cost effective. A three-year Norplant has just been introduced onto the market. It was developed because the five-year implants were considered too long an interval for many women. At this writing, not enough data are available on the three-year version, but the side effects and benefits are the same. The only change is in costs.

Any family physician should be able to insert and remove Norplant. The manufacturer, Wyeth-Ayerst, markets the implant as a kit to doctors, with detailed instructions for insertion and removal. Doctors can also take a course on inserting and removing Norplant through the Association of Reproductive Health Professionals. Before you allow your doctor to insert Norplant, ask the doctor if he or she has ever done it before, and if he or she has taken this course.

The New Controversy: Depo-Provera

Depo-Provera is an injection that works exactly the same way as Norplant—as a time-release progesterone. One injection of Depo-Provera in the muscle of the arm or buttocks protects you against pregnancy for three months. The FDA approved Depo-Provera in October 1992, and the contraceptive is manufactured by the Upjohn Company in Kalamazoo, Michigan. The active ingredient in Depo-Provera is, again, a synthetic progestin hormone. Depo-Provera is considered as effective as Norplant in preventing pregnancy and is rated as 99% effective. More than 11 million women worldwide have used it so far.

The amount of Depo-Provera in the bloodstream is at the highest level just after injection. Over time, the level drops and after three months the level may no longer offer enough protection. It's important to be on time for your next injection and to use a backup method, such as condoms, in the last week before you're due for another shot. If the time between injections is more than 14 weeks, you should request a pregnancy test before you get your next injection. Again, like Norplant, you can't use Depo-Provera if you either are or suspect you're pregnant.

You'll need to get your first injection within five days after your period. Depo-Provera is effective immediately after the injection. If you've just had a baby and want to wait a while before having your next child, you should get your shot within five days after giving birth if you're not breastfeeding. Otherwise, like Norplant, you'll need to wait six weeks after delivery. If you decide that you want to get pregnant, don't go back for another injection.

Depo-Provera differs vastly from Norplant in that it takes at least 10 months before you can conceive again. The reason why isn't clear. Here's the official answer: "Since Depo-Provera does not accumulate in the body, the return to fertility is independent of the number of injections received, but may be affected by a woman's age or weight." Translation: We don't know. Until the dosage can be perfected for each individual woman, immediate fertility after three months won't be possible. Depo-Provera costs less than $200 per year.

What are the Side Effects?

The side effects of Depo-Provera are exactly the same as those of Norplant: irregular menstrual cycles and bleeding. Only this time, after being on Depo-Provera for a year, between 50 and 80% of users will have no periods at all. Once you go off Depo-Provera, your menstrual cycle will return to normal after a few months. If you continue to menstruate while on Depo-Provera, your periods will be easier: lighter flow, fewer cramps, and reduced PMS symptoms. About 25% of Depo-Provera users also complain of pregnancy symptoms, such as breast tenderness and nausea, but these symptoms go away after about two months on Depo-Provera.

Like Norplant, weight gain is another side effect that affects about two-thirds of the users. It's not clear why this happens; it could be water retention or a change in appetite. Finally, headaches, nervousness, hair loss, abdominal pain, dizziness, weakness, and fatigue have also been reported. In general, use the Norplant guidelines above to decide whether you are an ideal Depo-Provera candidate. Women at risk for breast cancer and osteoporosis may want to look for an alternative (see below).

Unlike Norplant, Depo-Provera has a tainted past. It is possibly linked to breast cancer. This suspicion hinges on an early 1970s' study in which breast cancers were found in beagles treated for more than three years with Depo-Provera injections. However, the dose was equal to *25 times* that of the human contraceptive dose, and beagles are considerably smaller than human females. The study was discounted by the FDA, which said the beagles were not "appropriate animal models" for determining Depo-Provera side effects. In the 1980s, another study was conducted by the World Health Organization (WHO) on 11,000 Depo-Provera users worldwide. The study found that women were *not* at risk for breast cancer on Depo-Provera, which is now available in 90 countries. Herein lies the controversy. The National Women's Health Network in the United States is very unhappy with the FDA's conclusions. It counters that the WHO study was done on women who lived in countries where breast cancer rates are *half* that of the United States, and argues that the study is totally inaccurate. Again, stay alert and watch the medical headlines for more news on this.

There is another strike against Depo-Provera. A July 1991 study published in the *British Medical Journal* found that bone density significantly decreased in 30 women who had been using Depo-Provera for at least five years. If you are already at risk for osteoporosis due to your family history or due to the fact that you smoke or are underweight, or if you are are of European or Asian origin, you should look for another contraceptive. In response, the FDA has asked Upjohn to continue research on the connection between Depo-Provera and osteoporosis.

Oral Contraceptives

When the Pill first came on the market in 1960, it seemed like the answer to our prayers. However, in the early 1970s, concerns developed that there were serious risks linked to oral contraceptive use. Most of the problems with the early pills had to do with their high estrogen content. To counteract the problem, combination pills were developed with lower amounts of estrogen. Among these were triphasic pills, which released different amounts of hormones throughout the cycle. Also introduced was the "mini-Pill," or progesterone-only pill. There is also something known as the abortion pill, RU 486, which is discussed in chapter 11.

Over 56 million women worldwide are using OCs, and over 10 million of them are in the United States. OCs are very effective and have a success rate of 98%. The 2% failure rate is due to human error, such as forgetting to take the Pill. However, women on OCs have a higher chance of contracting an STD. Why? They simply have sex more often because of the spontaneity OCs allow, and OCs offer absolutely no protection against STDs. Used in conjunction with a condom, however, OCs are an ideal contraceptive/prophylactic system for millions of women.

Even though the estrogen content of the Pill has been reduced by at least half, the Pill is still a very potent contraceptive that carries risks. The Pill affects every system in the body, and some of its side effects can persist even after you go off it. For example, the risks are substantial for women over 35 who smoke.

OCs work by preventing ovulation and causing the cervical mucus to thicken. It's almost exactly the same as Norplant and Depo-Provera (which are modeled after OCs), except that with combination OCs, the estrogen causes the uterine lining to thicken, which means that it *needs* to shed. The difference between combination OCs and the new timed-release hormonal contraceptives is that your periods are induced on OCs. All OCs come in a packet or case containing either a 21-day or 28-day supply of pills. For the 28-pack, the last week of your supply contains only sugar pills; the 21-day supply requires a little more thought. You'll need to remember to start your next package seven days later. Because you're off the synthetic hormones for seven days, you will get a period, known in clinicalspeak as "withdrawal bleeding." These periods are incredibly punctual and usually come on exactly the same day at the same time, every month. You'll have less cramping, and a briefer, lighter flow. You need to take the pills at exactly the same time every day in order to keep the hormone levels in your body consistent.

The induced period is what makes OCs so popular. Anyone who suffers from irregular cycles, painful periods, PMS, or heavy flows will benefit from oral contraceptives, as long as they are using it to prevent pregnancy and not STDs. OCs are also known to guard against fibrocystic breast disease, benign ovarian cysts, and PID (discussed in chapter 6).

The mini-Pill has *exactly* the same advantages and disadvantages as Norplant because it is the same thing, except it is taken orally. Mini-Pill users will therefore experience irregular menstrual cycles, but these pills are an option for smokers, older women, women who are breastfeeding, and other women for whom traditional pills are a risk. Unless you smoke, are over 35, have high blood pressure, a heart condition, a personal history of breast cancer, or certain cancers of the reproductive organs, you'll be prescribed one of the low-dose combination pills. Then, if you suffer from too many adverse side effects, your doctor will put you on the mini-Pill.

What are the Side Effects and Risks of Combination OCs?

Combination OCs now have far less estrogen or progestin than those of the 1960s and 1970s; women today are exposed to about 1/25th of the estrogen they once were. However, the side effects of estrogen in OCs are numerous: nausea, breast tenderness, swelling, increased breast size (which some women enjoy), weight gain, vaginal discharge, headaches, and blood clots. Serious risks include cardiovascular problems, which increase the chances of heart attacks and strokes. A careful family history and personal medical history should be taken by whoever prescribes OCs to you. The side effects caused by the progesterone in OCs are increased appetite and weight gain, depression, fatigue, decreased sex drive, acne and oily skin, decreased carbohydrate tolerance, increased risk for diabetes, and increased cholesterol levels. The combination of both estrogen and progesterone can cause headaches, high blood pressure, heart problems, and cervical dysplasia. Both triphasic and monophasic OCs can cause breakthrough bleeding (bleeding between periods). Persistent breakthrough bleeding can usually be treated with supplemental estrogen without stopping the oral contraceptive.

We've all read the long list of risks associated with combination OCs. In general, if you're under 35, don't smoke, and don't have any chronic medical illnesses, then your risk of suffering from any of the "fine print" risks listed on your OC package is low. That being said, here is the fine print:

Blood clots are the most common serious risk linked to OCs. Clots can form in the brain and heart, which translates into heart attacks and strokes. Smokers on OCs are more likely to have a heart attack than non-Pill users. Women who don't smoke are more likely to develop heart disease than non-OC users, and increase their chances of a heart attack. They are also more likely to have a stroke than non-OC users. Women on OCs are also more likely to rupture a blood vessel in the brain than a non-OC user, and more likely to develop a blood clot in the leg or arm, which can mean amputation. They are more likely to suffer a pulmonary embolus, and the risk of blood clots in the lungs is higher. A woman planning to have major surgery will need to discontinue the OC about six weeks prior to the surgery. In addition, the chances of developing gallbladder disease increase. Short-term and long-term use of the OC has been linked to benign and cancerous growths on the liver, but this is rare.

The risk of cervical cancer is four times greater on OCs than off; but the risk of uterine and ovarian cancer is decreased. Combination OCs are not yet technically linked to breast cancer, but a 1989 Boston study showed that OC users under 45 had twice the incidence of breast cancer as nonusers; the risk of breast cancer was doubled for women who had used OCs for less than 10 years, and quadrupled for women who used OCs for more than 10 years. Another study showed that the rate of breast cancer in former OC users ages 30–34 tripled, compared to nonusers in the same age group; for women who had been on OCs and had had a child in this age group, the risk of breast cancer was *five times* greater.

Finally, one study reported that urinary tract cancer, thyroid cancer, and one type of skin cancer occurs more often in OC users than in nonusers. Yeast infections are also more common on OCs than off, as is gum disease for some women. (Gums are also known to swell during pregnancy, however.)

Obviously, all of these risks are scary. That's why when you begin using OCs, you may be given only a three-month supply at first. Then, if you *do* suffer any serious or unpleasant side effects, your dose can be re-evaluated and your doctor may suggest either mini-Pills or another form of birth control altogether. If you've been using OCs for more than three months and don't suffer any serious side effects, you probably never will, but you still have the above health risks to contend with. When you decide to get pregnant, it takes between 3 and 6 months for your menstrual cycle to return to normal. (See chapter 2 for details on menstrual cycles after the OC.) Only 1% of OC users suffer from infertility. Depending on what you read, some sources will say the risks are greater or less than others, and these statistics vary from country to country and year to year.

Stay away from OCs if you have a history of the following:

- blood clots in the legs or eyes
- cardiovascular problems
- heart disease or coronary heart disease
- breast cancer

- liver tumors
- abnormal vaginal bleeding
- migraine headaches
- high blood pressure
- diabetes
- active gallbladder disease
- sickle cell disease
- any major injury to your leg(s) that required a cast

You should also avoid combination OCs if you smoke or are over 35. OCs can't be taken when you're pregnant, and they also shouldn't be taken if you're breastfeeding.

How to Use Combination OCs

Below is a set of guidelines for using OCs:

1. There are several ways to start taking your OC; use the method your doctor suggests, or the method suggested in the instruction booklet that comes with your OC:
   METHOD A: Start your first pack of pills on the first day of bleeding, when you get your period;
   METHOD B: Start your first pack of pills on the first *Sunday* after your period begins;
   METHOD C: Start your first pack on the fifth day of or after your period;
   METHOD D: Start your pill today if there is absolutely no chance that you could be pregnant.
2. For the first month, use a backup method of birth control. OCs don't take full effect until the second month. Furthermore, use your backup method if you run out of pills, forget to take one, experience danger signals (discussed below), and, of course, to protect yourself against STDs.
3. Read the pamphlet that comes with your pills. Each pamphlet is FDA approved and tells you about warning signs and risks of your particular brand.
4. If you're on a 28-day pack, swallow one pill a day until you finish the pack, and then start a new package immediately. If you're on a 21-day pack, swallow one pill a day until you finish the pack. Wait

one week and start a new package. You will always start your new pack on *the same day* every month.

5. Take your pill at the same time every day to keep the hormone levels in your body stable. It doesn't matter what time of day you take them.
6. Check your pack of pills each morning to make sure you took one the day before.
7. If you miss two pills in a row, take the two pills as soon as you remember. Then, take two pills the next day. Use a backup method of birth control until the next month. (Missing two pills may also cause some spotting.) If you've missed three or more pills in a row, discard the pack. Use your backup method, and start a new pack the following Sunday, even if you're bleeding.
8. If you miss one pill, take the forgotten one as soon as you remember it, and then carry on.
9. If you have bleeding between periods, it probably means you're not taking your pills at the same time every day. If you *are* taking them at the same time every day and you still have bleeding, see your doctor. Spotting is not serious and will probably go away after your system is used to the OC. If it doesn't go away, the bleeding can be stopped with supplemental estrogen.
10. If you get sick and have either diarrhea or vomiting for several days in a row, use a backup method. You might have expelled the pills before they've had a chance to work.
11. To remember the danger signals of OCs, remember the word *ACHES:* **A**bdominal pain, **C**hest pain, **H**eadaches, **E**ye problems, and **S**evere leg pain are signs to watch out for. Stop taking the pills if you experience any of these symptoms.

Finally, it's important to remember that periods on combination OCs can be scanty. Even if your blood is brown and you just spot slightly, this *is* considered a period.

A word about the mini-Pill.

Follow the same instructions outlined above. You will not be getting regular periods, however, so just keep track of when you do get them. If you go for more than 45 days without a period, go to your doctor for a pregnancy test just in case. You'll also need to take your pill religiously at the same time each day. *If you're even 3 hours off, you'll need a backup method of birth control for the next 48 hours.*

Intrauterine Devices

IUDs are tiny devices that are fitted inside the uterus. A thin, silky thread hangs down through the cervix, just barely into the vagina, in a tamponlike fashion, to indicate that the device is in place correctly. Some IUDs are shaped like rings, with a thread attached; some are shaped like tiny sewing scissors with a thread extending from the base; some are shaped like a capital T, with a thread extended from the base; the earlier IUDs were loop-shaped. The amazing thing about IUDs is that no one really knows *why* they prevent pregnancy. The main theory is that as a foreign object in the uterus, it interferes with the sperm's reaching the egg and the egg's implanting itself in the uterus. Its failure rate ranges between 3% and 6%.

The first IUD was developed in 1909 by a German gynecologist and sex researcher named Ernst Grafenberg. It was a ring-shaped device that wasn't widely used until the 1920s. In 1934, Tenrei Ota, a Japanese physician, came up with another design. Both designs had no strings, and both physicians were reluctant to use the device because of the fear of uterine infection. Once antibiotics were discovered, physicians felt comfortable using the IUD.

The most extensive IUD study was done in Israel between 1930 and 1957, where one doctor reported his success with the 1909 model. The Israeli results were promising, and IUDs were being engineered in the United States by the 1960s. One of the key figures in American IUD engineering was Jack Lippes, a gynecologist from Buffalo, New York. He tried both the Grafenberg and Ota rings but found they were difficult to remove. He ingeniously attached a simple blue string and changed the ring to a loop instead. The string would allow women to check to see if the device was still in place, and would enable the doctor to remove it more easily. This string has been the springboard for IUD engineering ever since. The Lippes Loop became the best known and most widely used IUD in developing countries outside of China. Currently 85 million women use IUDs, and 59 million of them are in China (where the stringless IUD is still used).

After the Lippes Loop came out, several IUD series were soon developed, including the Saf-T-Coil and copper-bearing IUDs in the late 1960s. In the 1970s, a second generation of IUDs was born, and usage shifted toward copper IUDs, which yielded fewer complications, and hormone-containing IUDs, which released progestin into the bloodstream. (Today, Progestasert, a hormone-releasing IUD, is the only one widely available in the United

States.) By the mid-1970s, everyone wanted to get in on the IUD market. Untested devices went out, and IUDs have been followed by lawsuits and controversy ever since.

The IUD Disaster

The most controversial IUD was the Dalkon Shield, which was banned in 1975 and "recalled" in 1980. This was a badly designed, untested IUD that was rushed onto the market by the pharmaceutical firm A. H. Robins Company. At that time, IUDs did not require FDA approval. A. H. Robins purchased the rights to the Dalkon Shield from Dr. Hugh Davis in 1970, but the pharmaceutical company didn't conduct any tests on the IUD. Instead it relied solely on the research of Doctor Davis, which was faulty. Furthermore, since Davis was both testing and marketing the device *himself,* he was in violation of professional ethics.

Insertion of the Dalkon Shield was painful, and there was a very high rate of infection among users. This was due to a braided tail, which was a haven for bacteria. As a result, the device was banned in 1975. By 1976, 17 deaths had been linked to its use, but Robins took no action until 1980, when it finally recalled the shield, advising physicians to remove it from all users. The company's failure to act quickly resulted in several lawsuits, and A. H. Robins eventually went bankrupt in 1985. As of that date, 10,000 lawsuits had been brought against it. By 1986, several U.S. pharmaceutical companies, fearing the same predicament, discontinued their IUD lines.

In the post–Dalkon Shield era, however, IUDs were—and still are—alive and well in Canada and the rest of the world. The reason why they were virtually banned in the United States had more to with liability insurance, since U.S. health care is all private. Since the Dalkon Disaster, IUDs must now pass FDA approval before they're marketed.

How Do You Get an IUD?

IUDs are not that widely available in the United States, but it depends on the hospital, clinic, or doctor. The FDA *has* approved a few new ones since 1988, but distribution varies. If you're American and can't find a doctor who will recommend one or insert it, you could go to Canada to get one prescribed and inserted there, and pay for it through Blue Cross insurance. Regardless of *where* you get it done, it's important that whoever inserts it is an experienced gynecologist who has at least *15 IUD insertions under his or her belt.* Your doctor will perform a pelvic exam, take a detailed medical history, and describe other contraceptive options to you. Then, if your doctor still feels an IUD is the right thing for you, he or she will prescribe one that best suits your history and physical contours. Insertion requires the utmost skill and sensitivity. If your doctor isn't experienced or won't disclose his or her experience, find another doctor who will, or find another contraceptive method. If you want it removed, these same credentials aren't necessary; it simply involves pulling on the string. If the device is imbedded in the muscle, most gynecologists can remove it. Improper removal can result in perforation, however.

What are the Risks and Side Effects?

IUDs increase your risk of PID, an infection in the upper genital tract that can cause infertility. Recent studies show that the risk is highest in the first four months after insertion. Basically, the infection results because the IUD needs to go through the cervix when it's inserted. The risk of infection is highest in the first four months, as bacteria transfer from the vagina to the cervix to the uterus, hitchhiking up the IUD string. You're also at a higher risk of getting PID if you have been exposed to an STD. In other words: *STD + IUD = PID!* Another potential risk is an ectopic pregnancy, or tubal pregnancy. If you do get pregnant with an IUD in place, an ectopic pregnancy should be ruled out. Since IUDs prevent the egg from implanting in the uterus, the egg decides to stay in the fallopian tube, which is very dangerous. Periods may also be much heavier with IUDs, and you'll either get more severe cramps or *develop* cramps. Because of this, anemia is common in IUD users. IUDs have also been linked to uterine and cervical cancer, but this area is still murky. About 15% of IUD users have them removed because of bleeding, spotting, hemorrhaging, or anemia.

Other complications arise when the IUD partially expels (comes out), which means lots of cramping, painful intercourse, unusual discharge, and spotting. Often, though, expulsion is painless. Lost strings are another problem, making removal difficult. Full-term pregnancies have been reported with an IUD in place, but if you do get pregnant while you have an IUD, there's a 30% chance you'll miscarry. If a miscarriage does occur, there's an increased risk of infection. Some of these infections can be fatal. Punctures in the uterus or cervix are another drawback to IUDs and can lead to pelvic infections.

Don't go anywhere *near* an IUD if you:

- have PID, an active pelvic or vaginal infection, or an STD;
- suspect you're pregnant;
- have multiple sexual partners;
- have hemophilia or a blood coagulation disorder; or
- have an allergy to copper (many IUDs are copper but you could still use Progestasert).

In addition, avoid IUDs if you have a history of heavy and/or painful periods, diabetes, any kind of benign or malignant pelvic tumors, or STDs.

If you choose to use an IUD, keep in mind these important guidelines:

1. Insertion can be very painful. Bring along a friend or spouse. Don't walk home or drive home yourself. Take an Advil, Nuprin, or Anaprox before you have it done.
2. Always read the package insert for your IUD. It will tell you about the risks and warning signs for removal.
3. Make sure your doctor shows you how to find the string. Check the string every other day, especially after intercourse. If your string is missing, longer, or shorter, or if you can feel the IUD through your cervix, see your doctor immediately. These are indications that your IUD is not in place correctly. Copper 7 strings can get *really* long and dangle down to the opening of the vagina. Whatever you do, don't pull on it. Get yourself to your doctor's office as soon as possible. Always use a backup contraceptive when you have string problems.
4. The danger signals for IUDs spell the word *PAINS:* **P**eriod problems (lateness, spotting, bleeding in-between); **A**bdominal pain, or intercourse pain; **I**nfections of any kind; **N**ot feeling well (fever, chills); **S**tring problems (missing, longer, or shorter). See your doctor immediately if you have any of these symptoms.
5. Use a backup method of birth control for the first three months after insertion, just in case. IUDs do not protect you from STDs, and furthermore, exposure to an STD could be aggravated by an IUD. If you are concerned, use a latex condom in conjunction with your IUD.

Barrier Methods

Barrier methods are the oldest types of contraception. They involve simply placing some kind of obstacle inside the vagina that prevents the sperm from entering the uterus. Many women, weary of the risks associated with hormonal contraception and IUDs, are returning to barrier methods.

Not much has really changed in barrier method designs other than the materials. In the past, women in Sumatra molded opium into a cuplike shape and inserted it into the vagina to cover the cervix. Chinese and Japanese women covered the cervix with oiled silky paper. Hungarian women used beeswax melted into small disks. Some barrier devices recorded were particularly ingenious: Casanova recommended women squeeze half a lemon and then insert the lemon rind into their vaginas, fitting it over the cervix. The citric acid from the lemon acted as a spermicide, while the rind served as a diaphragm, covering the cervix. Natural sea sponges have been used since antiquity for contraception and did much the same thing as a contraceptive sponge does today. Barrier methods are also very safe and pose fewer risks to the user. However, unless they're combined with spermicide and a condom, they offer no protection against STDs. The only risk considered significant with barrier contraceptives is that of toxic shock syndrome (TSS), discussed in chapter 2. TSS occurs in 10 out of every 100,000 barrier users, a very low occurrence rate. The reasons why TSS would occur are the same reasons as for tampon use. Whatever barrier method you decide on, here are some rules to follow that will greatly reduce your risk of TSS:

1. Wash your hands with soap and water before inserting or removing a barrier (diaphragm, cervical cap, or contraceptive sponge).
2. Do not leave your barrier in place longer than 24 hours (cervical caps can be left in up to 48 hours).
3. Don't use your barrier during your period, when you're bleeding for any other reason, or if you have any abnormal vaginal discharge. (The menstrual flow may also break the suction.)
4. After full-term pregnancy, wait 6–12 weeks before using your barrier again. (The cervix may still be dilated.)
5. If you think you may have TSS (see symptoms in chapter 2), remove your barrier immediately and see your doctor.
6. If you have a history of TSS, choose another method of birth control.

The Diaphragm

The diaphragm is a dome-shaped cup with a flexible rim that fits over your cervix and rests behind your pubic bone. It looks like a tiny rubber flying saucer. Inserted before intercourse, it blocks the sperm from entering the uterus through the cervix. Rubber diaphragms have been around since the early 1880s and were introduced into the United States by Margaret Sanger. Not much happened to diaphragm technology until the 1950s, when spermicides were introduced and used in conjunction with the diaphragm. Typically, you place spermicidal jelly inside the diaphragm before you put it in. The jelly helps to hold the diaphragm in place.

The most recent development in the history of the diaphragm was the introduction of a new model in 1983. This product incorporates a soft latex flange attached to the rim. The flange is intended to create a seal with the vaginal wall. In addition to the new model, the same manufacturer introduced a spermicide packaged in foil in premeasured amounts for convenient, one-time use and portability. Disposable spermicidal diaphragms are also being developed and haven't yet passed FDA approval.

The failure rate ranges between 10% and 20%. This is considerably higher than hormonal methods, but much of the failure has to do with improper use and insertion. Diaphragms come in different sizes and styles. You'll need to be fitted for one by either your family doctor (who probably does it all the time) or, of course, your gynecologist. Once you're fitted, you'll be given a prescription and can purchase the diaphragm at any drugstore. Then you'll need to go back to your doctor and be shown how to use it yourself. Sometimes you'll need a plastic inserter, sometimes you won't. Go home and practice and see your doctor one more time before you use it so that he or she can make sure you're putting it in correctly. (See below for instructions.)

There are three basic types of diaphragms on the market. The Arcing Spring has a double spring in the rim, which applies pressure against the vaginal walls. It's most suitable for women with poor vaginal muscle tone or mild uterine prolapse. This style tends to flip in place by itself and is almost impossible *not* to fit correctly. Many physicians recommend this type to new users. The Coil Spring Rim is the most common style in North America. It's suitable for women who have strong vaginal muscles, no displacement of the uterus, and a normal size and contour of the vagina. It can be inserted by hand without an inserter. The Flat Spring Rim has a thin, delicate rim with gentle springs. It's most useful for women who haven't had children.

Before your doctor recommends a diaphragm, he or she should perform a pelvic exam to make sure you don't have any physical abnormalities that would prevent you from using one in the first place. It's important to get a diaphragm that fits well. If it's too small, it will expose the cervix; if it's too big, it will buckle. You should also be refitted if you've gained or lost more than 15 pounds, had pelvic surgery, had a child or an abortion, or if you found the first fitting uncomfortable. If you just can't get the hang of a diaphragm, it's probably not for you.

What are the Side Effects?

Aside from the low risk of TSS, there is evidence that suggests a link between urinary tract infections and diaphragm use. If you have a history of urinary tract infections, don't use a diaphragm. Some women are also allergic to rubber or spermicide. Again, don't use a diaphragm if you have these allergies. Other side effects include an irritation caused by the spermicide, foul-smelling discharge associated with prolonged wearing of the diaphragm, pelvic discomfort, cramps, or pressure on the rectum or bladder (usually caused by poor fit).

There *is* a benefit to diaphragm use. Women who use them have lower rates of STDs and PID. This may be because the diaphragm helps block bacteria from entering the cervix, and the spermicide helps to kill them.

How to Use a Diaphragm

Hold the diaphragm as if it were a cup. Apply one teaspoon of spermicide in the center, making a circle about the size of a quarter. Spermicide may be applied to the rim of the diaphragm to ease insertion. Squeeze the diaphragm firmly between your thumb and forefinger into an even fold. This should make it narrow enough to fit inside the vagina. Then assume a comfortable position: Stand with one foot on a chair, bed, or toilet seat, squat on the floor, or lie back on the bed with your knees up. Then insert the folded diaphragm into the vagina and push it up as far as it will go. When you release the diaphragm, the rim will regain its round shape and fit around the cervix. When it's in place comfortably, you shouldn't be able to feel it. If you do, take it out and reinsert it. You might also want to incorporate the diaphragm insertion into your foreplay. Partners can insert and check the diaphragm as well.

To remove it, hook your finger or thumb over the rim toward the front, and pull the diaphragm down and out. Use the same position to remove it as you did to insert it. You may also try breaking the suction by slipping a finger between the diaphragm and the sides of the vaginal wall, and then pulling the diaphragm out. Don't panic if you can't get it out at first. It just means you're tensing up. Wait a while and try again. There's no way it can "get lost" inside your body. You'll need to take it out after 24 hours or else you may get a foul smell as the bacteria grow on it. The bacteria can also cause irritations and discharge.

If you use a diaphragm, keep the following in mind:

1. Be sure to use the diaphragm with spermicidal cream or jelly *every time you have intercourse.*
2. After intercourse, leave your diaphragm in place for at least 6–8 hours before removing it. Don't douche during that time (or ever, in fact!).
3. If you are going to have intercourse again *after* 8 hours, wash the diaphragm with mild soap and water, dry it with a clean towel, apply new spermicidal jelly or cream, and reinsert it. Try to remove your diaphragm at least once every 24 hours.
4. If you have intercourse more than once within the 6–8 hour period, you can leave the diaphragm in, but insert more spermicide with an applicator into your vagina each time you have intercourse.
5. Make sure you always have a "diaphragm supply kit" on hand, either at home or when you travel: a diaphragm in a plastic case, one or two tubes of spermicidal jelly or cream, and a plastic applicator for inserting extra spermicide.
6. *Each time you use your diaphragm, check for holes!* Diaphragms wear out after about two years. Hold your diaphragm up to the light to see if there are any defects, and stretch it a little bit. Then, pour water into it and see if any water leaks out. If it does have holes, *don't use it.* You'll need a new one.
7. Your diaphragm shouldn't interfere with normal activities. Urination or bowel movements shouldn't be affected, and you should be able to bathe and shower normally. If it is interfering with these activities, it may not be in properly or might be the wrong size.
8. Keep your diaphragm away from petroleum jelly, which can erode the rubber. For lubricants, try K-Y Jelly, Personal Lubricant, H-R Lubricating Jelly, or Surgilube.
9. Although this may sound like a broken record, diaphragms do not offer any protection against STDs. If this is a concern, you'll need to use a latex condom with it.

The Cervical Cap

The cervical cap is a small, thimble-shaped cap that blocks only the cervix and *not* the entire upper part of the vaginal canal, the way a diaphragm does. In essence, the cervical cap is a "mini-diaphragm" with a tall dome. It was actually invented 44 years before the diaphragm. Dr. Adolphe Wilde of Germany took an individual impression of a woman's cervix and then made a custom-fitted cap out of rubber to wear over it. At about the same time, a New York physician, Dr. E. B. Foote, invented his own version. The cervical cap has always been widely available in Europe. The caps that were popular in North America 30–40 years ago were actually made out of silver or copper (more recently of plastic) and were left in place for up to four weeks. The caps that are currently available in North America are manufactured in England and are now made of soft rubber.

The *same instructions apply to the cap as to the diaphragm.* The only difference between the cervical cap and the diaphragm is that the cap doesn't need to be squeezed or folded to fit in; you simply insert the cap with your forefinger and place it over the cervix yourself. You can also leave the cervical cap on for a longer time frame—36–48 hours instead of 24 hours. Because it is smaller, you need far less spermicide inside it.

The device was not available in North America until 1988. Although the cap was popular at the beginning of the century, it became unpopular because it is a little more difficult to fit than a diaphragm (although many women do report that it is easier and less messy than a diaphragm). The main problem with the cap was that it required women to be very "comfortable" with their bodies. In the early 1970s, feminist health organizations lobbied for its return to the U.S. market. By 1976, all contraceptive manufacturers had to provide the FDA with data on the safety and failure rates of their products. Lamberts Ltd., the British manufacturer of the cap, for some reason failed to provide the necessary data to the FDA. As a result, the FDA put the cervical cap on its Class III list, banning its use. Finally, after much protesting, tests were done, data were provided, and the ban was lifted in 1988. The FDA approved one type of cap, the Prentif cavity-rim cervical cap for general use. Like the diaphragm it must be fitted, and it has a failure rate of about 17%. The cap also has the same side effects and advantages as the diaphragm, except that there's no risk of bladder infections, but there can be some irritation to the cervical lining, due to improper use. About 6% of cervical cap candidates will not be able to find one that fits (shorter or longer cervixes are a problem, apparently). Obviously, as with a diaphragm, until you're using it correctly, use a backup method of birth control.

The only women who shouldn't use the cervical cap are those who have a history of abnormal Pap tests, cervical or vaginal infections, or PID; those who have had a cervical biopsy or cryosurgery within the past 6–12 weeks; those who have an allergic reaction to rubber (plastic caps are also available); and those who have difficulty using it properly.

Cervical cap users will need to follow the general rules under "Barrier Methods," as well as the diaphragm instructions above.

The Vaginal Contraceptive Sponge

As of this writing (1995), the contraceptive sponge is no longer on the market. I'll keep you updated in future editions!

Permanent Contraception: Sterilization

Thousands of couples in North America deliberately *seek out* sterilization, otherwise known as permanent contraception. Many single adults will also seek out permanent contraception if they are certain they do not want children. It is also an option for many HIV-positive adults who do not wish to pass on the virus to their offspring. (See chapter 5.)

Permanent contraception is an alternative for couples who have chosen a child-free lifestyle (see above), and for couples who already *have* children and do not want to have any more.

Two procedures are involved in sterilization: a vasectomy for a man, and what's called tubal ligation (tying the tubes) for the woman. As a couple, only *one* of you needs to be sterilized, but a vasectomy is a far simpler procedure that involves fewer risks and that *can be reversed* about 90% of the time. The vasectomy procedure is discussed further below.

If you're a single woman who wants permanent protection against pregnancy, the *only* procedure you should consent to is tubal ligation. Shockingly, and as recently as 10 years ago, hysterectomies and oophorectomies were recommended to many women as "sterilization" procedures. Women were told that having "everything out" would protect them from other problems such as fibroids and cancer. Tubal ligation *should* never *be done for this reason!* As discussed in chapter 7, women need their reproductive organs for *all kinds* of functions other than pregnancy and childbirth. Tubal ligation is a safe procedure that preserves all of your reproductive functions except for one: having open tubes where the egg and sperm can meet. This procedure requires a general anesthetic and it should be considered *irreversible.* Again, I'll discuss the male procedure only briefly, and discuss the female procedure in more detail.

The Vasectomy Procedure: Male Sterilization

A vasectomy is simple to do and can be done under a local anesthetic. During this procedure, the vas deferens, which normally carries the sperm from the testicle, is cut on each side. Period. It can then be resewn at any point and be reversed. This procedure should be done by a urologist who knows his or her way around the area a little better than perhaps a family doctor, and who certainly has more experience with it. The procedure can be done in a hospital on an outpatient basis or, depending on how well the urologist's office is equipped, as an in-office procedure. There is a three-month waiting period involved before the man becomes absolutely sterile. During this time you'll need to use a backup method of birth control.

The pregnancy rate in couples who have *reversed* a vasectomy is 18–60%. There are no long-term side effects from a vasectomy procedure.

Tubal Ligation: Female Sterilization

Tubal ligation cuts the fallopian tubes, burns the ends with electrocautery, and blocks them so that the sperm can't get inside to meet the egg. The egg is then absorbed by the body. For this procedure, you'll need the services of a gynecologist trained in microsurgery (laparoscopy and laparotomy) and an anesthesiologist. Although 30–60% of fallopian tubes can be successfully reconstructed in the event that a woman changes her mind and wants it reversed, there's now only a 12–20% chance of her ever becoming pregnant. Therefore, this procedure is really irreversible for all intents and purposes.

In the past this procedure involved major abdominal surgery. Today it's done via laparoscopy, just as any pelvic microsurgery. After you go under a general anesthetic, your bladder is emptied and your vagina and abdomen are cleaned with an antiseptic solution. Your doctor will then make one small incision about ¼ to ½ inch long, just above the pubic bone. Next, the laparoscope is inserted into the incision and the instrument used to block your tubes is inserted through the telescope. While looking through the laparoscope, the doctor will proceed to block your tubes using cauterization, clips, rings, or bands (these squeeze the tubes together, which successfully blocks them), and may even remove a section of the tube. (There are various procedures your doctor can use; each about as effective as the next.) Ask your doctor to tell you which method he or she is using, and whether the procedure has any chance of reversal. The operation takes about 30 minutes and can be done on an outpatient basis. You can usually go home the same day and resume normal activities after about a week.

After the procedure, the incision is covered with a fairly small bandage. You should refrain from heavy lifting and may need a couple of days to recover from the anesthetic. This procedure is effective immediately and does not require you to wait three months. Since this procedure does not affect your menstrual cycle, your periods will resume as usual, and you'll go into menopause naturally. About 2 in 1,000 women will still become pregnant after a tubal ligation, some of whom will have ectopics.

Although tubal ligation is a safe procedure, no pelvic surgery is free of complications, and there are potential long-term side effects. Some women report heavier menstrual periods and painful cramps. Some women go into ovarian failure because the surgery may interfere with the blood supply to the ovaries (see chapter 7). Some women develop scar tissue from the procedure and have pelvic infections or recurrent abdominal pain. A 1989 Australian study showed that sterilized women had 40% less estrogen in their systems and 20% less progesterone, caused by damage to the ovaries' blood supply.

Other women can become depressed after the procedure, but this may have more to do with being in conflict with the decision. In general, because the fear of pregnancy is alleviated by sterilization, sex lives between couples can become freer. Fifty percent of couples reported that they had a better sex life after tubal ligation, and 75% reported a better sex life after a vasectomy.

Deciding on sterilization is not an easy decision. If you have a family, here are some questions to ask yourself:

1. Am I satisfied with the number of children I have?
2. Would I want another child if, for example, one of my children died in childhood?
3. Have I asked my partner to consider a vasectomy?
4. If my partner is uncomfortable with a vasectomy, have I explained the risks involved with tubal ligation?
5. If my partner died or we divorced, would I want the option of having children with a second partner?

If you're single, you might consider these questions:

1. Is it likely I'll meet a man in the future with whom I'd want children?
2. If my choice of career or poor financial resources is influencing my decision, would I feel the same if I changed careers or suddenly became more comfortable financially?
3. Have I discussed my decision with my significant other?

The purpose of this chapter was to cover safe-sex practices and contraceptive products. There is one more effective method of contraception: natural methods, known as fertility awareness techniques, that one can use to plan or prevent pregnancy. These techniques are discussed in chapter 12. The next chapter, "Women and AIDS," covers HIV exposure and the unique risks HIV-positive women face. It should be read by all women.

CHAPTER 5

Women and AIDS

When it affects women, acquired immunodeficiency syndrome (AIDS) is a *gynecological* disease. Not only is the virus transmitted to women through heterosexual intercourse—in addition to intravenous (IV) drug use or transfusion—but women with AIDS or HIV (human immunodeficiency virus)-related illnesses will develop far more gynecological infections than healthy women. As a result, they will need to undergo more pelvic exams, Pap smears, and gynecological treatments or procedures than healthy women.

Women who are HIV positive will also need to practice meticulous birth control and abstain from any mucus-sharing sexual activity. The HIV virus may be passed on to the fetus through the placenta, amniotic fluid, or via maternal blood at delivery. As a result, some HIV-positive women may want to consider therapeutic abortions. The risk of transmitting the virus to the fetus is approximately 35%. Finally, women with AIDS need to practice stricter gynecological hygiene.

In the previous chapter, considerable space was devoted to the discussion of safe sex, high-risk behavior, and preventing the spread of HIV and AIDS. It also discussed who should get an AIDS test by outlining the risk assessment guidelines every woman should consider. The purpose of chapter 5 is not only to discuss the actual AIDS test itself and where to get one, but also to discuss the consequences, implications, and unique concerns women who test *positive* face. Also outlined is the HIV-positive woman's responsibilities to herself and others, as well the kinds of symptoms and treatments she can expect.

AIDS 101: A Refresher Course

AIDS is a general label that refers to a collection of *opportunistic infections (OIs)* that people with intact immune systems don't get. HIV is the only virus known to cause AIDS. The virus attacks a particular kind of white blood cell that "commands" our immune system. The cell is called a *T4 or cD4 cell.* But before you can understand what goes wrong, it's important to know how a healthy immune system works.

T4 cells are the "generals"—they keep a strict, 24-hour watch to make sure that the body isn't invaded. When enemy viruses or bacteria *do* invade, T4 cells multiply and spread out all over the body. They then train other cells for combat, preparing them for aggressive attack strategies that will render helpless the enemy viruses or bacteria. This is done through the production of *antibodies,* a kind of "germ warfare" designed to specifically match the genetic material of the viruses or bacteria. When the antibody is sprung on the germ, the germ dies, and the battle is won. That's how we recover from colds, flus, measles, chicken pox, and so forth. There is no such thing as just one general, however. Several thousand generals are needed in the body to do the job.

T4 generals also have the amazing capability *to reproduce at will* so that they can never be overwhelmed by the enemy. They can turn themselves into hundreds of battalions to get the job done. When the infection is destroyed and the war is over, the T4 cells contact "diplomat" cells to negotiate a cease fire and the withdrawal of troops. Otherwise, the cells would continue to fight and might start to attack healthy tissue, which happens in an *autoimmune,* or self-attacking, disorder. The diplomat cells are called *T8 cells* or *cD8 cells* (also known as *T-suppressor cells*).

HIV is to our immune system what a nuclear invasion is to a country like the United States: *There is no way to fight, and no way to win.* After the missile is dropped, the military *itself* is virtually destroyed. All that's left is a skeleton military, consisting mainly of diplomats—T8 cells, who have no understanding of strategic combat. This isn't the end of the damage, though. Not only are the remaining generals, or T4 cells, sick from "fallout" and hence considerably weaker, they are captured by the invading HIV enemy and brainwashed into "serving" them. The T4 cells' unique ability to reproduce is completely perverted by the HIV enemy, and instead of making more healthy T4 cells, they become factories for the production of HIV! T4 cells that *have* managed to avoid capture are still quite sick from fallout. Although they try to help the body make HIV antibodies, these antibodies are not effective; the generals are simply too weak and sick to perfect them. The HIV fallout eats away at them and their numbers decrease rapidly.

Thus, your body's "citizens" are essentially left without an army. All they have now are a bunch of babbling diplomats who negotiate in vain with HIV. In fact, HIV is so fearless of the T8 cells that it leaves them alone. Worse, any effective generals still alive are outnumbered by the Diplomats at a 2:1 ratio (normally, T4 cells outnumber T8 cells 2:1) and can't seem to convince them that what they need to do is get organized and mobilize.

In the aftermath, chaos erupts in the body. Simple diseases that were once child's play for the powerful and intelligent T4 generals infest the body, taking over whole communities. These simple-minded, primitive enemies are known as opportunistic infections, and a healthy immune system can destroy them in the blink of an eye. The body situation deteriorates, and HIV is said to have then progressed to AIDS.

Because of the higher ratio of T8-suppressor cells, a person with HIV is described as being *immunosuppressed.* The immune system can decay over many years. Some people can be infected with HIV for more than 10 years and not show signs of immune suppression. Perhaps their generals take longer to die out or are better at resisting HIV brainwashing, or perhaps everyone has a different number of generals to begin with. Nobody really knows why some people can progress to AIDS in a six-month period, while others take six years and still others take *16 years*. This is part of the great mystery surrounding HIV.

Organized Resistance and Outside Aid

In HIV-infected persons, organized resistance movements from within and *outside* the body can help prevent opportunistic infections from raiding its communities and raping its citizens. "U.N. forces," in the form of *prophylaxis* (preventative medicine) can be called in to help keep order. With aid from doctors, multivitamins, information on better nutrition, hygiene, herbal remedies, and sophisticated, preventative drugs, citizens within the HIV-infected body can survive for long periods of time. For example, vitamins, minerals, and exercise combined with good nutrition and prophylaxis, can help these vulnerable, armyless communities protect themselves from falling prey to opportunistic infections. For now, there isn't an HIV vaccine. Basically, nobody *understands* the virus enough to develop either a treatment or a vaccine that works. But research is continuing, and there will probably be more advanced treatment drugs available by the time you read this, perhaps even the glimpse of a vaccine. Vaccines are currently being investigated in two areas: The first involves developing a vaccine that will prevent people from acquiring the HIV virus to begin with; the second involves developing a vaccine that will prevent disease progression to AIDS in HIV-positive persons. The difficulty with developing a vaccine is that the virus is continuously mutating. This is a bit like trying to hit a moving target.

The AIDS Picture

In terms of age, AIDS is in its "early teens," first discovered in 1981 among the homosexual population. By the year 2000, roughly 6 million people will have died from AIDS worldwide. Nobody really knows where HIV came from. It's believed to have originated in Central Africa, transported to Haiti, then to the United States, and from there, to the rest of the world. This travel route is suspected for two reasons: (1) HIV is extremely prevalent in Uganda, Zaire, Rwanda, Malawi, and Zambia at a male-to-female ratio of 2:1; and (2) a "sibling" virus to HIV was discovered in the African green monkey. Although the green monkeys don't suffer from immunosuppression, when their virus is transmitted to *other* monkey species, an AIDS-like condition develops.

How did this green monkey virus get into the human population? No one really knows. Theories range from someone being bitten by the green monkey to someone *eating* green monkey meat. It's *crucial* to understand that in the countries where HIV first appeared, it was a nondiscriminating virus, infecting mostly heterosexuals. Why has it come to be known as the "gay plague"? It just so happened that the first infected American was a homosexual male. Since anal sex results in the exchange of *both* semen and blood (discussed in Chapter 4), it provides an *optimum* transmission route for HIV. This is why HIV attacked the homosexual population more viciously. To aggravate matters, the homosexual population at the time of this first contact was an extremely promiscuous community.

Chapter 4 discusses this in more detail and outlines every conceivable route of HIV transmission. But for most women, HIV is transmitted through IV drug use or vaginal, heterosexual intercourse. There are three categories of HIV infection:

1. *Asymptomatic:* You can be infected with the HIV virus but not show any symptoms whatever of immune suppression. You will appear to

be outwardly as healthy as anyone else, but capable of infecting someone else with the virus, who, in turn, can show symptoms or be asymptomatic for a time.

2. *HIV Disease:* You can be infected with HIV and display common symptoms seen in HIV-infected persons, such as fatigue, weight loss, persistent swollen lymph nodes, yeast infections, and so on, but still have enough T4 cells left to ward off opportunistic infections categorized as being AIDS-defining illnesses. In other words, you may get sick a lot and take longer to get better, but you'll respond to treatment for the specific illness. Over the years, people in this category were defined as having *AIDS-related complex (ARC).* This terminology has been upgraded to *HIV disease,* considered a less harsh and more accurate phrase.
3. *Full-blown AIDS:* Your immune system has deteriorated to the point where you have virtually no T4 cells left. As a result, you frequently fall prey to opportunistic infections. Many people don't find out that they have been exposed to HIV until they develop an AIDS-defining illness.

Getting Tested

In the 1990s, it's not enough to know your partner; you need to know your "serostatus" (whether your blood shows the presence or absence of HIV antibodies, discussed below). The number of women diagnosed with AIDS has increased dramatically in recent years and is expected to rise. Although in North America men still account for a far greater portion of AIDS cases than women, the U.S. Centers for Disease Control (CDC) reports a 33% rate of increase in women with AIDS in 1990 compared to 1989. The rate of increase among men for the same time period was 22%. However, the number of AIDS cases *reported* reflects a very small portion of women who are actually *infected* with HIV. In 1992, the CDC estimated that about one million Americans are infected with HIV but have not yet developed AIDS. Of those infected, it is estimated that 140,000 are women. In Canada, of the estimated 30,000 Canadians who have tested positive for HIV, 10% are thought to be women.

Unfortunately, many HIV-positive women remain undiagnosed and unreported. In the United States, more women in racial and ethnic minority groups are exposed to HIV than white women due to socioeconomic risk factors, not race. For example, although African-American and Hispanic women represent 19% of all U.S. women, they represent 72% of all U.S. women diagnosed with AIDS—a shocking statistic. In 1988, the death rate from HIV infection was *nine times* higher for black women than for white women. In Canada, the rate of infection is far higher among the Native Canadian population for the same reasons.

Until recently, most AIDS cases among women were related to IV drug use, either by sharing needles and syringes or by sexual contact with a male IV drug user. This is what accounts for such a disproportionate number of AIDS cases in minority women; there's simply more drug use in lower income communities. However, AIDS in women resulting from casual, unprotected heterosexual intercourse is rising at an alarming rate. In Canada, for example, 60% of women with AIDS got infected by having unprotected heterosexual intercourse. By the year 2000, according to World Health Organization estimates, 6 million people will have died from AIDS, 90% of all new AIDS cases will be due to heterosexual contact, *and more women than men will be infected.* But for the most part, HIV infection in women resulting from heterosexual intercourse is not accurately tracked because of certain biases that still exist about who is at risk.

In a March 1993 study published in the *American Journal of Public Health*, it was found that women who become infected with HIV from sexual intercourse often go undiagnosed until the later stages of their disease. Why does this happen? The study concluded that doctors seldom ask questions about sexual behavior; 92.5% of the time, they asked women patients only about IV drug use. Doctors were also found to do an HIV blood test only on women who had either symptoms of HIV disease or AIDS-defining illnesses, or on those who revealed to their doctors that they were engaging in high-risk behavior. Yet women are just as likely to pick up HIV from unprotected sexual intercourse as they are from IV drug use. Obviously, this fact isn't yet recognized by many doctors. For example, the study surveyed medical charts of 2,102 consecutive patients aged 13 or older who were treated at a Bronx emergency room. For 855 patients who received blood tests, additional specimens were checked anonymously at an independent lab for HIV testing. Emergency-room doctors recognized or suggested HIV infection in only 30% of the patients who later tested positive for HIV exposure, and most of them were male. Indeed, 20 of the 50 men with positive blood tests were identified by doctors as being possibly HIV positive prior to testing, *but the same doctors identified only 7 of the 40 women infected with the virus as being possibly HIV positive!* Translation: *Approximately 83% of HIV-infected women utilizing that emergency room were not being tested.* This is an appalling revelation. It also means that thousands of children are at risk for HIV exposure in the womb (perinatally) from their unsuspecting infected mothers.

It all comes down to personal responsibility. Every woman who answers yes to any of the risk questions outlined in chapter 4, pg. 97, should be tested for HIV exposure and encourage her partner(s) to test also.

Low Risk Versus High Risk

Women who feel uneasy about possible HIV exposure are often considered to be in an extremely low-risk group. In the health industry, low risk means any of the following:

- You're white
- You're a professional or homemaker
- You're in (or have been in) a long-term monogamous relationship
- You're suburban, upper middle-class, or wealthy

Women in all of the above categories can be just as much at risk for HIV exposure as women who are:

- of color
- in a lower income bracket
- single mothers
- living in a high-crime area

The bottom line is all women are at risk for HIV infection. Currently, the problem with getting tested is the stigma of taking the test. This may change radically in the near future. If anonymous testing becomes mandatory for *everyone*, regardless of age, race, marital status, or income, the information that would result would become a social "AIDS vaccine."

This raises some thorny questions. Can mandatory testing be anonymous? If not, when would HIV testing cross the line and become an instrument of discrimination? Will being branded HIV positive stimulate the kind of Nazi-occupied, yellow-star environment that Jews experienced during the Holocaust? Once employers, insurance companies, or immigration officials begin demanding HIV testing, will there be enough sensitivity to use the information wisely, simply as a tracking of the epidemic?

In 1986, accusations of racial discrimination soared when the British government suggested screening African visitors to Britain for HIV. But in the U.S. military, mandatory HIV testing has been in place since 1985. The

U.S. CDC has considered introducing mandatory testing of people who are in drug programs, who visit family planning clinics, who apply for marriage licenses, and who are pregnant. These proposals were overwhelmingly rejected by public health officials in 1987. The argument against mandatory testing is that unless it absolutely guarantees anonymity or at least strict confidentiality, the information would badly compromise many people's basic civil rights. For what it's worth, infectious disease screening for immigrants was widely practiced in many countries for decades, particularly at Ellis Island. But HIV is different because it *cannot* be spread through casual contact, the way tuberculosis can, for example (coughing spreads tuberculosis).

For now, HIV-positive people are guaranteed their civil rights in exchange for following an "honor code," in which they self-govern: practicing safer sex and appropriate hygiene and refraining from high-risk activities (including condomed sex) as much as possible. If you're wondering whether you should get an HIV test, you should *definitely* be tested. The test is free at most anonymous test centers in the United States, and covered by government health plans elsewhere in the developed world. The cost of not taking the test is higher. Don't let the words *low risk* fool you. It's not who you are but what you do that matters.

Anonymous Testing

As of this writing, a home HIV test, similar to a home pregnancy test, is in the process of being debated and developed. If home HIV testing is approved, skip to the "Testing Positive" section. Until that day comes, read on. After much thought, I've decided against endorsing any kind of AIDS testing that can't guarantee anonymity. First of all, no matter where you live, anonymous testing is available to anyone; it's not a privilege, it's a right. The stress of living with HIV exposure and AIDS is enough of a burden without having to combat the cruelty that's inflicted by society on persons with AIDS. There are several good reasons why you should get an HIV test:

1. If you do test positive, early diagnosis permits early access to therapies that may prolong your health.
2. If you're planning a pregnancy or facing an accidental pregnancy, getting tested will tell you whether your fetus is at risk for HIV-exposure. Then you can consider options to either prevent pregnancy or terminate the pregnancy before it progresses too far.
3. Knowing your HIV status means that you take the necessary steps to protect other people from exposure.
4. Testing negative will alleviate your anxieties about exposure.

There are two fundamental reasons why you should get an *anonymous* test:

1. *Privacy.* You control who finds out about your results. Test results that are "confidential" wind up in your medical records, which in turn can wind up anywhere.
2. *Protection.* A positive result gets around. You don't want to lose your friends, your job, or your health insurance, or be asked to vacate your apartment if you rent. (Much of this is illegal, but legal remedies take time and money, which not all infected people have.)

Any hospital, clinic, AIDS hotline, or primary care physician will have lists of anonymous testing centers in or near your area. In fact, many AIDS networks and hotlines report that the majority of their calls are from people asking about anonymous testing. *Every* major city in North America and Europe, for example, has local AIDS hotlines set up specifically to refer people to anonymous test centers as well as primary care physicians who specialize in treating women with AIDS or HIV. AIDS hotlines also provide pre-test and post-test counseling, education, literature, and support to HIV-infected persons and their families. Major cities also have specific AIDS support organizations or hotlines for women. You can also go to women's health centers to find out about anonymous testing. These centers usually dedicate phone lines or staff to issues concerning HIV infection and AIDS. Some doctors will even do an anonymous test for you. They will draw your blood and send it off to an anonymous lab under either a pseudonym or a number. Beware the word *confidential—it* doesn't mean anonymous, it simply means "only you *and* your doctor/clinic know for sure."

An anonymous test center will give you a number that only you have access to. Often the number is a double-letter/double-digit combination, such as AB12. That number is used to identify your blood specimen, but there is no way that number can be linked to your name or address. When you call the test center, you'll usually need to make an appointment (some of the test centers operate on a walk-in basis). When you arrive, you'll be led to a private room. Someone will come in and discuss the nature of the test and explain the meaning behind a positive and negative result (see below). They will also ask you why you feel a need to be tested. Are you simply being cautious? Do you suspect infection? Once the pre-test counselor is satisfied that you understand what the test is all about and what the results mean, someone will come into the room to take your blood, or you might be shown to a different room for a blood test. You'll then be asked to come back to the test center (usually two weeks later) and will be given your results in person. Regardless of whether you've tested negative or positive, *no test results are ever given over the phone.*

What is an AIDS test?

The AIDS test reveals whether or not HIV antibodies are present in your blood; if they are, it means you've been infected with the HIV virus and are likely to develop either ARC (HIV disease) or full-blown AIDS. However, you can have HIV for years without developing AIDS or any of the AIDS-related symptoms, as discussed earlier. In essence, the test cannot tell you if or when you'll develop AIDS, only that you have been exposed to HIV.

The most common test to detect HIV antibodies is the ELISA. A positive test result usually means that since antibodies are present, the virus has been in the body for at least a few months and has therefore had some time to react to it. People who test positive are known as "antibody positive," "seropositive," or "HIV positive." This means you are capable of passing on the virus to someone else. In fact, whether or not you display any symptoms has nothing to with the impact your HIV virus will have on another person. Jane Doe, who is HIV positive and asymptomatic, can sleep with John Doe, infect him with HIV, and one year later discover that he has died from full-blown AIDS, even though she herself is still healthy and asymptomatic.

Occasionally, an HIV antibody test can produce a false positive. This means that the test shows you've been infected with HIV, when in fact you haven't been. False positives tend to occur more often in women, for reasons not really clear. For the most part, however, HIV antibody tests are 97% accurate.

A negative test means there are no HIV antibodies present in your *blood at the time of the test; it does not mean you* haven't *been exposed to HIV.* Since it takes a few months for your body to produce HIV antibodies, the test will tell you only whether you were exposed to the virus in the time period ending six months prior to the test. For example, a negative test result in July 1995 means that up until January 1995 you were not infected with the virus. If you slept with an infected person in March 1995, the test could be negative and may not tell you whether that encounter exposed you to HIV. To find out for certain, you'd need to retest in September 1995. If you've been celibate for at least six months prior to taking the test and have not engaged in any other high-risk activities, you would only need to take the test once. For the best accuracy, anyone considering taking the HIV antibody test should abstain from all high-risk behavior for at least six months before taking the test. That would eliminate the need for retesting.

Some people make the mistake of assuming that a negative HIV antibody test means they are somehow *immune* to the HIV virus. Being HIV negative simply means that, while you haven't been infected with HIV, you remain unprotected from it unless you practice safe sex and abstain from other high-risk behavior.

Not all states provide anonymous testing. Prior to taking the test, your pre-test counselor will go over the confidentiality of your test results in relation to office/clinic procedures and state reporting requirements. In Colorado for example, all persons who test positive must be reported to the state's health department. This may seem cruel, but reporting requirements are designed to control the spread of HIV. The health department would then contact that individual and ask him or her about his or her sexual history, then contact each partner of that individual. All the partners would be advised to test and refrain from sexual activity until they were aware of their serostatus.

In Canada, there aren't very many anonymous testing sites. The Hassle-Free Clinic in Toronto, Ontario (416-922-0566), has a list of all the anonymous testing facilities throughout Canada. If you have the test done by your family doctor, he or she will also be required to report a positive test to the provincial Ministry of Health. Again, this requirement is in place to help control the epidemic; it's important to track the source of infection, as well as warn other partners that they may also be infected. Anonymous testing is not as crucial for Canadians, however, since all of their health care is covered regardless of their HIV status. There are, of course, the social implications of having their serostatus in their medical records.

If you live in such a state or province, the best thing to do is to get your test done somewhere else, where your anonymity *is* guaranteed. If you live in Colorado, for example, go to California to get the test done; if you live in a smaller city in Canada where anonymous testing isn't available, go to a metropolitan center where anonymous testing is available. Even if it means taking time off work to go to another state or province, the cost of losing your anonymity may be higher, particularly for American women.

During your pre-test counseling session, your counselor will discuss the pros and cons of taking the test. He or she will point out the tremendous stress involved with waiting for test results and prepare you for possible emotional reactions should you test positive. The social consequences of a positive result will also be explained to you prior to taking the test. Your employment, housing, insurance, and personal relationships could be jeopardized by a positive result. Because people are scared of HIV and don't understand that the virus *cannot be transmitted through casual contact,* HIV-positive persons are discriminated against. Only when you understand the ramifications of a positive test will you be truly prepared to take the test. You'll then be asked to sign a consent form. Before your blood is taken, your counselor will book an appointment with you to discuss your test results.

Testing Positive

Whether you've secretly been expecting a positive result on some level or are taken by surprise, the first feelings you'll probably experience are numbness and shock over a positive test result. By law, your post-test counselor cannot let you go until you understand the meaning of testing positive: *You've been infected with HIV, but you do not necessarily have AIDS and may* never *develop AIDS.* Your counselor will then exhaustively review all the routes of HIV transmission (discussed thoroughly in chapter 4) and will assess your psychological condition. Most women who test positive benefit tremendously from women's support groups, private counseling, and, in some cases, psychiatric treatment.

Part of assessing your psychological health is determining whether you're going to act responsibly about your serostatus. For example, in anger, you might feel so hopeless about your condition that you may not *care* whether you transmit your virus to someone else. You might find yourself saying unthinkable things like "What good will safe sex do me now? I might as well have as much fun as I can with the time I have left!" You might be so angry at the person who gave you the virus that you may want to go out on an "infect-fest" and expose someone else to HIV. Angry, rash statements such as these are all *normal* reactions, and counselors are trained to hear them as pleas for help. If the counselor feels that you're not committed to reducing the risk of exposure to others, you'll definitely be sent for follow-up counseling and referred to experienced AIDS networks, hotlines, or organizations. Most of the people involved in AIDS organizations are either HIV positive themselves or are close to people who are. It's the kind of support that *really* will make a difference and bring your serostatus into a healthier perspective.

Your counselor will also take note of whether your depression over the news warrants psychiatric follow-up. Depression and anger are normal reactions to bad news, but are you on the verge of a breakdown? Will you not be able to function on your own? The bottom line is that psychological health and well-being is your key to a longer life span when you're living with HIV, just as it is for anyone living with cancer or any life-threatening condition.

After assessing your psychological health, you'll be instructed to do the following:

- See your primary care physician and/or gynecologist immediately for a full physical and pelvic examination. Inform the doctor about your serostatus. As an HIV-positive woman, you're prone not only to more general infections, but also to more *gynecological* infections, so whoever does your pelvic exams will need to be alerted. Anyone who comes in contact with your blood—a dentist, health care worker, and so on—needs to know that you're HIV positive. It is your moral and ethical duty to inform them. In other words, this responsibility goes beyond borders and legislation.
- If you're pregnant, see the section on pregnancy below. There are a number of options and special concerns.
- Do not donate blood or body organs (change your driver's license donor card as well).
- Try to abstain from sex or at *least* practice ultra-safe sex (double-bagging condoms and so forth) from here on. But even condoms aren't 100%!
- Do not share needles with anyone if you're an IV drug user.
- Do not share any of your personal hygiene or makeup items, such as razors, mascara, toothbrushes, and dental floss.
- Contact all of your past sexual partners and/or people you've shared needles with and advise them of your serostatus. Suggest that they, too, be tested.

Virtually no woman is emotionally "fine" after hearing that she is HIV positive. Most women are given phone numbers of AIDS organizations and are encouraged to contact them as soon as they find out. AIDS organizations have lists of primary care physicians and infectious disease specialists who work exclusively with HIV-positive and AIDS patients. The organizations have several support groups women can join to air their concerns, feelings, and frustrations. AIDS organizations also have the most up-to-date information on prophylaxis treatments.

Gynecological Health and HIV

In 1982, the CDC defined AIDS by pulling together a list of life-threatening disorders indicating severe immune deficiency from HIV disease or ARC.

Since then, the definition of AIDS has been revised twice. Unfortunately, this list continues to exclude many HIV-related conditions common in women, which means that doctors may not recognize conditions that indicate HIV *disease* in women.

All gynecological disorders related to HIV are considered to be HIV symptomatic but *not* AIDS. There are also several other disorders that fit into this class, including endocarditis (inflammation of the lining of the heart), tuberculosis, clotting disorders, kidney failure, and bacterial infections such as pneumonia, bronchitis, sinusitis, and sepsis (bacteria in the blood). These are all common conditions in women with HIV. This chapter will concentrate on gynecological disorders in HIV-positive women but will also include a brief checklist of other conditions classified as AIDS-defining illnesses.

Female hormones such as estrogen and progesterone have always had a strong effect on women's immune systems. For example, healthy women seem to be more resistant to a variety of viral, bacterial, and fungal infections than men. By contrast, women seem more likely to fall prey to far more autoimmune disorders such as lupus, rheumatoid arthritis, and thyroid disease. Women are also more likely to reject transplant organs or grafts. Researchers believe that women tend to live longer because of this apparently superior ability to fight off infection. Does this mean that HIV-infected women are stronger than HIV-infected men? Perhaps. The positive effects of estrogen and progesterone on HIV-positive women haven't yet been researched, but there could definitely be some answers by the end of this decade. The good news is that the possibility exists and HIV-positive women may be able to ward off opportunistic infections more effectively because of their hormonal makeup. Gynecological disorders are not considered opportunistic diseases, but they can badly aggravate and complicate HIV infection. This section contains what has been researched so far on HIV infection and gynecological problems.

Menstrual Problems

HIV-positive women do complain about changes in their menstrual cycles, which include irregular periods, changes in flow (either heavier or scantier), and an increase in PMS (premenstrual syndrome) symptoms. It's still not known whether this is due to HIV infection, opportunistic infections, or life-prolonging medications such as AZT (azidothymidine). Any chronic illness, for example, can affect weight. When women lose a lot of weight, their menstrual periods can stop, for the same reasons covered in chapter 2. New data from an unpublished pilot survey of 46 HIV-positive women attending a clinic in Brooklyn found that most women experienced a variety of menstrual disorders after HIV infection was discovered. In fact, 89% of the 46 women surveyed who *complained* of menstrual irregularities were taking AZT; only 34% of women not taking AZT had menstrual complaints. Also significant is that 66% of the women who had menstrual problems also had T4 cell counts under 500.

Obviously, certain menstrual changes, such as a heavier flow, can predispose even the healthiest woman to anemia. Anemia is already a chronic problem in HIV-positive women. If the problem is amenorrhea (no periods), a HIV-positive woman should definitely rule out pregnancy after two missed periods and try to correct the underlying cause of her amenorrhea. (She may need to have her period induced to prevent a buildup of endometrial lining that can predispose her to endometrial cancer; see chapters 2 and 8.) Amenorrhea can be caused by ovarian failure, hypothalamic failure to stimulate FSH (follicle stimulating hormone) production, or severe weight loss. At any rate, the course of treatment for menstrual irregularities is the same for women who are HIV positive as it is for healthy women. If amenorrhea is due to severe weight loss, weight-gain strategies can put your periods back on track. They include taking appetite stimulants, marijuana therapy (Marinol), or tube feeding. See chapter 2 on the menstrual cycle for more details about menstrual irregularities.

Premature Menopause

Many HIV-positive women seem to suffer from premature menopause, which is more common in immune-suppressed women. The symptoms and effects of premature menopause are no worse or different from general menopausal symptoms, discussed in chapter 13. However, HIV-positive women who experience hot flashes at night may be misdiagnosed as having night sweats, common to other HIV-related diseases such as TB or diseases that cause "wasting"—an involuntary loss of 10% or more of a person's usual body weight. Vaginitis (irritation or inflammation of the vagina caused by dryness) is also a common menopausal complaint that can be mistaken for yeast. Furthermore, menstrual irregularities could be caused by this early menopause. It's important to keep track of your cycles and report your suspicions to your doctor to avoid misdiagnosis or hormonal treatments that may not be necessary.

Pregnancy

There are a number of factors that pregnant HIV-positive women need to consider. First, progesterone during pregnancy induces a state of natural immunosuppression. This happens naturally in order to prevent the mother from "rejecting" the fetus, which is really a "foreign" object potentially presenting danger to the immune system. Interestingly, during the last months of pregnancy, there is a decrease in the number of T4 cells in the body, which also occurs in HIV infection. It is not known whether a further reduction in T4 cells in an already immunosuppressed woman speeds up the progression of HIV to AIDS. It is suspected, however, because disease progression in HIV-positive women advances in pregnancy.

Ironically, HIV infection does not seem to affect the course of pregnancy itself; the risks of complication are the same for both healthy women and HIV-positive women except that HIV-positive women are at greater risk for infections in general. The most profound impact of HIV infection on pregnancy is the outcome. Children born to HIV-positive women have between a *30 to 50% chance of being infected with HIV*. If by some miracle an HIV-positive woman delivers a baby who has not been infected, the child can be infected through breast milk. A 1995 study found that when AZT was taken by an HIV positive mother during pregnancy, the risk of passing on the virus to her child dropped from roughly 25-30% down to 8%. This is a huge clue that mandatory HIV testing in pregnancy may prove to be of enormous benefit to children at risk.

If you are HIV positive and in your first trimester or fourth month, you should definitely consider having a therapeutic abortion (in this case, the abortion would be performed for medical reasons). If your pregnancy has progressed beyond this, consult your obstetrician for options. So far, amniocentesis does not detect HIV infection in the fetus. Ultimately, whether you terminate a pregnancy or carry it full term, you should consider *permanent* forms of contraception to prevent a future tragedy. HIV-infected children can be subjected to extremely sorrowful lives, particularly when they're given up for adoption (which happens a lot) or are orphaned. It's found that many HIV-positive women progress to AIDS shortly after delivery. If the children are survived by their parent(s), the impact of their suffering and deaths deeply affects the family. Chapter 10 discusses pregnancy in more detail, chapter 11 discusses abortion in detail, and chapter 4 discusses permanent contraception. Amazingly, studies show that being HIV positive does not seem to affect a woman's decision about abortion. Studies from the

Bronx, Brooklyn, and Scotland have found that 50% of 28 HIV-positive women and 44% of 36 HIV-negative women who learned about their serostatus 24 weeks prior to conception, chose to abort.

Contraception

Contraception is far more crucial for HIV-positive women than for healthy women because of the risk of passing on the virus to the fetus. The unfortunate truth is that very little research has been done on the pros and cons of various contraceptive methods and HIV infection. Technically, the risks for hormonal contraceptives (the Pill, Norplant, Depo-Provera) are said to be the *same* for HIV-positive or -negative women. This is because there are no studies that indicate otherwise. HIV-positive women should be aware of the following factors about hormonal contraceptives:

1. Nobody knows how they interact with HIV medications such as AZT.
2. Hormonal contraceptives can trigger vaginitis and urinary tract infections.
3. Nobody knows how they will affect the HIV virus and whether they will further compromise immunity, although data so far suggest their immune effects are negligible.
4. Hormonal contraceptives may exacerbate liver dysfunction and further reduce immunity.

All that being said, the risk of pregnancy if you're HIV positive is worse than any of the unknown risks of oral contraceptives. In short, the benefits of OCs in this case outweigh the risks of pregnancy.

A disadvantage of Norplant, mini-Pills, and Depo-Provera may be the changes in the menstrual cycle. In addition, Norplant requires surgical implantation, which can pose hazards to the health care provider. Depo-Provera also involves monthly injections and, like Norplant, carries risks. Intrauterine devices (IUDs) are also not wise for HIV-positive women because they increase the risk of all kinds of pelvic infections, which may progress to PID. To date, the best *reversible* contraceptive methods for HIV-positive women are diaphragms and cervical caps, used with spermicide (see chapter 4). Whether HIV-positive women will suffer from urinary tract infections or TSS *more* than HIV-negative women as a result of barrier contraceptives is still not known.

Tubal ligation (sterilization) is still the best method of contraception and should be considered by HIV-positive women to prevent pregnancies. Nonetheless, whichever method of contraception is chosen, *HIV-positive women must always insist on condoms to prevent HIV transmission, or wear the Fe-*

male Condom. See chapter 4 for a detailed discussion of safe sex, contraception, and side effects of various contraceptives. Infectious-disease specialists recommend the best choices for HIV-positive women are safe sex combined with permanent sterilization.

Traditional STDS

Although chapter 6 discusses the symptoms, diagnosis, and treatment of STDs *other than HIV*, as well as other infections, there are a number of considerations regarding "traditional" STDs that HIV-positive women need to be aware of.

First, there already is an epidemic of traditional STDs in HIV-negative women. For HIV-positive women, an STD can do a lot of damage: It is more difficult to treat and can cause HIV disease to progress more quickly. It's crucial that HIV-positive women do everything they can to prevent contracting an STD. Abstinence or the Female Condom, *combined* with the male condom, is probably the best course of prevention at this stage, since some STDs can be transmitted from the base of the penis, not covered by the male condom. And, of course, condoms break.

Herpes

Herpes outbreaks are more persistent in HIV-infected persons, *regardless* of whether you contracted herpes prior to or since HIV exposure. If you're HIV positive with herpes, doctors recommend that you wear loose clothing and cotton underwear, take warm sitz baths, and keep your sores dry with either a blow dryer or by towel drying. See chapter 6 for more details. Acyclovir (zovirax) may be helpful.

Chlamydia

Chlamydia is a weird STD classified as neither a virus nor bacteria. It is rampant in single women under age 30. *In fact, 50% of all single women in this age group (in some studies) have chlamydia whether it's diagnosed or not.* Chlamydia is tricky because it may be asymptomatic; nevertheless, it may do a lot of damage to the reproductive organs. It's also not as easily detected by lab analyses as are other STDs. Every sexually active woman is at risk for chlamydia, but evidence suggests that chlamydia is more severe in HIV-positive women. Chlamydia *is* curable with simple antibiotics; however, HIV-positive women may need a higher dose of antibiotics or may need to take them for longer periods of time.

If you're HIV positive, you should *assume* that you also have chlamydia. Why? Since chlamydia is so much more common an STD than HIV, if you've already been exposed to HIV, your chances are increased manyfold of also having chlamydia. And since it's asymptomatic, there's no way of knowing whether you have it. This chlamydia "assumption" is also made in women diagnosed with gonorrhea. In fact, when women are treated for gonorrhea, doctors will automatically treat them for chlamydia whether it is diagnosed or not. If by chance chlamydia is *not* present, the treatment is harmless. It's better to err on the side of overtreatment. See chapter 6 for more information.

Gonorrhea

Gonorrhea is an extremely common bacterial infection, transmitted exclusively through sexual contact. HIV-positive women are, again, more at risk of contracting it than healthy women. About 80% of the time, gonorrhea is asymptomatic but is easily diagnosed through a swab taken from the cervix, anus, or mouth. If you're not practicing abstinence and are HIV-positive, get swabbed regularly for gonorrhea. Gonorrhea is curable with antibiotics. See chapter 6 for more details.

Syphilis

Syphilis is also known as the "Great Masquerader" because syphilis mimics many kinds of illnesses. This is especially deadly if you're HIV positive, because syphilis is a serious disease and can progress to the brain (see more in chapter 6). Syphilis diagnosis increased 105% in 1987, and there was a 150% increase in diagnosis in that same year for women. Syphilis is diagnosed through either a blood test or spinal fluid. If you're HIV positive, you should request a syphilis test regularly, because treatment doses are still not perfected for HIV-positive persons. If you're seeing a doctor who deals with HIV infection on a regular basis, chances are he or she has already done battle with numerous syphilis cases.

Pelvic Inflammatory Disease

PID, also covered in chapter 6, occurs when an STD remains undiagnosed and invades the pelvic region, damaging the reproductive organs. It can be extremely painful and often difficult to diagnose. HIV-positive women are more likely to develop PID. Again, HIV-positive women need to be proactive about this illness. If you experience lower adominal pain, lower back pain, pain during a pelvic exam, or chronic fevers, request that your doctor put you on an antibiotic regimen for PID caused by chlamydia or gonorrhea. Antibiotic therapy, although not considered to be a definitive cure, is still the best treatment. Since there is no set dosage for HIV-positive women, they are always purposely *over*medicated, which can cause nausea and yeast infections. PID is discussed in chapter 6; hysterectomies are discussed in chapter 7.

HPV, Cervical Cancer, and Paps

HIV-positive women are more likely to contract the human papillomavirus (HPV), which causes genital warts, which can lead to cervical cancer. Some studies report as many as 95% of HIV-positive women have HPV, while HIV-positive women are developing cervical cancer at an alarming rate. Because of this, HIV-positive women must get a Pap test done *at least* every six months for the rest of their lives. Smoking can put women more at risk in general to cervical cancer, so if you're HIV positive, avoid smoking like the plague. Pap smears detect whether the cells on the cervical lining are abnormal. The test is about 70% accurate, and false positives do occur more frequently in HIV-positive women. To get the most out of your Pap test, refrain from intercourse, douching, vaginal medications, or tampons for at least two days before the Pap test. If your Pap test is positive, you may not necessarily have cervical cancer but a precancerous condition. You'll then be referred to a colposcopist, discussed in chapter 3, and will need to have colposcopies every three months after treatment. Since HPV treatment is less successful in HIV-positive women, a Pap smear and a follow-up colposcopy should be done every three months for life. Treatments for cervical cancer are discussed in chapter 9. Some HIV-positive women are using 5-Fluorouracil—5 FU (a cervical "sloughing" cream, discussed in chapter 3) on a weekly basis, which has been shown to decrease the recurrence of cervical abnormalities and cervical cancer.

Candidiasis: Yeast

Candidiasis is the medical term used to describe the overproduction of the yeast *Candida albicans*. It is said to be the most common initial symptom of HIV infection in women. The symptoms, diagnosis, and treatment of vaginal yeast or candidiasis is the same for *all* women, regardless of their serostatus. However, both vaginal candidiasis and oral candidiasis (called *thrush)* tend to be chronic in HIV-positive women, while vaginal candidiasis is common only in HIV-negative women. When thrush develops, the tongue and skin lining the inside of the mouth are coated in a milky white goop. It's very unsettling, but it is not life-threatening. Fortunately, there are a number of things HIV-positive women can do to control candidiasis, which are covered in the next chapter.

Many women who are not HIV positive suffer from chronic vaginal yeast infections as well, and it is notorious in diabetic women. HIV-positive women are generally found to have nutritional deficiencies, which can complicate the yeast scenario. Seeing a doctor, nutritionist, or naturopath for vitamin or herbal supplements will really help. Recommended vitamin supplements include a multivitamin, additional zinc, beta carotene, selenium, vitamins C, E, and B, iron, calcium, magnesium, and essential fatty acids. (Many of these vitamins can be obtained through natural fruit and vegetable juices.) There are good, specific prophylactic treatments available to prevent oral and vaginal candidiasis.

AIDS-Defining Illnesses

As discussed at the beginning of this chapter, HIV-positive persons can live many years without developing AIDS. The information below is intended as a brief description of the groups of illnesses that people with AIDS are prone to. AIDS-defining illnesses are what we refer to as opportunistic diseases, as discussed at the beginning of this chapter. When you have an AIDS-defining illness, it means that your HIV infection has progressed to AIDS. Many women are not even diagnosed as being HIV positive until they develop an AIDS-defining illness. However, many of these illnesses can be prevented, treated, and controlled, to prolong life for several years. It might be a good idea to keep a log of your health each day (not unlike a menstrual chart). Then, as soon as you notice particular symptoms, you can try to treat them as soon as possible to prevent the disease from progressing further and weakening your immune system.

Pneumocystis Carinii Pneumonia (PCP)

PCP is an infection of the lungs that is caused by an organism known as *P. carinii.* Symptoms include shortness of breath, dry cough, and fever. PCP seems to occur very frequently in women as a first or second AIDS-defining illness, but diagnosis is often delayed until the PCP becomes severe. In other words, PCP is often the first sign that a woman has developed AIDS. All HIV-positive women with less than 200 T4 cells should take specific PCP prophylaxis to help prevent it. *PCP is an opportunistic infection that can be prevented in 90% of the people who take appropriate prophylaxis.* A distressing study showed that only 52% of women with under 200 T4 cells were taking PCP prophylaxis, while only 70% of HIV-positive women with a history of PCP were taking PCP prophylaxis. Certainly, all women with a history of the disease should be on medication to prevent it from coming back!

Esophageal Candidiasis

Also an opportunistic infection, esophageal candidiasis is the same yeast infection that occurs vaginally or orally, but it develops in the esophagus. This is another AIDS-defining illness that can be controlled in the same way as vaginal yeast infections, through diet, exercise, antifungals, and so forth. Symptoms include painful swallowing, weight loss, and vomiting. There is an excellent article on preventing fungal infections in *Treatment Issues,* available through the Gay Men's Health Crisis (GMHC), 212-807-7035. The publication is mailed out free. Ask for Vol. 5, No. 7, and Vol. 6, No. 4.

Mycobacterium Aviumintracellular Complex (MAC)

MAC is a serious AIDS-defining infection that tends to occur later on in the disease. Symptoms include wasting, fever, diarrhea, fatigue, anemia, and diseases of the bone marrow, liver, lung, adrenal glands, and gut. Usually MAC doesn't occur unless you have fewer than 50 T4 cells. There are some promising drugs such as clarithromycin and rifabutin that offer hope, but prophylaxis is difficult because of the wide variety of symptoms. Call the

GMHC at the number above and request *Treatment Issues*, Vol. 6, No. 2, for more information on MAC treatment and prevention.

Tuberculosis (TB)

There are two kinds of TB. Pulmonary TB (in the lungs) is a HIV-related disease; widespread or disseminated TB is an AIDS-defining illness that affects the liver, central nervous system, adrenal glands, lymph nodes, skin, reproductive organs, and heart. Both forms of TB develop while the immune system is still intact with a T4 cell count of 300–500. It's aggravated by urban smog and pollution and places with poor ventilation. It may result from a new infection or the reactivation of an old infection. Make sure you're living in a properly ventilated area, and if you have the opportunity to move into a more rural community with less pollution, you should consider it. Find out if any of your close friends or family have had TB or have ever been exposed to it. If they have, you can be tested for TB before symptoms develop. Symptoms include fever, cough, and chest pain. TB in HIV-infected people can be cured, but it may take a while. There is a simple test that diagnoses it. If you have TB, you'll need to be on multiple medications for over a year. Obviously, the sooner it's discovered, the greater the chance of recovery.

Kaposi's Sarcoma (KS)

KS is the classic AIDS-defining illness in men but develops far less frequently in women. KS was once thought of as a rare form of skin cancer. It is now described as a collection of abnormal blood vessels caused by a variety of body chemicals interacting with immune suppression. KS symptoms are hard, not-very-painful, purplish splotches found on the skin and also on internal organs. A recent study in London of KS in bisexual and homosexual men with AIDS indicated that men who came into contact with each other's feces (via anal sex) were more at risk for KS. Currently, only about 3% of women with AIDS develop KS. For more information about KS, call any AIDS hotline and request the May 1, 1991, edition of *AIDS Treatment News* (No. 122).

Wasting

As mentioned earlier, wasting is an involuntary weight loss of 10% or more of a person's usual body weight. Wasting often occurs as a symptom of other diseases but can occur in the absence of major infection as well. In women, wasting can be misdiagnosed as anorexia nervosa, bulimia, or crash-dieting, but it is a serious AIDS-defining illness that leads to severe malnutrition. Diarrhea is the major symptom. Specific infections such as parasites should be ruled out first before any of the weight-gain strategies described above (for amenorrhea) are investigated. Any doctor or nutritionist can prescribe a weight-gain diet.

Serious HIV-Related Illnesses

There are a number of HIV-related conditions that are not considered AIDS-defining.

Endocarditis

Endocarditis is a bacterial infection that causes inflammation of the heart valves. If left untreated, it could lead to heart failure and death. This occurs most often in IV drug users. The most common symptoms are fever, heart murmurs, irregular heartbeat, chills, headache, back and chest pain, stomachache, nausea, and vomiting. It can be treated successfully with antibiotics. Keep a health chart and record all of your symptoms.

Blood Disorders

There are several blood disorders that HIV-positive women are prone to. They include anemia (low red-blood-cell count), common in all HIV-positive women, and a garden variety of disorders that interfere with blood clotting, to which drug users and persons with hemophilia are prone. Anemia can seriously complicate HIV infection. One study of HIV-negative women found that anemia was more prevalent among African-American black women and women in low-income brackets. Anemia can be easily controlled with proper nutrition and vitamin supplements.

Thrombocytopenia is another serious blood condition that occurs in 40% of people with AIDS. Steroid treatment is available and is usually successful. Finally, there is a condition known as *neutropenia,* caused by a low number of a certain white blood cell. Drugs that damage the bone marrow, such as AZT, can trigger it, but it is rarely life-threatening. Good nutrition and vitamin supplements help prevent it.

Ongoing Care and HIV Hygiene

All HIV-infected persons need to be referred to a primary care physician experienced with HIV, or to an infectious-disease specialist, usually an internist who specializes in infectious diseases. In most cases, HIV disease can be managed for years by a primary care physician. He or she will monitor your overall health, which might include blood tests, diagnostic procedures, antibiotic treatments, and prophylaxes for various infections. He or she can also treat most symptoms resulting from HIV disease. However, once you develop an AIDS-defining illness, it's better to seek a referral to an infectious-disease specialist. In addition, women will need to see a gynecologist experienced in treating HIV-positive women. To find one, call an AIDS organization to get names of gynecologists you can interview. There are also some specific hygiene habits HIV-positive women need to follow religiously.

If you're HIV positive, you're more vulnerable to bacteria than someone who is HIV negative. There are a number of ways you can reduce the bacterial risk by modifying your diet and lifestyle:

- *Avoid raw meat, raw fish, and raw eggs.* Salmonella flourishes in these things. First, don't touch or prepare raw meat, fish, or eggs. The bacteria can be transferred through utensils, bowls, cutting boards, and so forth. Second, don't *eat* anything containing these raw ingredients. Avoid caesar salads, mayonnaise, meringue, sushi, steak tartare, and so on. Avoid fried eggs or anything that has soft yolks. Well-cooked scrambled eggs are fine, though. Similarly any time you eat meat, make sure it is thoroughly cooked. If you must prepare raw meats, wear rubber gloves and wash the dishes in *very* hot water to kill the bacteria. Carefully dry the dishes afterward before you use them again. If you don't have a dishwasher, blow-dry your dishes or even "nuke" them for a minute in the microwave after you've washed them. The point is to kill the salmonella with heat.
- *Avoid alcohol, drugs, and smoking.* All these damage your immune system and can contribute to advancing your illness.
- *Make sure you get a lot of rest.* Listen to your body. If you feel tired, rest—don't fight it. Go to sleep earlier if you need to in order to get up early. Try to get at least 10 hours of sleep each night, and if you can, take a nap during the day.
- *Practice safe sex to protect* yourself *from any other STDs mentioned above.* And, of course, you'll want to prevent passing on HIV to someone else.
- *Avoid going places where the sanitary conditions are poor and where there is a high*

risk of developing infections. Movie theaters are fine, but rethink truck stops, fast-food restaurants off highways, and so forth. Don't visit *anyone* who's sick. If your friends have children, make sure the child is *well* before you visit. "Just getting over a cold" won't do! Things like chickenpox and measles can be deadly, even if you already had them as a child yourself.

Here are other health and hygiene musts for persons who are HIV infected:

- *Don't go near any cat litter boxes.* Cat feces carry protozoan called toxoplasmosis, and can be very dangerous. Cats *are* wonderful pets, however, which can have a calming and positive effect on your health. If you have a yard, you can easily train the cat to go outside. You should also wash your hands *each time* after you touch your cat. If you don't have a cat, try to avoid places that do—the litter may not be clean! If you don't have any litter "helpers," find another home for your cat. If you don't have a yard, you'll need to send your cat to "boarding school." Using rubber gloves to change the litter will not protect you from infection because the infectious material may get into the air and be inhaled when the litter is disturbed.
- *Don't accept any kind of vaccination unless your doctor knows that you're HIV positive.* Killed viruses in the vaccine are fine, but avoid viruses that are *altered.*
- *Don't donate blood, plasma, body organs, or other tissue.* Men should not donate sperm!
- *Don't engage in high-risk behavior* (see chapter 4).
- *Avoid getting pregnant.*
- *Do not breastfeed your child if you've just delivered.*
- *Cover any cuts or grazes with a waterproof bandage.*
- *Avoid sharing toothbrushes (gums bleed) or razors to reduce transferring contaminated blood to someone else.*
- *Clean up any spilled blood, vomit, or other bodily fluids immediately.* Wash the surface down with one part bleach, 10 parts water.
- *Dirty clothes, linen, towels, and so forth should be washed in the hot wash cycle in an ordinary washing machine.*
- *Used sanitary napkins and tampons should be burned or put into a sealed plastic bag and disposed of safely.*

HIV and AIDS are clearly enormous topics that can't possibly be covered in the scope of one chapter. Appendix A contains a list of excellent organizations you can contact for more information. If you are HIV positive, you'll need to continue practicing safe sex to reduce the risk of aggravating your condition by contracting a STD. The next chapter discusses other STDs in detail.

CHAPTER 6

Other Viruses and Infections

Women are vulnerable to a long list of gynecological infections. Some are caused by viruses or bacteria that are sexually transmitted, but many infections are spontaneous, meaning, for the purposes of *this* chapter, they are *not* transmitted sexually; they develop for reasons that have nothing to do with one's sexual behavior. Spontaneous infections may be caused by diet or irritation, or the cause may be unknown. Yeast infections, for example, are classic spontaneous infections.

Many of you may be reading this chapter to find information on a specific infection you're suffering from *now.* In lieu of this, I've added a bracketed label for each heading below that will immediately identify each infection or group of infections as either a sexually transmitted disease (STD) or a spontaneous infection. Another label identifies an infection that can be both an STD and spontaneous. In other words, while the infection can suddenly develop for no reason, the same infection can also be transmitted sexually.

The one STD you *won't* find discussed below is HIV. HIV and AIDS are discussed in chapter 5. Prevention of STDs is discussed in chapter 4. The human papillomavirus (HPV), also known as venereal or genital warts, is discussed briefly below and extensively in chapter 3.

No matter how old you are or what kind of background you have, chances are you've had, have, or will develop a gynecological infection at some point in your life. For instance, yeast infections and urinary tract infections are so common that virtually every woman has one in her history, or will experience one. If you're sexually active, chances are you have already been exposed to an STD of some kind. You may have been treated for it long ago, or you may not even know you have it. Chlamydia, for example, is asymptomatic, and can exist for years before it's detected. In some studies, the prevalence of chlamydia in women 18–30 years old is as high as 50%. Chlamydia is currently the number-one cause of infertility. Pelvic inflammatory disease (PID), which is most often caused by an untreated STD (most often chlamydia and gonorrhea), affects over one million North American women each year. Gynecological infections are a fact of life for almost every woman across the globe. If you're sexually active, live in an urban community, are between the ages of 15 and 24, and have had more than one partner, you're at the highest risk of contracting an STD.

Since the advent of AIDS, however, many of us feel tremendous panic and fear over any unusual discharge or obvious symptoms of gynecological infection. The irony is that HIV is *still* less common than *most* gynecological infections. The purpose of this chapter is to calm you down and give you the plain facts about the other viruses and infections—the ones that most of us get.

Sexually Transmitted Disease [STDs]

The term *sexually transmitted disease* is relatively new and has come to replace the now archaic term *venereal disease* (VD). STD refers to any disease that can be transmitted through sexual contact: viruses, bacteria, lice, and other parasites. Since HIV emerged in 1981, there has been more acceptance of "traditional VD," which includes gonorrhea, syphilis, herpes, genital warts, crabs, and scabies. There is a hidden, misguided morality that tells women: "As long as a partner is not HIV positive, unprotected sex is fine, because the *other* diseases are curable and can't kill you the way AIDS can!" There is a long list of "other" STDs that were not part of the VD families of the 1950s, 1960s, or 1970s. Although many of the "other" diseases are indeed curable with antibiotics, they *can* remain asymptomatic for years. Some—such as "traditional" herpes or genital warts—are not curable.

Chlamydia

Chlamydia was discovered in the late 1970s and is neither a typical bacteria nor a virus. It is very small in size, like a virus, and has some characteristics of bacteria but can't manufacture its own energy the way bacteria or viruses can. Instead, it acts like a parasite, entering cells and using *their* energy. It is caused by an organism known as *Chlamydia trachomatis*, but it is not always easy to detect. Ten percent of the time, people who have chlamydia will test negative for it.

Chlamydia is one of the most common STDs in North America. In the sexually active 18–30 crowd, 50% have chlamydia. Chlamydia is particularly nasty because it is asymptomatic. In one year, about 4.5 million women in North America will be infected with chlamydia, and 60% of them will not have any symptoms. The disease can do a lot of damage, though. Some experts estimate that chlamydia causes 50% of all pelvic infections and 25% of all tubal pregnancies due to scarring of the fallopian tubes. It can also cause urethral infections, cervicitis (inflammation of the cervix), and PID, which can lead to infertility or complications during pregnancy or birth.

In men, chlamydia can cause *nongonococcal urethritis (NGU)*. Nongonococcal means the infection is not caused by gonorrhea; urethritis means inflammation of the urethra. If a man with NGU has sex with a healthy woman, she will probably get chlamydia. Finally, chlamydia can also cause *proctitis*, which is inflammation of the rectum.

The symptoms of early-stage chlamydia are usually nonexistent for four out of five women. The most common symptom, if any, is increased or abnormal vaginal discharge, which usually develops about 14 days after infection. Sometimes a strong, rather foul vaginal odor develops as well. Painful urination, unusual vaginal bleeding, bleeding after sex, and low abdominal pain may also be signs, and the cervix may become inflamed (noticeable when you are examined by a doctor). If your cervix bleeds easily after a Pap smear, this is also a major clue. If chlamydia spreads to your uterus and fallopian tubes, it will have progressed to PID, and you may develop some of the symptoms discussed below.

One way to find out whether you have chlamydia is to ask your partner whether he has symptoms of NGU. Painful urination or urethral discharge that appear one to three weeks after infection are telltale signs. About 10% of the time, men show no symptoms of chlamydia either. The best thing you can do if you're sexually active is to be regularly screened for chlamydia by your family doctor. The test is 90% accurate. The screening is simple: Your doctor takes a culture swab of cervical mucus. It can be done in conjunction with a Pap test. How regularly should you be swabbed? Every time you have a new partner. If you test negative but still suspect it, request antibiotic treatment for it anyway. Even if you are treated for nonexistent chlamydia, the treatment is relatively harmless to you, other than the mild side effects of antibiotics discussed below.

NGU can also be caused by *Ureaplasma urealyticum (T-Mycoplasma)*, another STD. Some practitioners feel that this can also cause PID in women. However, culturing for ureaplasma is very difficult. If your doctor suspects it, it's easier for him or her to just treat it and not bother culturing.

The good news about chlamydia is that it is *extremely* easy to treat: Tetracycline will cure both chlamydia and ureaplasma infections. The drug usually prescribed is called *doxycycline* (Vibramycin), a derivative of *tetracycline (Achromycin* and many other brands). Two doxycycline capsules per day for 10 days will do the trick. Tetracycline is cheaper and must be taken four times a day, but many people forget to take that many pills; that's why the doxycycline is better. If you're pregnant or cannot be on tetracycline, you'll be given *erythromycin* (*ERYC, PCE, Ery-Tab*, and many others). *Penicillin*, on the other hand, is not effective here.

As many as 10% of all pregnant women are believed to be infected with chlamydia. This can lead to all kinds of complications during pregnancy or at birth, including miscarriage, infant pneumonia, *conjunctivitis* (severe eye infection), and even blindness. If you're pregnant, request a screening for chlamydia as soon as you can. If you have it, you can be treated with erythromycin. The antibiotics should be taken as prescribed, or the infection could resurface. The typical treatment regimen for a *nonpregnant* woman is either two doxycycline capsules for 10 days, or a tetracycline derivative four times a day for 7 days. See the section below on antibiotic treatment. After you've finished your antibiotics, you will need to be rescreened to make sure that the infection is gone. Abstain from all sexual activity until you're *sure* that you are cured.

A final note on chlamydia: The best way to avoid chlamydia is to practice safe sex, discussed in chapter 4. It is also believed that hormonal contraceptives increase your risks of exposure because the cervical mucus changes and is therefore a better "host" for chlamydia. The most disturbing fact about chlamydia is that it is a leading cause of infertility. Physicians believe that if more attention were paid to preventing chlamydia, infertility clinics would lose revenue, and the infertility "epidemic" going on today in North America would dramatically decrease.

Gonorrhea

Gonorrhea is caused by the bacteria *gonococcus*. This bacteria makes a home for itself in genitals and urinary organs and affects the cervix, urethra, and anus. You can transmit the virus through oral sex, anal sex, and regular intercourse. If an infected person has gonorrhea discharge on his or her fingers and then touches your eyes, you can also get gonorrhea and develop conjunctivitis.

Gonorrhea is fairly common and does more damage to women than to men. However, it is *less* common than chlamydia. If you're diagnosed with gonorrhea, you'll also be treated for chlamydia. The reasoning is that if you managed to contract gonorrhea, there's an enormous chance you already have chlamydia. In fact, women can often be simultaneously infected with both chlamydia and gonorrhea if the partner is a carrier of both infections. Women are thought to have a 30% chance of contracting gonorrhea after one sexual contact with an infected partner, and almost 100% if they are on hormonal contraception. Like chlamydia, early-stage gonorrhea is asymptomatic about 80% of the time. Symptoms depend on where the gonococcal bacteria are "living."

Gonococci (plural for gonococcus) love the cervix most of all, so cervical infection is the most common. About three days after infection, a discharge develops, caused by an irritant released when the gonococci die. You may notice it yourself, or your doctor may be able to see redness on the cervix. If your urethra was infected, you'll experience painful and more frequent urination. Conjunctivitis, menstrual irregularites, spotting after intercourse, and swelling of the vulva (vulvitis) are also symptoms. If gonorrhea spreads to your fallopian tubes, it will have progressed to PID, and you may have PID symptoms, discussed below. Most PID is caused by gonorrhea or chlamydia.

If you contracted gonorrhea in your throat through oral sex, you may have a sore throat and swollen glands. When gonorrhea progresses into something called *disseminated gonococcal infection (DGI)*, symptoms can get really nasty: rashes, chills, fever, painful joints and tendons in the wrists and fingers, and sores on the hands, fingers, feet, and toes. During your annual pelvic exam, your doctor will check your cervix for any unusual discharge and may take a culture as a routine screening. Usually, gonorrhea tests are 90% accurate if a culture test is done; if only a "gram stain" is performed, in which the discharge is smeared onto a slide and stained, the test is only 50% accurate for women but very accurate for *men with symptoms*. The best thing to do if you suspect gonorrhea is to request two culture tests one week apart.

If you *do* have gonorrhea, you will be either screened for chlamydia or automatically treated for it. Gonorrhea is easily treated with antibiotics: one dose of *ceftriaxone* (Rocephin) and a follow-up prescription of doxycycline to cure the probable chlamydia. The Centers for Disease Control (CDC) may revise recommended treatment to include certain oral antibiotics. If you're pregnant, you should be routinely screened for gonorrhea, but double check! All hospitals now treat the eyes of newborns with silver nitrate or antibiotic drops to prevent gonococcal infection just in case.

A crucial point is that many women self-diagnose gonorrhea discharge as *yeast.* They then self-treat with over-the-counter yeast infection medication such as Monostat 7. Never self-diagnose! Vaginal discharge can mean *anything,* including the presence of tumors. Whenever you notice unusual discharge, always get it checked by a qualified primary care physician or gynecologist.

Herpes

Herpes is caused by the herpes simplex virus. The virus enters the body through the skin and mucous membranes of the mouth and genitals and then permanently sets up shop at the base of the spine. Herpes was the "AIDS" of the 1960s and 1970s and it was the STD everyone feared most because it was permanent. There are two types of herpes: Herpes Simplex Virus Type I (HSV I), which is characterized by cold sores and fever blisters on the mouth and face, and Herpes Simplex Virus Type II (HSV II), the dreaded genital herpes. HSV I can be transmitted through kissing. You can also contract both HSV I and HSV II if you have oral sex and intercourse with an infected partner. Herpes *is* contagious whether the sores are active or not; it is most contagious, however, when the sores are active, but most infection takes place when the sores are *inactive.* This is when herpes is known to be asymptomatic. When the sores are active, they're visible and stand as a warning to the other partner "not to touch." Indeed, touching the sores with your fingers and then touching the skin of a healthy person may transmit the virus. That's how potent the sores are. However, when there are no visible sores, the virus can be transmitted.

The herpes sores are called vesicles, and they are painful, watery blisters that occur anywhere from 2 to 20 days after infection. Just before the vesicles appear, a herpes outbreak can be preceded by a tingling or itching sensation on the skin surrounding the outbreak. This is known as the *prodromal* period. The vesicles that women get in HSV II are most commonly found on the labia, clitoris, vaginal opening, perineum, and sometimes on the vaginal walls, buttocks, thighs, anus, and navel. Women can also have sores on the cervix, but these are not painful. Within a few days, the vesicles rupture, leaving behind shallow blisters that may ooze or bleed. After three or four days, scabs form and the vesicles fall off, healing by themselves without treatment.

There is no cure for herpes, but there are some antiviral medications (pills) that can help alleviate the pain of the vesicles. The initial herpes outbreaks are by far the worst. You may find it painful to urinate. Filling an empty shampoo bottle or squeeze-top bottle with warm water and simultaneously pouring it on the sores as you urinate will help. (The urine burns the sores, which is very painful.) You can also urinate in the shower or bath if it gets really bad. You may experience dull aches or burning sensations on your vulva or might develop vulvitis, which is inflammation of your vulva. Fever, headaches, and swollen lymph nodes around the groin are also common with the first outbreaks. The initial outbreaks also take longer to heal, lasting about two to three weeks. Then, the virus will start to taper off, and you may go from monthly initial outbreaks to just annual outbreaks. The usual pattern is nasty initial outbreaks, and milder recurrent episodes within 3 to 12 months after the first herpes outbreak. Then, recurrences become milder and far more sporadic, perhaps once every two years. Factors such as stress, poor diet, caffeine, and hormonal elements trigger herpes outbreaks. The presence of other infections, such as vaginitis, genital warts, or yeast can also trigger a recurrence.

Recurrences of HSV I are less frequent. Previous infection with HSV I may provide some resistance to HSV II or make HSV II less severe. About 25% of people with HSV II may also never experience a recurrence. To obtain a definite diagnosis, a culture is recommended. A blood test can also detect whether you have herpes antibodies present. The problem with this test is that it can only tell you that there has been an infection at some point. It doesn't tell you when the initial infection occurred.

There are a number of homeopathic treatments women use for recurrent herpes that include oils and vitamins. It's also important to keep the sores dry. Blow-dry them or towel dry, take warm sitz baths with baking soda every few hours, and wear all-cotton clothing and underwear. Controlling your diet is also important. Foods high in caffeine (such as coffee, chocolate, and colas) can trigger outbreaks, and *acyclovir* capsules (Zovirax) can help prevent frequent outbreaks. For more information on natural therapies, contact the Herpes Resource Center (HRC), which operates a hotline: 919-361-8488 or The Herpes Advice Center at 212-213-6150. Also refer to Appendix A. Over 30 million North Americans are currently infected with herpes, but only about 25% of them know they have it. Preventing herpes is easily done by practicing safe sex, discussed in chapter 4. It's estimated that roughly 30% of the general population have been exposed to HSV II.

If you have herpes:

1. Don't have sex when you have active sores, and insist your partner wears a condom, even when there are no sores present. (Or, you can wear the Female Condom.) If you're in a monogamous relationship and wish to conceive, ask your primary care physician for advice. The risk of passing on herpes to your spouse or partner years after an initial outbreak may be quite low if you don't suffer from recurrent herpes. Many women with herpes go on to have normal, healthy pregnancies and deliveries.
2. Don't donate blood during an initial outbreak. (Men should not donate sperm.)
3. If you're pregnant, make sure your obstetrician is aware you have herpes. Depending on how frequent and severe your outbreaks are, you may need a cesarean section to avoid transmitting herpes to your child. Cesarean section is recommended only if visible lesions are present or if there are symptoms of a recurrence during delivery. Most women won't need a C-section because of herpes.

Human Papillomavirus (Genital Warts)

Genital warts (also referred to as venereal warts) are caused by HPV. This virus is very similar to the one that causes skin warts, but there are several types of HPV floating around. Warts are painless and can appear on the vulva, cervix, or penis. Unless the warts are on the cervix, your doctor can usually spot them and treat them with a solution that will burn the wart off. HPV on the cervix can take the form of raised or flat lesions. Both types of lesions will be picked up by a Pap smear. If left untreated, HPV can cause the cells on the lining of your cervix to change, which can lead to cervical cancer. Detection of HPV by Pap smear, colposcopy, and treatment is discussed in chapter 3. HPV is currently *the* most common STD in North America. It is rampant in sexually active women ages 18–35. Practicing safe sex, discussed in chapter 4, can prevent HPV.

HPV can be treated but never technically cured. Once the warts are removed, the virus may not cause any further problems. However, recurrences are common. It's also possible to be infected with another strain of the virus, since infection with *one strain* doesn't protect you from another. Follow-up Pap smears for the first couple of years after HPV diagnosis, and annual Pap smears after that will enable you to nip HPV in the bud should it decide to erupt again.

Syphilis

In the past, syphilis was a very serious, incurable disease that often resulted in madness. Today, it's easily treated with antibiotics. Syphilis is caused by a bacterium known as *spirochete.* There are three stages of syphilis: primary, secondary, and tertiary (late stage). It's transmitted through sexual or skin contact with someone who is already infected. A pregnant woman can also transmit the disease to her unborn child. Syphilis spreads through open sores called *chancres,* or rashes that pass through the mucous membrane lining the mouth, genitals, anus, or broken skin.

During the 1970s, syphilis was virtually eliminated as an STD because it had been treated so aggressively in previous decades. In 1985, however, the incidence of syphilis began skyrocketing in the United States and has continued to rise since.

Diagnosing syphilis is tricky. Known as the "Great Masquerader," syphilis symptoms imitate other symptoms and can be misdiagnosed. Syphilis is diagnosed through a blood test that checks for antibodies to spirochetes in the bloodstream. Syphilis is a miserable, damaging disease. The first three stages of syphilis can be completely cured, leaving no permanent damage. Tertiary syphilis and subsequent neurosyphilis (when the disease spreads to the brain) can be cured, preventing any *further* damage. Once damage is done, however, the damage can't be repaired. Amazingly, syphilis is treated with simple antibiotics, either penicillin or tetracycline. After you've been treated for syphilis at any stage, you'll need to have a follow-up test to make sure you've been cured.

Primary syphilis.

In primary syphilis, a chancre will develop. Chancres can look like pimples, open sores, or blisters, and are generally painless. It can take between 9 and 90 days for a chancre to develop after infection. Chancres usually appear on the genitals, but they can also show up on the fingertips, lips, breast, anus, or mouth. Ninety percent of the people with chancres don't notice them. This is unfortunate, since it is at the primary stage that syphilis is most infectious. If left untreated, syphilis progresses to the secondary stage within six weeks to three months after infection.

Secondary syphilis.

Secondary syphilis can last for months, even years. Symptoms include hair loss, sore joints, widespread rashes including the palms or soles, swollen lymph nodes, and weight loss. (It can also be possibly misdiagnosed as HIV or a severely complicated HIV infection!) Flu-like symptoms are also common. There may also be a raised area around the genitals and anus. At this point, syphilis can be transmitted through mucus and contact with the raised patches. If it's still not treated here, syphilis will go into a type of "remission" known as a *latent stage.* Here, someone with syphilis will feel fine and experience no symptoms at all. When syphilis goes into a latent stage, it can last for up to 20 years. The disease is also no longer infectious by this stage, but it can do a lot of damage to both men or women and attack the body at full force at the late or tertiary stage.

Tertiary syphilis (late stage).

If the syphilis remains untreated, it will move to the tertiary stage where it can attack the heart, eyes, nervous system, or brain. It's extremely rare for anyone to get to this stage, but HIV-positive persons are less likely to be successfully treated for primary syphilis and may in fact wind up with tertiary syphilis. Request a syphilis screening if you suspect it or have been having unprotected sex with numerous partners. Tertiary syphilis is not contagious.

Neurosyphilis.

Neurosyphilis is an advanced form of syphilis that can cause serious problems in the brain and nervous system. It is diagnosed through a spinal tap. Symptoms are headaches, stiffness in the neck, confusion, blurred vision, blindness, abnormal eye movements, facial weakness, hearing loss, or loss of balance. This stage is not contagious.

Congenital syphilis.

No matter what stage of syphilis you're in, you can *always* pass it on to your unborn child. The number of congenital syphilis cases reported in 1988 was the highest since the early 1950s, and in New York City alone, that number increased more than 500%! All pregnant women should request a syphilis test, particularly if they're HIV positive.

Hepatitis B

Hepatitis B is a virus that causes inflammation of the liver. It is a serious STD that is on the rise. It is transmitted through contaminated needles or blood and also through mucus-sharing activities that include saliva, semen, or vaginal fluid, which enter the bloodstream of an uninfected person. Like HIV, hepatitis B can flourish in an anal-sex "environment" and among drug users. Tattooing and ear piercing are also common routes of infection. Mothers can also pass on this virus to newborns during childbirth. Those at highest risk for hepatitis B are intravenous (IV) drug users, gay men, health care workers, and prostitutes.

Hepatitis B can take up to 180 days after infection for any hepatitis symptoms to develop. In an extreme case of hepatitis B, symptoms are nasty and include skin lesions, arthritis, fever, fatigue, nausea, diarrhea, vomiting, and so on. The second phase of the illness is characterized by jaundice, dark urine, pale stools, and a tender, enlarged liver.

Most people who get hepatitis B remain well, have no symptoms, and completely recover. However, even if you're asymptomatic, the virus can cause damage to the liver, which can lead to serious illness and even death. Those who *do* get sick generally experience flulike symptoms, jaundice, darker urine, and lighter stools. Generally, you will recover from hepatitis, but if you're unlucky, the illness can overwhelm you for several months; you don't want to get hepatitis if you can avoid it. Some people will always carry the hepatitis B virus and will remain infectious to others.

There is no cure for hepatitis B, *but there is a vaccine!* In fact, safe sex is *not* considered adequate protection from hepatitis B; only a hepatitis B vaccine will protect you. The vaccine is given by injection, three doses over a six-month period. The second shot is given one month after the first shot; the third shot is given five months after the second. Side effects from the vaccine are rare, other than a sore arm for a day or two. If you do suffer from any side effects, you'll experience general feelings of unwellness and fatigue. Contact the physician or clinic that administered the vaccine.

Mycoplasma

Mycoplasma (a.k.a. *Ureaplasma urealyticum)* is an asymptomatic bacterial infection that is more often than not, an STD. (In other words, virgins don't usually get mycoplasma!) Your doctor can detect mycoplasma by culturing cervical mucus during a routine Pap smear. It's important to be screened for mycoplasma prior to pregnancy because if left untreated, mycoplasma can travel to the endometrium, causing inflammation. This is known as *endometritis*—not to be confused with endometriosis. If you were pregnant with endometritis, the embryo may not implant in the uterus, and you would miscarry.

Infestations

Crabs or Pubic Lice

The name of this particular lice is *Phthirus pubis,* round, pinhead-size bugs that look like crabs. If you look hard enough, you can actually see them. They live in pubic hair, chest hair, armpit hair, and even eyelashes and eyebrows. You generally get crabs by having pubic-hair-to-pubic-hair contact with someone else who has them. But you can also get them from sleeping on infested bedding, using towels, or borrowing clothing from someone who has them (like a roommate). Crabs are also bloodsuckers, and the main health danger to you is that they can give you other diseases such as typhus. You can't have crabs and not know it: You'll have an intolerable itching in the infested area, and you can see the crabs yourself without a microscope. Unfortunately, scratching the itch makes it worse and can transfer the lice to other parts of your body.

Treatment involves pesticide lotions: *permethrin 5%* (Elimite) and *lindane 1%* (Kwell), both of which should be used very carefully. If you're pregnant, you shouldn't use it. There are safer nonprescription drugs you can ask your pharmacist about. None of these drugs can be used around the eyes, however. If you do have crabs in this area, petroleum jelly is recommended; it will smother the crabs. You can also see an ophthalmologist (eye specialist) who can prescribe a pesticide lotion that is safe for this area.

Once you're treated, you'll need to wash all your clothing, bedding, and towels in hot water, or just dry-clean them. The reason for this is because the eggs can live up to six days, and you can reinfest yourself or someone else.

Scabies

Scabies are mites that live under the skin. They're trickier than crabs because they cause skin irritations that resemble eczema, allergies, or even poison ivy. The eggs and feces of the scabies will cause tremendous irritation and itching as well. You may find raised bumps or ridges on the skin between fingers, under the breasts, around the waist, wrists, genitals, or buttocks. You can get scabies through both sexual contact and contact with infested clothing, bedding, towels, or even furniture. Lindane 1% is about the only treatment there is. For pregnant women, *crotamiton* (Eurax)is prescribed.

For both crabs and scabies, see a dermatologist in addition to your primary care physician. Because both the infestations and the treatments irritate the skin, it's wise to have soothing lotions on hand to apply after treatment.

Rare STDs

The STDs discussed in this section are extremely rare, and some of them affect only men.

Chancroid

Chancroid is very similar to herpes and is caused by the bacterium *Hemophilus ducreyi.* It begins as a dark spot on the genitals, called a *macule.* The macule enlarges, fills with pus, and develops into a painful ulcerlike sore. Unlike herpes, chancroid can be cured with antibiotics, and a "sibling" bacterium also causes one of the vaginal infections described below. Chancroid is rare and definitely not on the top 10 list of common STDs. Like herpes, you can get chancroid through intimate contact with an infected person, or by touching the pus and then touching your mucous membrane. This is usually a "just for men" STD. Chancroid is also known as "soft chancre" or "mixed chancre."

Lymphogranuloma Venereum (Frei's Disease)

Lymphogranuloma venereum, also known as "fifth venereal disease" in medicalspeak, is actually a strain of chlamydia. It is characterized by three stages: the first stage manifests with open sores or ulcers around the genitals; in the second stage, enlarged lymph nodes develop around the genital area; the third stage is a kind of genital "elephantiasis" where the lymph nodes fill with lymph fluid and become noticeably large and obstructed. The rectal opening can also narrow due to scarring, which makes bowel movements painful. This disease is quite rare, transmitted sexually, and cured with antibiotics.

Granuloma Inguinale (or Granuloma Venereum)

Again very rare, granuloma inguinale is an STD that is similar to chancroid but attacks only women. It is characterized by deep ulcers on the vulva, and they're found mainly on the mons, pubis, and labia. It is caused by the bacterium *Calymmatobacterium granulomatis* and tends to affect persons with darker pigment. It is also known as "fourth venereal disease" in medicalspeak. It is treated with antibiotics and transmitted through direct contact with an infected person.

Vaginal Infections

Trichomoniasis [often an STD]

Trichomoniasis is caused by a one-cell parasite called *Trichomonas vaginalis.* This parasite is very common in both men and women, and many women have trich organisms inside their vagina without knowing it. In fact, about 50% of all women infected with trich are asymptomatic. When there are symptoms, you'll notice itching, irritation, painful intercourse, and thin, foamy vaginal discharge that is yellowish green or even gray in color and has a foul odor. If there is another infection present as well, the discharge can be thicker and whiter.

Trich is diagnosed by swabbing the vaginal discharge and examining it under the microscope. But trich can also cause urinary tract infections, discussed below. Usually, trich is contracted through vaginal intercourse, but it can be passed on by moist towels, bathing suits, underwear, washcloths, and, yes, *toilet seats*. Emotional stress can cause "friendly trich" to flare up and cause symptoms. Many practitioners suggest a drug called *metronidazole (Flagyl)* to treat trich. Sixty percent of women with trich are cured with an antifungal medication called *clotrimazole (Lotrimin, Mycelex)* as well. Generally, if you're taking medication for trich, make sure your partner gets treated as well. It can be passed back to you again and again.

A natural remedy that may help relieve the symptoms of trich and other vaginal infections, including yeast, is a garlic suppository. Just take an ordinary peeled (but not pierced) garlic clove, wrap it in gauze, and insert one into the vagina every 12 hours. *This is a harmless way to relieve the* symptoms, *but it doesn't* cure *trich!* To prevent recurrences, take frequent warm baths, wear loose clothing (exposure to air will destroy parasites) and avoid tampons, douches, and vaginal sprays.

Bacterial Vaginosis [can be spontaneous]

In the past, this infection was also called *Gardinerella hemophilus* or *Corynebacterium vaginale*. Bacterial vaginosis is actually one of the most common caused by the bacterium *Gardinerella*, which tends to thrive when the normal pH balance of the vagina is "off." No one really knows how it develops, but it's been suggested that you can get this bacteria through sexual intercourse, and some believe that washcloths may also transfer it. The symptoms are the same for this infection as for trich, but the discharge is creamier or grayer and very fishy smelling. The treatment is either oral or vaginal metronidazole or clindamycin suppositories. If your partner has it, he should be treated with metronidazole, and if he doesn't, make sure he wears a condom until you're cured. You can also try the garlic here as well and follow the "natural remedy" suggestions outlined in the section on yeast infections below.

Yeast Infections [usually spontaneous]

Yeast infections are *not* STDs. There are currently some theories that suggest yeast *can* be transmitted sexually, but they are not yet proven, nor has yeast *ever* been classified as an STD. *In short, safe sex will not prevent yeast infections.*

Yeast infections are caused by a yeast known as *Candida albicans*, a type of one-cell fungus that belongs to the plant kingdom. Under normal circumstances, candida is always in your vagina, mouth, and digestive tract. It is a "friendly" fungus. For a variety of reasons, candida will overgrow and reproduce too much of itself, changing from a harmless one-cell fungus into long branches of yeast cells, called mycelia. This is known as candidiasis.

Causes.

Generally, any changes to your vagina's normal acidic environment can make you vulnerable to yeast infections. The list of factors that affect your vaginal environment is actually quite long. The most common factor is pregnancy, because it makes the vagina less acidic and increases the amount of sugar stored in the vaginal cell walls. And yeast *love* sugar! In fact, diabetic women often suffer from chronic yeast infections because of their blood sugar levels. Sometimes the first sign of diabetes is a stubborn vaginal yeast infection. If you suffer from chronic yeast infections, get screened for diabetes.

Hormonal changes and contraception are other factors. In order to work, hormonal contraceptives change the cervical secretions that bathe the vagina, discussed in chapter 4. This can change the vaginal environment drastically and make it vulnerable to yeast. Menopause also causes the cervical mucus to change, which again predisposes you to yeast infections.

Anything that interferes with the immune system will make yeast thrive. Antibiotics, for example, kill not only the harmful bacteria, but also the friendly bacteria that are always in the vagina, necessary to fend off infection. If you're prone to yeast infections and your doctor prescribes antibiotics for, let's say, chlamydia, tell your doctor that you're prone to yeast before you fill the prescription. He or she can recommend some preventive measures (some of which are discussed below) you can take to ward off yeast.

Immune deficiency is another common factor that causes yeast infections for the same reasons. In addition to HIV infection (yeast and HIV infection are discussed in chapter 5), steroid drugs and anticancer drugs and therapies (such as radiation or chemotherapy) also destroy the body's natural immune system, which leaves the vagina vulnerable to yeast. In addition, whenever you're fighting another infection, your immune system is involved and not as responsive to nipping candidiasis in the bud.

Menstruation is always a factor that affects the vagina. Yeast love the warm, moist conditions that menstruation provides. Wearing tampons will make the conditions even better for yeast to grow, so avoiding tampons is a good idea if you're suffering from chronic or frequent yeast infections.

A number of overall health factors affect the vagina: stress, fatigue, too much sugar or fruits, anemia, and low levels of thyroid hormone (which will affect your whole metabolism and slow down your menstrual cycle).

Following are guidelines to help you avoid yeast infections:

1. *Don't wear tight clothing around your vagina.* Tight pants, panties, and nylon pantyhose prevent your vagina from breathing and make it warmer and moister for yeast. Wear looser pants that allow your vagina to breathe, switch to knee-highs or stockings, or limit your pantyhose wearing to special occasions. Go to bed "bottomless" to let air into your vagina.
2. *Wear only 100% cotton clothing and/or natural fibers around your vagina.* Synthetic underwear and polyester pants are not a good idea. All-cotton underwear, denim, wool, or rayon pants that are loose-fitting are fine.
3. *Don't* ever *use vaginal deodorants or sprays.* These are unnecessary and disturb the vagina's natural environment, which is fully designed to self-clean.
4. *Don't douche unless it's purely for medicinal purposes.* Douching can push harmful bacteria up higher into the vagina, disturb the vagina's natural ecosystem, or interfere with a pregnancy.
5. *Watch your toilet habits.* Always wipe from front to back with toilet paper. When you do it the other way around, you can introduce rectal material and germs into your vagina. After a looser bowel movement, wet the toilet paper and clean your rectal area thoroughly so that fecal material doesn't stay on your underwear and wind up in your vagina. To be prepared for less hygienic circumstances, consider carrying some moist wipes, the kind that are safe for babies' bottoms.
6. *Don't insert* anything *into a dry vagina.* Whether it's a penis or tampon, make sure your vagina is well lubricated before insertion. Dry vaginas can be cut during insertion which creates an excellent home for yeast.
7. *Avoid sex "feasting."* After long periods of abstinence, continuous sex can predispose you to yeast infections. This is common in new relationships when two thirsty people drink from a well. Basically, the vagina doesn't adjust quickly enough to its new visitor, and its environment is upset. Cuts or abrasions from post-abstinence sex are also common.
8. *Avoid long car trips on vinyl seats.* New research indicates that vinyl seats increase a woman's risk of developing a yeast infection. The vinyl traps moisture and doesn't allow the crotch area to breath.

Symptoms.

Severe itching and a curdlike or cottage-cheesy discharge are classic symptoms of a vaginal yeast infection. The discharge, interestingly, may also smell like baking bread, fermenting yeast, or even brewing beer. The discharge may also be thinner and mucoid. Other symptoms are swelling, redness and irritation of the outer and inner vaginal lips, painful sex, and painful urination due to an irritation of the urethra. Women who have candidiasis may *not* have symptoms.

When yeast is in the throat, it is called thrush and usually occurs in immune-deficient women (they may be HIV positive or undergoing cancer treatment). Thrush is unsettling because the mouth and throat are coated with a milky white goop. It can also be present in newborns when yeast-infected mothers give birth. Thrush is treated orally with nystatin drops. Finally, since yeast is present in the intestines, HIV-positive women can develop severe, life-threatening esophageal yeast infections, discussed in chapter 5.

Treatment for single vaginal yeast episodes.

Vaginal yeast infections are so common that in the U.S., over-the-counter medications such as *miconazole* (Monistat), *Terconazole* (Terazol), *nystatin* (Mycostatin and many others), and even an herbal product, *Yeaststat,* are readily available. *Don't ever self-treat without consulting your doctor and confirming that what you have is* indeed *yeast.* Again, by self-diagnosing, you could be misdiagnosing gonorrhea, trich, chlamydia, or bacterial vaginosis for candidiasis. A doctor will confirm yeast by doing a "wet prep". Generally, all over-the-counter vaginal yeast medications are antifungal creams or suppositories. There are numerous brands that are equally effective.

Other over-the-counter treatments include boric acid. This is really cheap, and you can put it in gelatin capsules and insert it high into the vagina as a suppository. Boric acid can also be used as a douche: two tablespoons to two quarts of lukewarm water once a day for a week (when douching is medicinal, such as this case, it's fine). Caution: Keep boric acid out of your child's reach. It is very toxic if taken orally. *Betadine* is also helpful. It's a concentrated antiseptic iodine solution that kills yeast, trich, and bacterial vaginosis (gardinerella). Betadine is really messy, however, and stains everything brown. Pregnant women should not use it.

The old garlic suppository routine mentioned above is also helpful for symptoms of yeast but will not cure it. You can follow up the garlic treatment with a vinegar solution douche (which, again, is OK to do in this case). The garlic routine can be continued for three days. The only side effect may be a garlicky taste in your mouth.

Plain yogurt is reportedly helpful for symptoms of yeast as well. Eat 8 ounces of yogurt daily containing active yogurt cultures.

For unbearable itching, 1% hydrocortisone cream, available in the United States over-the-counter, is also helpful. Here are some home remedies that have been reported to relieve symptoms: witch hazel compresses, warm water baths with epsom salts or baking soda, or a poultice (compress) of cottage cheese on a sanitary napkin. Then, blow dry your vagina and dust it with cornstarch.

Other medications are in the imidazole family of drugs. They include *clotrimazole* (Mycelex), *terazole,* and *econozole* (Ecostatin). Nystatin, which comes in the form of vaginal tablets that are inserted as suppositories twice a day for 14 days, can also be used but it's less effective. It also comes in a cream, which is inserted with an applicator, and in oral tablets, liquids, and powder form.

For more severe cases, using a Q-tip to paint the vagina, cervix, and vulva with *gentian violet,* a purple, antifungal stain does the trick. You'll need to wear a sanitary napkin to avoid dripping the stain onto your clothes. The only time this stain is not helpful is when you're allergic to the stain itself.

Treatment for recurrent or chronic vaginal yeast infections.

If you have four or more episodes of vaginal yeast infections per year, you have recurrent yeast infections. You should confirm that the problem really is yeast and not serial infections with different organisms (that is, one month gonorrhea, the next month trichomoniasis, and so on). If you have frequent episodes of vaginal infections, it's especially important to confirm the exact diagnosis. If you seem to "always" be getting rid of a yeast infection, you suffer from chronic yeast infections. For recurrent episodes, it's important to try to do as much prevention as you can by following some of the dietary guidelines below.

Miconazole in vaginal cream or boric acid in gelatin capsules every night for seven days, then every other night for four weeks, and then monthly during menstruation, is one recommended route for recurrent episodes. At the same time, taking one teaspoon of lactobacillus acidophilus powder orally with meals is recommended.

You can also take *caprylic acid* and *myocidin,* both fatty acids derived from oils that are excellent antifungal agents. You can get them at health food stores in capsule form. Two capsules three times a day will help fend off yeast. *Citrus seed extract* (Citricidal) and *Tea-tree oil* can be used as a gargle for thrush (common in HIV-positive women). Drinking *Pau D'Arco tea* (Taheebo) will also help.

Diet and prevention.

You can do a lot to keep yeast out of your vagina, and much of it involves dietary prevention. Eliminating sugar will help enormously. Reacidifying your vagina is also an important preventive measure. Certain foods will help; check with your doctor or nutritionist. (Note: cranberry juice, associated with reacidifying in the past, is not helpful in preventing yeast.) If you suffer from severe, chronic yeast infections, in addition to eliminating sugar in your diet you should also avoid the following: honey, maple syrup, molasses, and any foods that contain it; alcoholic beverages; vinegars and foods containing vinegar such as pickled foods, salad dressings, mustard, ketchup, and mayonnaise; moldy nuts, such as peanuts, pistachios, and cashews; soy sauce, miso, and other fermented products; dairy foods with the exception of butter, buttermilk, and yogurt; coffee, black tea, or sweetened soda; dried fruits; and processed foods.

Instead, eat more of these foods: whole grains such as rice, millet, barley, and buckwheat; breads, crackers, muffins that are yeast-free and preferably wheat-free; raw or cooked fresh vegetables; fish, chicken, and lean meats (organically fed and hormone- and antibiotic-free); nuts and seeds that are not moldy; fruit in moderation (limiting sweeter fruits).

If you're immune-deficient for any reason, you can try strengthening your immune system through vitamin supplements (see chapter 5) and exercising (which reduces stress and anxiety). You can also avoid exposing yourself to bathroom and kitchen mold in general (in other words, keep your bathroom and kitchen very clean).

Genital Inflammations [can be caused by STDs]

The result of various STDs or vaginal infections, such as yeast, are often inflammations of the vagina, cervix, or vulva. In fact, anything with the suffix *-itis* means that you have an inflammation of some sort, as in *tonsillitis, hepatitis,* and *thyroiditis.*

Gynecological inflammations, however, are tricky. In these cases, the inflammations themselves are not the infection; they are only *symptoms* of an infection. For example, when your doctor tells you that you have vaginitis (inflammation of the vagina), you may think it is the name of an actual infection that's causing your itching or other symptoms. It isn't. It is simply the name of a *symptom*, which is in turn caused by something else. The purpose of this section is to explain the various causes behind each inflammation, and the symptoms characterized by the inflammation itself.

Vaginitis

Vaginitis is characterized by itching, redness, and a swollen vaginal opening. The three major causes of vaginitis are yeast infections, trich, and bacterial vaginosis. Vaginitis can also indicate the presence of other diseases. In addition, it can be caused by irritation as a result of insufficient lubrication due to hormonal changes that affect vaginal secretions. Menopausal women frequently complain of vaginitis, which is aggravated by intercourse. Lubricating the vagina artificially should clear up vaginitis caused by dryness. The next time your doctor tells you that you have vaginitis, respond by asking, "And what's *causing* it?"

Cervicitis

Again, cervicitis is not a disease in and of itself. Cervicitis is characterized by a swollen, red cervix that is not usually noticed until a doctor examines your cervix with a speculum. What you may notice is bleeding between periods, after intercourse and painful intercourse, unusual cervical mucus or tenderness when you touch your cervix for any reason (inserting a diaphragm, for example), or unusual discharge that comes from the cervix. Gonorrhea, chlamydia, PID, and other STDs can all cause cervicitis. Cervicitis can also result after IUD insertion, abortion, or childbirth. If cervicitis is caused by an STD, it will get better when the STD is treated. If it's the result of childbirth or IUD insertion, it will usually get better without treatment. In any case, you should have a pelvic exam whenever you have cervicitis. After it's been treated, a Pap smear should be performed as well as a thorough STD screening to isolate the disease that may be causing the cervicitis.

Vulvitis

Vulvitis is characterized by an itchy, red, swollen vulva and may include blistering. Diabetic women often suffer from vulvitis because of a sugar imbalance that predisposes them to infection. Postmenopausal women can develop vulvitis because their tissue in this area becomes less elastic, thinner and drier, *and* more susceptible to irritation. Scratching only makes it worse.

A number of factors cause vulvitis. External irritants, such as allergies to certain fabrics, powders, soaps, or perfumes are common causes. Oral sex, sanitary napkins, medications, diet, stress, or the presence of STDs or other infections can trigger it.

The best way to deal with vulvitis is to isolate the cause first, especially if it's an allergy or a bacterial infection. If you're predisposed to vulvitis as a result of menopause or diabetes, avoid overcleaning your vulva, and use either Crisco or mineral oil to clean it. Treat your vulva like you would your face: Keep it moisturized. The extra lubrication will really help.

Endometritis, Salpingitis, and Oophoritis

Endometritis means "inflammation of the uterine lining (or endometrium)" and is not to be confused with endometriosis. It's caused by a bacterial infection that gets inside your uterus. Salpingitis is an inflammation of the fallopian tubes and is caused by a bacterial infection that invades your tubes. Oophoritis, inflammation of the ovaries, is also caused by bacteria. Like both tubal and uterine inflammations, oophoritis is also a manifestation of PID. Endometritis, salpingitis, and oophoritis are discussed below.

Pelvic Inflammatory Disease

PID is a general term that refers to infection and inflammation of one or more of your pelvic organs: your cervix, uterus, fallopian tubes, or ovaries (known as your upper genital tract). These infections can also spread to other parts of your body, infecting your abdominal cavity, kidneys, liver, lungs, and so on. PID is a serious condition that affects more than one million women each year in North America. It's been more easily diagnosed since the availability of laparoscopy in the 1970s. Prior to laparoscopy, women with chronic pelvic pain were hard to diagnose. As a result, women with chronic PID were often misdiagnosed, or branded hypochondriacs when they complained of chronic pelvic pain or other PID symptoms, outlined below.

What Causes PID?

Bacteria. Normally, the cervix acts as a barrier and prevents bacteria from getting inside the upper pelvic region. But when the uterus is invaded by an STD or dilated for any reason, bacteria can enter the uterus and do a lot of damage. For example, when certain bacterial STDs—primarily gonorrhea and chlamydia—remain untreated, the infection can spread higher inside your pelvis and cause PID.

Bacteria can also get inside your pelvis through IUD insertion, the second major cause of PID in countries that use IUDs; douching; certain pelvic surgical procedures such as abortions, D & Cs, and amniocentesis; and natural phenomena such as miscarriages and childbirth. Smoking has also been linked to PID. Both current and past smokers were found to be *twice* as likely to develop PID. The reasons why are not known, however.

In many cases, PID can be avoided by an accurate diagnosis of the initial STD that causes PID in the first place. Often, the "diagnostic" blame is placed on the female patient who doesn't visit her doctor soon enough after noticing symptoms of an STD. Too often, she is misdiagnosed by her doctor, who may not have sufficient training in STD diagnosis. In 1980, fewer than one in six American medical schools had a specific STD clinic available for STD training. A 1985 survey showed that only one in five medical schools provided even half its students with STD clinical training. Worse, fewer than *one in ten* clinicians takes adequate sexual histories of patients. This sexual history is crucial in preventing STDs and PID in the first place. Questions should be asked about number of partners, lifestyle, and sexual practices that indicate high-risk behavior. A past STD history needs to be taken as well. If this were done by all clinicians, prevention of STDs could be more widely practiced, which would eliminate a significant portion of all PID cases. More thorough histories would also prompt clinicians to routinely screen and treat women for asymptomatic STDs such as chlamydia and gonorrhea, eliminating another significant portion of PID cases. The irony is that in the majority of cases, PID is actually preventable.

Symptoms of PID

Because PID is a general label that doesn't tell you where the infection is, the symptoms can vary depending on what's infected. Although there are several symptoms associated with PID, the common pattern is to experience only one or two of them. Some women have only mild symptoms, some women have symptoms so severe they can't function, and some women experience no symptoms at all and may discover they have PID only when they investigate infertility.

The most common symptom is lower abdominal pain. This pain may be sporadic or chronic and may occur only during or after intercourse, menstruation, or ovulation. Often the pain is on one side of the abdomen and increases with movement: walking, climbing, and so forth. This pain is always present during a pelvic examination, when your doctor feels your pelvic region manually to check for enlargements or abnormalities. Sometimes the pain is present when you urinate or have a bowel movement.

Other symptoms include lower back pain, nausea and dizziness, a low fever, chills, bleeding between periods, bleeding after intercourse, heavier menstrual cramps and flows, frequent urination, burning during urination or an inability to empty the bladder, unusual vaginal discharge with a foul odor, feeling like you have to constantly move your bowels, a general feeling of ill health, and abdominal bloating.

PID most commonly localizes in the fallopian tubes, causing salpingitis, or inflammation of the fallopian tubes. The tubes close up or scar as a result, leading to infertility (this is often reversible, however). Ectopic pregnancy can also result from PID for the same reasons. PID is divided into four categories of infection: *acute,* meaning severe; *subacute,* meaning less severe; and *chronic,* meaning that you have a fresh acute infection, or that scarring has developed as a result of a previous infection.

Diagnosing PID

First, during the speculum examination, your doctor will look for pus that might be coming out of the cervix, a symptom of cervicitis. If there is pus, a sample will be taken and sent to a lab. During a normal pelvic exam, your doctor should always perform what's known as a *bimanual examination.* Here, two fingers are inserted into your vagina, while your abdomen is felt on the outside simultaneously with the other hand. This procedure is comparable to fitting a comforter inside its cover: one hand on the inside, the other on the outside to adjust and feel for contours and abnormalities. Pain and swelling are classic signs of PID that an experienced gynecologist or primary care physician will immediately notice.

At this point, the appropriate antibiotic medication will be prescribed. You could conceivably be cured at this point. Your partner will also need to be treated for infection to prevent reinfecting you or someone else. (Treatment is discussed below.) After treatment a followup exam and repeat cultures are necessary.

A blood test can also indicate whether you're fighting an infection of some sort. If you are, you'll have increased levels of white blood cells.

An ultrasound test may also be helpful. It is most useful in determining whether an abscess has formed on the organs. However, frequently the ultrasound will be normal. In women with chronic PID and extensive tubal damage, there may be abnormal findings on the ultrasound.

Finally, if all else fails, a laparoscopy can be performed, which will definitely confirm a PID diagnosis. A laparoscopy might also be done if it's suspected you have abscesses (resulting from severe inflammation) that have burst—a potentially life-threatening situation. Laparoscopy is discussed in chapter 2 (under endometriosis).

Once your PID is diagnosed, successfully treating PID depends on identifying the right bacteria responsible for the infection in the first place so that you can be treated with the *right* antibiotic! This isn't always easy. There are three procedures used to obtain a culture of the PID bacteria. The first is obtaining a cervical culture, mentioned above. The second procedure is called a *culdocentesis,* similar to amniocentesis, where fluid is taken out of the cul-de-sac, an area in your pelvic cavity where fluid tends to collect. A long needle is used to withdraw the fluid, and the fluid is sent to a lab for investigation. This is done in a hospital under a local anesthetic. Another technique used is a *tubal sample.* Here, fluid and tissue samples from your fallopian tubes are obtained during a laparoscopy procedure and sent to a lab for bacterial analysis.

Antibiotic Therapy: The PID Treatment

The beauty about bacterial infections is that they can be destroyed with antibiotics. Antibiotic therapy is the most common treatment regimen for acute and subacute PID. Even chronic and recurrent PID can be treated successfully with antibiotics. Since PID indicates such a serious infection, antibiotics are given intravenously as a therapy; they're more potent this way and work faster. Sometimes there are several different types of bacteria identified in PID. This is known as a *polymicrobial* infection. If this is the case, you may be treated with more than one kind of antibiotic simultaneously, or you may be treated with a single, broad-spectrum antibiotic, which is less effective.

By far the best treatment approach is intravenous antibiotic therapy followed by bed rest. To receive intravenous antibiotics, you'll need to be admitted into the hospital for about four days, the usual treatment duration. Oral antibiotics for 10–14 days may follow in conjunction with rest. In some communities, it may be possible to receive intravenous medications at home. This helps reduce the cost of hospital stays.

There are many different kinds of antibiotic regimens that work. The following is just a sample regimen. For PID caused by gonorrhea and/or chlamydia, 100 milligrams of doxycycline by IV twice a day, plus 2 grams of cefoxitin (the pill that cures gonorrhea) four times a day by IV, is the standard treatment for about four days, followed by 100 milligrams of doxycline prescribed twice a day for about 14 days.

For PID caused by chlamydia and/or anaerobic bacteria (a certain strain of bacteria), the regimen is 100 milligrams of doxycycline by IV, plus 1 gram of metronidazole (Flagyl) twice a day for about four days, followed by the same dosages of both drugs orally, twice a day for about 14 days.

For PID caused by anaerobic bacteria or facultative gram-negative rods (other strains of bacteria), the prescription is 600 milligrams of clindamycin (Cleocin) four times a day by IV, plus gentamicin or tobramycin at a dosage of 2 milligrams for each kilogram of body weight, followed by 1.5 milligrams per kilogram three times a day for four days; then, 450 milligrams of clindamycin orally four times a day for about 14 days.

If you're pregnant or have other health problems, other antibiotics will be recommended. The above are prescription-only and are doses generally recommended for women who aren't pregnant and are otherwise healthy.

What are the side effects of these antibiotics?

Yeast infections are one side effect, for reasons discussed earlier. But each antibiotic carries individual side effects. *Doxycycline* can cause nausea, yeast infections, allergies, liver damage (particularly in pregnant women), and brown discoloration of teeth in children and fetuses. *Cefoxitin* (fine for pregnant women; not always recommended for women allergic to penicillin) can bring on allergies and kidney damage. Metronidazole can cause nausea, headache, loss of appetite, metallic taste in the mouth, dark urine, abdominal pain, constipation, inflammation of the tongue or mouth, yeast infections, and deposits in breast milk (*making it unsafe for pregnant women*), and cannot be combined with alcohol. Clindamycin brings on diarrhea, colitis (which disappears after usage), allergies, and temporary abnormalities in liver function.

What should I do after my antibiotic treatment?

Get rechecked by your doctor to make sure you are indeed cured. Request another culture to make sure the bacteria have been destroyed, and make sure your partner is treated for the same bacterial infection. Then, make sure you take time off work for complete bed rest for at least two days until you feel no pain whatsoever. You should also abstain from intercourse until you are pronounced cured. Intercourse can spread pus around your pelvic cavity while you're healing.

Surgical Treatment for PID

Inflammation is one thing, abscesses are another. An abscess is when the inflamed tissue forms a collection of pus. The abscess can then rupture and spread the bacterial infection elsewhere, causing your PID to move to other parts of your pelvic region. Even though severe PID often involves inflammation with no abscesses, when there are abscesses, surgically removing the abscess may be necessary, and surgically removing the badly abscessed *organ* may be an option. In either case, surgery is an emergency decision, made on-the-spot by your doctor as a necessary life-preserving step, or an elective decision, in which you choose surgery as a treatment option in *advance* and have time to prepare for it. If your abscesses have ruptured or are about to rupture, your doctor will schedule emergency surgery. Some patients may need more extensive surgery, which requires about a four-inch incision (laparotomy) in the abdomen. At this point, the surgical procedure performed will depend on the severity of PID and your desire for future fertility. It's crucial that you discuss exactly what kind of surgery to expect and take every precaution to preserve your reproductive organs if possible.

Both laparoscopy and laparotomy procedures are considered major surgery and are performed under a general anesthetic. A laparotomy is also performed if a *salpingectomy,* surgical removal of the fallopian tubes, is necessary. Depending on the severity of your PID and the location of the infection, this might actually be the best option for you. As mentioned above, it's most common for PID to localize in the fallopian tubes, which can cause a host of uncomfortable and painful symptoms for you. If the tubes are badly infected and have abscessed, removing them may just be the answer. This is often done to preserve your ovaries and uterus and prevent the PID from spreading further. Although the consequence of a salpingectomy is infertility, you can still have a child through assisted conception techniques, discussed in chapter 12. If abscesses have formed in the uterus or on the ovaries, more drastic surgery may be necessary in the form of either a *hysterectomy,* surgical removal of the uterus, *oophorectomy,* surgical removal of the ovaries, or both. Both procedures are discussed in chapter 7.

If surgery is being recommended to relieve your pain but there are no active infections, abscesses, or inflammations present, a procedure known as a *presacral neurectomy* is an option. In this operation, the sensory messages from the organs of the pelvis, carried along the presacral nerve, are eliminated by removing the nerve itself. Hence, the pain is also eliminated. This is also major surgery and requires a very skilled surgeon, since the nerve is close to large blood vessels. A presacral neurectomy is a more difficult operation to perform than a hysterectomy, but the surgery is about 75% effective in eliminating pelvic pain (a very promising statistic), and it does not affect fertility. One interesting side effect is that if a woman gets pregnant after the procedure, she will experience no pain during labor or childbirth! The procedure can also interfere with bowel and bladder function, which usually clears up on its own. To what extent this procedure affects sexual sensation, or even menstrual cramps has not yet been statistically tracked. In any event, this operation is considered a last resort for relieving pelvic pain associated with PID and is only a *palliative* (treating the symptoms rather than the disease) solution, not a cure for PID.

Prevention of PID

The good news is that in almost all cases, *PID is a completely preventable disease.*

The number-one cause of PID in North America is an untreated STD; chlamydia and gonorrhea are the two STDs that are considered principally implicated in causing PID. Translation: You can prevent STDs by practicing safe sex, discussed in chapter 4. If you're not practicing safe sex, request a screening for chlamydia and gonorrhea every time you have sex with a new partner. Currently, vaccines for chlamydia and gonorrhea are being researched and may be introduced as standard vaccines to the general public in the next century. In addition to choosing uninfected partners, postponing intercourse with new partners for as long as possible, using barrier methods, and notifying sex partners after discovering any STD are important steps in primary prevention. In fact, women are not considered cured of PID *unless* their partners are treated for the initial PID-causing STD as well. Partners of women with PID have infection rates as high as 53% with chlamydia and as high as 41% for gonorrhea, and a large percentage of these infections are asymptomatic.

Another crucial step in preventing PID is becoming more educated about the risks involved with certain contraceptives. It is an undisputed fact, for example, that women who use IUDs are *three to nine times* as likely to develop PID. Why? First, bacteria, normally screened by your cervix, can enter your uterus during IUD insertion. (Some experts counter that taking doxycycline prior to insertion will reduce the risk of infection.) Second, even if no bacteria enters during insertion, the IUD can irritate your uterus later on, causing a local infection.

If you're an IUD wearer in a mutually monogamous relationship, your risk of an IUD-related infection is small. However, if you're exposed to gonorrhea or chlamydia, you're more likely to develop PID. As a rule, whenever you have any cervical procedure, follow your doctor's advice before you resume having intercourse or using sex toys, douches, or tampons. See your doctor to make sure that the cervix has resumed its usual shape and appearance.

There is also evidence that hormonal contraceptives affecting your cervical mucus may increase your chances of contracting an STD during unprotected sex. Apparently, the mucus is not as effective in screening out harmful bacteria as "untampered" or natural mucus is.

Douching is also a factor in primary prevention. There are two reasons why it's a bad idea to douche: douching may alter the vaginal environment and make it less protective against harmful bacteria, and douching may flush vaginal and cervical bacteria into the upper pelvic region, causing infections.

Basic vaginal hygiene habits, discussed above in preventing yeast infections, can also help prevent PID in addition to practicing good overall nutrition. Even if you can't afford proper health insurance, you can improve your overall nutrition and hygiene.

In addition, if you notice any kind of unusual symptom that may indicate an STD, see your doctor and request a diagnosis or prompt antibiotic treatment for suspected STDs. Never self-diagnose! Treating an STD quickly will prevent it from causing PID.

Urinary Tract Infections (UTIs) [Can Be Caused by STDs]

UTIs, as they're called, are about as common as yeast infections. They are usually caused by the *Escherichia coli bacteria,* which travel from the colon to the urethra to the bladder. The most common UTI is *cystitis,* which can mean either inflammation or infection of the bladder. Classic cystitis symptoms include a painful or burning sensation coming from inside the urethra (known as *dysuria,* meaning "painful urination," as opposed to a burning caused by the urine touching an inflamed vagina or vulva), feeling like you have to urinate constantly (some women report that they have to urinate up to 60 times a day), and then finding that almost nothing comes out when you *do* try. It's estimated that between 10 and 20% of all women will or have already experienced a UTI of some sort. And 80% of women who have had a UTI will have another one within a year. Even severe UTIs are not usually serious, just miserable, and can be treated with antibiotics.

Other symptoms of UTI may include blood in the urine, known as *hematuria,* or pus in the urine, known as *pyuria.* Sometimes cystitis clears up on its own within about 24 hours. Because of this, wait one day before you see your doctor. If it doesn't clear up, report all your symptoms to your doctor and request a urinalysis (a urine test) to check for an infection. You may also need a urine culture; however, with a typical uncomplicated cystitis symptom, many doctors will treat it without a culture. At this point, your doctor may also perform a pelvic exam to check for the presence of other vaginal infections. For instance, women will often think they have a UTI when it's really vaginitis.

As you already know, a urine sample can be taken during your doctor appointment. What you might not know, however, is that there is a specific technique involved in getting the "most" out of your urine sample to avoid false positives due to contamination with skin or vaginal bacteria. Ask for the proper materials to do a "clean catch" or "midstream" urine. This will include a sterile container and moistened wipes for cleaning the outer vaginal area. To obtain the urine specimen, you may want to sit backward on the toilet and use the toilet lid as a shelf. Wash your hands before you begin and open the kit. Open the container, but do not touch the inside of the lid or the container. Using one hand, spread your vaginal lips apart and don't let go. Use the moistened wipes, wiping front to back one time with each wipe and dropping it in the toilet. Start the stream of urine, letting a small amount go into the toilet and then put the container under the stream. It's not necessary to fill the container completely. Put the lid on the container without touching the inside of the lid. At this point you may wash your hands to remove any urine from your fingers. Wipe the outside of the container with a moist paper towel. This may seem elaborate, but it's designed to keep normal vaginal and skin germs out of the culture. If your lab technician doesn't seem to know what a "clean catch" kit is, discuss this with your doctor. An alternative would be to carry your own sanitary wipes with you and use the above procedure.

If the urine culture is negative, meaning that no bacteria are present in your urine, your symptoms may be caused by another infection, probably an STD. In this case, you could be suffering from urethritis rather than cystitis. You would then need to be be screened for various STDs and treated accordingly.

A positive culture test means that bacteria is present in your urine. You can also have bacteria in your urine (found during a routine exam) but have no symptoms of UTI. This is more common in pregnancy. In either case, you'll be treated with an antibiotic.

Treatment for Cystitis [not an STD]

For a simple case of cystitis with no complications, you'll be prescribed either a single dose or a short-course treatment of an appropriate antibiotic, such as *trimethoprim/sulfamethoxazole,* or *TMP/SXT* (Septra) or Macrodantin. After the treatment, you'll need to give another urine sample to make sure the infection has cleared up.

If you're pregnant, diabetic, or elderly, or you have just had a UTI in the past six weeks, you'll be given the same antibiotic or other antibiotics for a longer period of time ranging from 10 to 14 days. Then, a follow-up urine culture will need to be done. If you do happen to suffer from recurrent UTIs, you can do a home urine test on your own, available through any pharmacy (only in the United States). This test is easy to do and comes equipped with a dipslide stick that turns color if it's positive.

Pyelonephritis [not an STD]

Pyelonephritis occurs when a bacterial infection has spread to your kidney, causing inflammation. The symptoms of pyelonephritis are similar to those of cystitis. Usually, you'll have a fever, pain in the flank (the fleshy side of your body between your ribs and hips), nausea, or vomiting *in conjunction* with cystitis symptoms. A urine culture may distinguish whether you have cystitis or pyelonephritis. To treat this infection, broad-spectrum antibiotics are used for 14 days: TMP/SXT or *ciprofloxacin* (Cipro) are the popular ones. With pyelonephritis, you'll need to be hospitalized and treated with intravenous antibiotics if nausea or vomiting is a problem, or if you're pregnant.

A new urine culture will be taken about 48 hours later. If you're *still* not well after this, further diagnostic procedures such as an ultrasound test will be done to get to the bottom of the problem. It will need to be taken care of to prevent more serious or even life-threatening consequences of severe kidney infection, and if you're not referred to a urologist or infectious disease specialist at this point, request it.

Recurrent or Chronic Cystitis [not caused by STDs]

Some women are more prone to cystitis than others, but the disease is triggered by several behavioral factors that you *can* control.

Intercourse can trigger cystitis. The term *honeymoon cystitis* refers to a woman who develops cystitis after her sexual "debut." The urethra can become irritated with intercourse, and more bacteria may get inside the urethra, which leads to the bladder. Also, during intercourse many women hold back their urge to urinate. Experts recommend that you should empty your bladder both before and immediately after sex. Urinating after sex will also help wash out the bacteria from the urethra. (See chapter 1 on the structure of the urethra and bladder.)

Diaphragm use is another trigger. Diaphragms that are too large can alter the angle of the bladder neck, making it difficult to empty the bladder completely. You can easily avoid this problem by making sure your diaphragm fits properly and by urinating before you put it in and after you remove it six hours later.

In addition, women in the habit of "holding it in" can be predisposed to cystitis. "When you gotta go, you gotta go"; don't hold it in. (The classic example is a teacher who can't leave her class to "go.")

Other reasons why you might be prone to cystitis include an obstruction or blockage, such as a stone anywhere along your urinary tract. This blockage may show up on a kidney X ray or an intravenous pyelography (IVP). An IVP is an X ray of your kidney and urinary tract. Iodine dye is injected into you, which makes the X ray easier to read.

Damage to your lower back area can affect the nerves that go to your bladder. This may prevent you from completely emptying your bladder, creating a breeding ground for bacteria, and is often a leading cause of chronic or recurrent cystitis. In addition, pelvic surgery such as a hysterectomy can damage nerves to the bladder. In this case, your cystitis bouts would have begun immediately after your surgery.

The general pattern of recurring cystitis is about three infections per year. If you suffer from more than three infections per year you should consult a urologist. If no specific abnormality is found, prophylactic antibiotics can be used to prevent recurrent cystitis. Since as many as 85% of women with recurrent cystitis notice the onset of infection within 24 hours after intercourse, postcoital antibiotics are often helpful. Usually, your doctor will get you on a self-treatment regimen for recurrent cystitis. This may involve using a home urine culture test kit (mentioned above), and taking one or two doses of antibiotics if the culture is positive.

Here are some tips for women with recurrent cystitis:

1. Never start your antibiotic until you know the results of your urine culture. If you have repeated cystitis symptoms with negative cultures, you may have another condition known as *interstitial cystitis (IC)*, discussed below.
2. Before you start self-treatment, make sure your doctor examines your urine under the microscope to check for blood and pus, which will help him or her make a more accurate diagnosis.
3. If bacteria show up in your urine more than three times in a row, request an IVP or an ultrasound of your kidneys. You may have kidney stones; your doctor will determine whether they need to come out.
4. Make sure you have a pelvic exam and an evaluation for yeast, trichimoniasis, chlamydia, and gonorrhea. Your symptoms could be caused or aggravated by these vaginal infections.
5. If all else fails, you should request a cystoscopy examination. Done under a general anesthetic, a cystoscopy checks your bladder for structural problems.

In the meantime, drinking plenty of water and cranberry juice while avoiding acidic foods will help. You can also try mixing one teaspoon of baking soda in a glass of water and drinking it. Do this only once, when symptoms first appear. This has been known to help.

Interstitial Cystitis [not an STD]

Many women with chronic cystitis are found to have IC, which is inflammation of the interstitium, the space between the bladder lining and bladder muscle. This can cause chronic pelvic pain, frequent urination, and a shrunken, ulcerated bladder. The bladder itself is lined with a protective layer that is secreted, like mucus, by the cells that line the bladder. This layer protects the inside of the bladder from acids and toxins in the urine and prevents bacteria from sticking to the bladder wall. If this layer is damaged, infection can result.

IC symptoms are the same as those of cystitis, but you may also feel bruised around your clitoral area. In addition, acidic foods, chocolate, red wine, old cheese, nuts, yogurt, avocados, and bananas, and sometimes antibiotics, seem to make the pain worse. IC starts out as normal bacterial cystitis, but if, after a few bouts, your urine cultures continue to be negative, you probably have IC.

There are several theories as to the causes of IC, including increased progesterone. In fact, menopausal women on progesterone may notice cystitis symptoms. If you have IC, you'll need to see a urologist (you should already be seeing one for recurrent cystitis anyway). Treatments include anti-inflammatory drugs and bladder relaxants. For more information on IC, contact the Interstitial Cystitis Foundation, 120 South Spalding Dr., Ste. 210, Beverly Hills, CA 90212, or the Interstitial Cystitis Association (ICA), P.O. Box 1553, Madison Square Station, New York, NY 10159.

Chapter 7 not only is devoted to the subject of fibroids, but it also discusses hysterectomies and oophorectomies in detail. Many of the infections you've read about in chapter 6 are preventable. Therefore, as you'll see, some of these surgical procedures are also preventable.

CHAPTER 7

All About Fibroids and Hysterectomies

Fibroids are quite harmless. They can be miserable to have, but they usually don't pose any danger to your gynecological health. Fibroids are benign—meaning *noncancerous*—tumors that grow inside your uterus. And, as you'll see, it is not the fibroids themselves that are extremely questionable and controversial; it is the method used to *treat* them. A *hysterectomy* is currently the treatment recommended for most women with fibroids. *In fact, fibroid tumors are the most common reason for hysterectomies in the United States, accounting for 30% of all hysterectomies performed in the country, about 200,000 hysterectomies per year.* Although there *are* some fibroid cases that *do* warrant a hysterectomy, with current technology many women with fibroids can avoid radical surgery. Studies estimate that 30–50% of all hysterectomies performed in general may have been clearly unnecessary, while another 10–20% may be avoided by using alternative approaches.

This chapter will explain exactly what fibroids are, point out how innocuous they can be, and explain treatment options for fibroids that will leave your reproductive organs intact. In addition, you will learn about hysterectomies, alternatives to them, and when a hysterectomy is necessary.

What Are Fibroids?

The term *fibroid* is actually medical slang. The correct medical term for what we've come to know as a "fibroid" is *leiomyoma uteri.* The word *fibroid* is really just an adjective that refers to anything fibrouslike or resemblng a *fibroma,* a benign tumor made of connective tissue, like muscle. So, describing a tumor as "fibroid" is like describing a sweater as "cotton"; it's simply referring to the *fabric* that the tumor is made of. (Tumors are discussed further in chapter 8). This means that a fibroid tumor can exist anywhere in the body, not just in the uterus.

Leiomyoma uteri is a benign tumor made of smooth uterine muscle. *Leio* means "smooth," *my* means "muscle," and *oma* means "benign growth." In general, muscle tumors called *leiomyoma* can also be found in the stomach and other parts of the body, but the uterus is the most common site. In fact, the uterus *consists* mainly of muscle. A *tumor* is essentially a clump of abnormal cells that form a lump, cyst, or mass. It usually starts with one cell that reproduces again and again. Why these cells develop in the first place is still a mystery. When these cells are *benign,* they are harmless. When these cells go awry, however, they develop into a clump within the *myometrium,* the smooth muscle coat of the uterus, which forms the main part of the organ. Fibroid tumors are therefore a collection of innocent uterine muscle cells that form a noticeable hard lump.

Fibroids develop most commonly in women who are in their 30s and 40s, but they can also develop earlier or later than this. In fact, about 30% of all women will develop fibroids by the time they reach 35, and fibroids are more common in black women. An estimated 20% of white women and 50% of black women over 30 years old have fibroids.

Fibroids are grayish white, firm, round, and ring-shaped. They come in all sizes, and it's common to have several fibroids growing at once. The main problem is that once fibroids develop, they may continue to grow, and even if they're surgically removed, there's a 10% chance they'll grow back. This is the main reason why so many doctors recommend hysterectomies for women with fibroids.

Fibroids are classified by location:

- *Intramural or interstitial:* fibroids in the outer or innermost layer of the uterus.
- *Subserous/serosal:* fibroids that protrude into the abdominal cavity and can be pedunculated (they grow on a stalk, like broccoli).
- *Submucous:* fibroids that invade the endometrium.
- *Parasitic:* fibroids that migrate out of the uterus and invade the cervix or other pelvic organs, developing their own blood supply.

What Causes Fibroids?

Nobody knows why fibroids develop. What we do know is that estrogen can trigger fibroids and may make the fibroids grow more quickly. Just as estrogen triggers the uterine lining, or endometrium, to grow and thicken during the estrogen peak in the menstrual cycle, it also triggers the myometrium to grow and thicken, which is where the fibroids are located. So, it's not surprising that the fibroids will grow too, since they consist of uterine muscle tissue.

After menopause, the fibroids will usually shrink. So if you're only a few years away from menopause and you've just developed fibroids, they may shrink on their own without treatment. If you're taking estrogen synthetically as a hormonal contraceptive, going off the contraceptive will often shrink your fibroids as well. A fibroid may not shrink after menopause (or first develop after menopause) if you are on hormone replacement therapy (HRT), discussed in chapter 13.

Are Fibroids Dangerous?

Not at all. Basically, a fibroid is to your uterus what a callus is to the heel of your foot. The callus will keep growing and getting thicker until you cut it off. Even after you cut it off, the callus sometimes grows back.

Imagine, though, what would happen if the callus grew so large that it interfered with your balance and walking. If this were the case, you would need treatment so you could walk properly again. Depending on their location within the myometrium, fibroids can grow so large that they can press against other reproductive organs and interfere with your pelvic functions. You might experience lower abdominal or back pain or even urinary problems. Menstruation can become heavier, with a gushing flow or clots that could predispose you to anemia. Sometimes these heavier periods are accompanied by more painful cramps, but cramps are often not a symptom. In some cases, the cause of the heavier bleeding is not completely understood. Although fibroids may cause abnormal bleeding between periods, this may be a symptom of another problem and should be evaluated before the bleeding is blamed on the fibroid. In other words, if you have fibroids, and are bleeding between periods, you should be checked for *other* causes of abnormal bleeding. An extremely large fibroid may interfere with a pregnancy simply because it takes up too much space. In fact, fibroids have been known to grow so large that they can make a woman appear to be in her 20th week of pregnancy. But for the most part, fibroids *that* large are also rare. The average "large" fibroid usually will *not* interfere with either conception or pregnancy.

Other symptoms of fibroids include a tender or achy feeling in your uterus or laborlike pains (sometimes the fibroid dies when its blood supply is cut off and the uterus tries to expel it). Pressure in your back legs or lower abdomen, backaches, painful intercourse, frequent urination, incontinence, and repeated urinary tract infections (UTIs) are other symptoms.

Just as you can have several calluses on your foot, you can also have several fibroids in your uterus. Keep in mind, though, that fibroids generally are of small to medium size and are *symptomless*. Women with symptomless fibroids can coexist peacefully with them and are not in any danger. Currently, about 40% of all reproductive-age women have one or more fibroid tumors, but only *half* of these women experience any symptoms.

Diagnosing and Treating Fibroids

If you do notice any of the symptoms described earlier, you have *symptomatic fibroids*. See your doctor and request a full pelvic exam that includes a rectal exam. Unless a rectal exam is done, your doctor can miss the fibroid. Large fibroids can usually be felt in a pelvic exam. Depending on where they're located, smaller fibroids can also cause these symptoms, particularly if you have numerous small fibroids. Generally, an ultrasound test or a laparoscopy will confirm whether or not you have smaller fibroids. If you have abnormal bleeding, then an endometrial biopsy should be done to rule out a hormonal deficiency. Hysteroscopy (in which a telescope is passed through the cervix) can determine whether there are more fibroids on or under the uterine lining. Sometimes these fibroids can be removed through the hysteroscope. Treatment for symptomatic fibroids is discussed further on.

What if you suspect you have fibroids but have no *symptoms?* If this is the case, you don't need to do anything until the fibroids start to bother you. If the fibroids grow larger and you develop symptoms later on, *then* you can see your doctor and confirm whether you have them.

Often, *symptomless* fibroids are discovered by your doctor accidentally during a routine pelvic exam. If this happens, just ask him or her to keep an eye on the fibroid(s). Then, see your doctor every six months instead of annually for a thorough pelvic exam. The bottom line is that if the fibroid isn't bothering *you*, you don't need to bother *it*.

The Symptomless Fibroid Controversy

In the past, if you had symptomless fibroids, once the uterus reached a certain size your doctor would have recommended either a myomectomy (surgical removal of the fibroids only) or, more likely, a hysterectomy. This was done because an enlarged uterus would prevent the doctor from feeling your ovaries and detecting potential problems. In addition, it was difficult to be certain that what he or she was feeling *was* in fact a fibroid. Back then, fibroid treatment was more radical because there really wasn't any way of absolutely diagnosing fibroids; there was no easy, inexpensive method of proving that the patient truly had only fibroids and not a more serious condition. The philosophy was, "Don't take chances."

Today, ultrasound is an accurate and relatively inexpensive method of confirming a fibroid diagnosis that can rule out ovarian abnormalities. In the United States, many gynecologists have ultrasound available in their offices. If there is still any doubt after the ultrasound, gynecologists today will continue on with a laparoscopy. Now, when a fibroid is confirmed and the patient doesn't have any symptoms, she has more options available to her. If you're told you have fibroids but you don't have any symptoms, and the diagnosis has been confirmed, seek a second opinion if any surgery, such as a myomectomy or hysterectomy, is recommended. In this situation, these procedures are very likely unnecessary.

Again, for fibroids of any size that are symptomless, *leave them be*. Removing them because of what they *may* do isn't a good enough reason to subject yourself to the expense (which includes lost time and income from your job), trauma, and consequences of major pelvic surgery. The fibroids may do *nothing*, and may naturally shrink after menopause anyway.

The Myths Behind Hysterectomies and Symptomless Fibroids

Medical opinion regarding treatment of symptomless fibroids once went like this: Fibroids grow larger with time and become symptomatic as they enlarge, so performing a hysterectomy when the tumors are small will prevent future problems and result in fewer post-operative complications.

But a new study, conducted by the Iowa College of Medicine and the UCLA School of Medicine and published in *Obstetrics and Gynecology*, yielded startling results. Researchers checked the medical records of 93 women who underwent hysterectomy procedures for fibroids. They found that women who had a uterus enlarged by fibroids to the size of a 12–20-week pregnancy suffered *no more* surgical complications than women who had smaller fibroids. The study also revealed that the so-called conventional reasoning behind performing a hysterectomy for symptomless fibroids was rooted in mythology rather than fact.

Here's the myth-by-myth breakdown:

MYTH: *Surgery will prevent the development of symptoms, which are inevitable as the fibroid grows larger.*

FACT: This is illogical. Not all large fibroids cause symptoms. Surgery can and should be avoided until symptoms develop. Women whose fibroids would *never* have caused problems would be spared the risk and expense of major surgery.

MYTH: *Large symptomless fibroids would interfere with early detection of ovarian cancer. Removing the fibroid can prevent a missed diagnosis of early ovarian cancer.*

FACT: As discussed above, ultrasound and laparoscopy are used to monitor the ovaries in the presence of an enlarged uterus. But it's important to be aware that even ultrasound may not detect early ovarian cancer, which is why more sophisticated screening methods are currently being developed.

MYTH: *If irregular or excessive bleeding is being caused by a fibroid, a hysterectomy will take care of the problem.*

FACT: Women with symptomless fibroids and irregular bleeding need to have their doctors rule out other causes for the bleeding first, before the fibroid is held responsible. When irregular bleeding is the only symptom present in women with fibroids, there may be another problem that's causing the bleeding, and it usually has nothing to do with the fibroid. An endometrial biopsy can rule out a hormonal cause, and for some patients, hysteroscopy might be useful.

MYTH: *There is a small but real possibility that a fibroid may develop into a cancerous tumor called a* leiomyosarcoma.

FACT: A woman's odds of dying of a hysterectomy (1 in 1,000) are much higher than her odds of developing a leiomyosarcoma. Therefore, it's not necessary to do a hysterectomy to prevent leiomyosarcoma. However, if a fibroid suddenly begins growing rapidly, then surgery would be indicated because the fibroid would become suspicious. In addition, leiomyosarcomas, rare as they are (occurring in less than 0.2–0.1% of all women), can be treated, even when they're discovered accidentally.

Treating Symptomatic Fibroids

The only reason *why* symptomatic fibroids need to be treated is to make you more comfortable and alleviate the symptoms. Technically, if you can live with the symptoms, the fibroids would not present any danger to your health. Symptomatic fibroids can make you extremely uncomfortable, however, and most women who have them will want to get rid of them. Unless you have enough information to make an informed decision about treatment, you might be railroaded into undergoing a hysterectomy, when in fact this procedure may not be necessary.

The first thing to do when you're diagnosed with symptomatic fibroids is to *triple-check* the diagnosis. Just because you have fibroids doesn't mean you don't have another condition at the same time: endometriosis, PID, sexually transmitted diseases (STDs), other tumors, and so on. Large fibroids will be felt in a pelvic exam; smaller fibroids are not that easy to diagnose. Before you undergo any kind of surgical diagnostic procedure (such as a laparoscopy to confirm small fibroids) or consent to any kind of treatment for larger, obvious fibroids, make sure you see, in addition to your gynecologist, a primary care physician as well as a *second* gynecologist. Have each of them do a full medical history and perform a pelvic exam to make sure that the original fibroid diagnosis is correct. Even if you do have fibroids, ask if there are any *other* reasons why you might have these symptoms. If there are, ask to be screened for these other conditions first.

If all three doctors suspect smaller fibroids are the problem, you may need to undergo a diagnostic procedure to confirm this. Before you consent to either a laparoscopy (chapter 2) or a D & C (dilation and curettage) procedure (see chapter 8), request an ultrasound *first.* Often, the fibroids are visible with ultrasound. *Transvaginal ultrasound* may be a better option for you since a full bladder is not necessary. In this test, a lubricated plastic probe is placed inside your vagina, producing a higher quality image. If this fails to confirm a diagnosis, ask about a procedure called *hysteroscopy.* Here, your doctor places a fiber-optic scope into the uterus, but the procedure can be done in his/her office. This is considered an advanced diagnostic tool for confirming fibroids. However, it can only identify those that impinge on the uterine cavity. A laparoscopy allows the surgeon to take a peek at the outer surface of the uterus. Sometimes, both procedures are combined and done under anesthesia. Ultrasound, hysteroscopy, or laparoscopy may tell you how many fibroids there are, their sizes, where they're located, and how fast they're growing. A hysteroscopy or laparoscopy will always confirm a fibroid diagnosis.

Other Treatment Options

Once you're satisfied with the diagnosis of symptomatic fibroids, *don't do anything yet.* How old are you? Do you have *that* much further to go until menopause? Can you live with the symptoms until then? For example, you could treat your fibroid symptoms with palliative measures, taking painkillers until the fibroids shrink naturally in menopause. Are you already *past* menopause and taking synthetic hormones? If so, tell your doctor that you want to go off any kind of synthetic estrogen product you might be taking (see chapter 13). Then, wait and see if your symptoms subside on their own. Are you taking oral contraceptives with estrogen? If you are, go off them for a while and see if the symptoms subside. (Other methods of contraception are discussed in chapter 4.)

Another treatment option involves laser surgery through hysteroscopy. During this procedure, fibroids under the uterine lining can be removed and the remaining uterine lining tissue destroyed. This will prevent bleeding, leaving you infertile, but will not interfere with your ovarian functions. Some women continue to have some bleeding, but it's usually much lighter. Because the endometrium may regrow, a tubal ligation at the same time may be necessary, since it's not known how damaging a pregnancy can be. There's also concern that the procedure could cause scarring of the uterine cavity that might complicate an endometrial cancer diagnosis. If your doctor considers you a high risk for endometrial cancer, then a hysterectomy may be more appropriate therapy after all.

If you're not taking synthetic estrogen and are more than a decade away from menopause, request a short trial period of *estrogen-blocking drugs,* such as *danazol,* also used to treat endometriosis. There's a good chance that these drugs may shrink your fibroids and your symptoms might improve. Although these drugs do have side effects (discussed in chapter 2), they are far less invasive than major surgery, and may work fine for a short period of time. Synthetic GnRH and LHRH are also helpful. The synthetic hormones take over your body's production of the hormone and help to inhibit estrogen. These hormones need to be injected daily, however, and are therefore inconvenient.

If you're under 45, you should definitely look into a myomectomy (really a "fibroidectomy"). Myomectomies *are* effective surgical procedures for removing fibroids. In this procedure, an incision is made through your abdomen and the fibroids removed while leaving your uterus and reproductive organs intact. Myomectomy has been around for years and was used to treat fibroids on younger women who still wanted children. But because it's a more time-consuming procedure than a hysterectomy, older women with fibroids are often not offered myomectomies as an option. A gynecologist experienced in reconstructive surgery is an appropriate myomectomy surgeon. Some fibroids can also be removed at the time of laparoscopy.

Your doctor might tell you that a myomectomy is more complicated than a hysterectomy and, if you're past menopause, may question your logic behind it. But studies show that when a surgeon is skilled in myomectomies, there are no more complications involved than in a hysterectomy, and none of the post-operative consequences of a hysterectomy either. In addition, a myomectomy can be performed with laser surgery, which involves far less bleeding.

If your doctor tells you that neither a myomectomy nor microsurgery is as effective as a hysterectomy, *get another opinion.* This response indicates that your doctor is unfamiliar with the procedures and prefers to rely on what he or she is *comfortable* doing, rather than on what's in *your* best interests.

Finding a Myomectomy Surgeon

If you live in the United States or Canada, call the Hysterectomy Educational Resources and Services (HERS) Foundation. This is a nationwide referral service that will provide you with lists of doctors who specialize in myomectomies and other alternatives to hysterectomies (they also have information for Canadians). The HERS Foundation is located at: 422 Bryn Mawr Ave., Bala-Cynwyd, PA 19004, 215-667-7757. The foundation also offers phone counseling.

Fertility surgeons are often skilled in both myomectomies and microsurgery. You can ask your gynecologist or primary care physician to refer you to a reproductive or fertility surgeon, who is usually a reproductive endocrinologist.

Hysterectomies

The latest statistics show that a hysterectomy is most likely to be performed for fibroids, uterine prolapse (discussed in chapter 13), and endometriosis (discussed in chapter 2). All three of these conditions can be successfully treated with alternative procedures or therapies.

Hysterectomies are performed primarily on women in their 30s and 40s, and about 40% of these women will wind up with their ovaries removed as well. In fact, one in three American women will not make it to the age of 60 with her uterus intact.

You might be interested to know that when the hysterectomy was first performed in the 19th century, it was an operation designed to cure excessive sexual desire. In short, a hysterectomy was designed to be a kind of sexual "lobotomy."

Well, in the 20th century, oophorectomies are performed for entirely different reasons and are often done as preventive surgery to reduce the risk of ovarian cancer, which is usually not diagnosed in time and has high mortality rates. If you elect to have a hysterectomy and are premenopausal, you should have a frank discussion with your gynecologist about your ovaries. He or she will take into consideration your family history, looking for family members not only with ovarian cancer, *but with colon and breast cancer*. Risk factors for ovarian cancer are discussed in chapter 8. Ultimately, it's your decision to keep your ovaries if they appear healthy at the time of surgery.

Many women don't wind up making an informed decision about an oophorectomy, and even when it's indicated they aren't prepared for the symptoms of surgical menopause. (What you need to know about oophorectomies is discussed in the next section.)

When an oophorectomy is performed in conjunction with a hysterectomy, some women experience a decrease in sexual function. For the majority of women, this can be relieved with hormonal replacement therapy, discussed in chapter 13. When women who know the consequences of oophorectomies are promised that their ovaries will remain intact and are then told that they will suffer no hormonal side effects of the surgery, as many as *half* of these women will go into ovarian failure anyway.

On the other hand, women who have hysterectomies (with or without an oophorectomy) to treat conditions that cause them chronic pelvic pain or heavy, chronic bleeding, will notice an improvement in their sex life because they'll be freer to enjoy it.

When Is a Hysterectomy Necessary?

You *will* need a hysterectomy if you have invasive cancer of the uterus, ovaries, cervix, vagina, and fallopian tubes (very rare). All of these cancers are discussed in chapter 9. You'll also need a hysterectomy for severe PID, severe, uncontrollable bleeding (rare but associated with childbirth, blood-clotting disorders, and endometriosis), life-threatening blockages of the bladder or bowels by the uterus or growths on the uterus, and rare childbirth complications, such as a uterine rupture. Finally, a fibroid condition that truly interferes with your quality of life will also warrant one. In 1990, Blue Cross/Blue Shield of Illinois found that one-third of the hysterectomies performed were "medically unnecessary." This appalling statistic means that since about 1 in 1,000 women die during a hysterectomy procedure as a result of complications, 200 women die each year because of an operation they may not have needed.

Because of this, it's important to investigate alternatives first before you agree. As for fibroids, if your fibroid is blocking the bladder or bowels, causing debilitating bleeding, or is the size of a Cadillac, you *may* need a hysterectomy—but only after investigating a myomectomy first.

There are several types of hysterectomies to choose from:

- *A total, complete, or simple hysterectomy (often called a partial hysterectomy)* removes the entire uterus with the cervix. The fallopian tubes and ovaries can be left intact, however. If they are, you will continue to ovulate, but you will not experience a menstrual period. The egg will just be absorbed by the body. It's important to note that the term *complete hysterectomy* is strictly a lay term. The medical description for this kind of hysterectomy is *salpingo-oophorectomy.*
- *A subtotal or partial hysterectomy* removes the uterus above the cervix but leaves the cervix intact. Fewer nerves are severed during this procedure, so the bladder, bowel, and sexual functions aren't as damaged. This proce-

dure does not make you immune to cervical cancer, however. The ovaries and tubes can be left intact as well.

- *A radical hysterectomy* is done only if there is invasive cancer. It removes the uterus, about one-third of the upper vagina, and lymph nodes around the groin for sampling. It can also mean removing the ovaries and tubes, but they can be left intact.
- *A modified or type II radical hysterectomy* is the same as above but tries to preserve nerve fibers to the bowel and bladder to preserve normal function. Again, the tubes and ovaries can be left intact.
- *A laparoscopically-assisted vaginal hysterectomy (LAVH)* is "hysterectomy by video." With the aid of a laparoscope and a video camera, the surgeon can make a small incision through the abdomen, view everything clearly on the video screen, maneuver various instruments inside the abdomen accordingly, and then complete the surgery through the vagina using traditional vaginal hysterectomy surgical techniques. The value of this procedure is that it may enable some women with fibroids, endometriosis, or PID to avoid the larger abdominal incision required for standard abdominal hysterectomy. In addition, recovery time is reduced.

The hysterectomy can be done either through an incision in the abdomen, where a 6–8 inch incision is made just below the pubic hairline (a bikini scar), or through the vagina, where an incision is made. But some conditions, including most cancers, require vertical incisions so that the surgeon can carefully examine the entire abdomen and remove large tumors. The benefit of a vaginal incision is that you'll have no visible scar. It also involves fewer complications and a shorter recovery period. The abdominal hysterectomy is done on women with large fibroids, invasive cancer, severe PID, or a history of abdominal surgery.

If your doctor suggests a hysterectomy for any of the following conditions, you should question the procedure and seek a second and even third opinion:

- fibroids
- uterine prolapse (see chapter 13)
- endometriosis (see chapter 2)
- pelvic pain
- ovarian cysts (see chapter 8)
- premenstrual syndrome (PMS) (see chapter 2)
- adenomyosis (see chapter 2)
- benign ovarian cysts (see chapter 8)

- inflammation
- hyperplasia (see chapter 8)

When your doctor recommends a hysterectomy, here are five questions you need to ask before you decide:

1. Who is performing the surgery? Make sure your surgeon is qualified.
2. What is being removed? (Many women don't know.) Be clear and comfortable about the fate of your ovaries.
3. When does this procedure need to be done? If it's not an emergency, use the time to get second and third opinions.
4. Will a vaginal or abdominal incision be done? Why is that particular incision being recommended?
5. Why do I need it? Invasive cancer, for example, is a valid reason (see other reasons above).

The Oophorectomy Issue

An oophorectomy means surgical removal of the ovaries and is usually done in conjunction with a hysterectomy of some sort. About 41% of all hysterectomy procedures involve oophorectomies as well. The main argument for removing the ovaries is that they can become cancerous later on, and since ovarian cancer is difficult to diagnose and treat, it's better to take them out. Women from some families have as high as a 50% risk of developing ovarian cancer. In this case, many doctors recommend that as soon as they're finished having children, they should strongly consider having a prophylactic oophorectomy. In one study, 28 women with a family history of ovarian cancer were given a prophylactic oophorectomy. Three of them went on to develop cancer in the *abdominal* cavity that was indistinguishable from ovarian cancer. However, this may have prevented the other 11 women from ever developing the disease.

In the general population, women with no history or family history of ovarian, colon, or breast cancer have only about a 1% chance of developing ovarian cancer. Therefore, if you don't have a family history of ovarian cancer, you and your doctor will need to decide whether removing your ovaries is premature.

Women who decide to take their ovaries out "just in case" or "while you're down there" are agreeing to what's known as a *prophylactic oophorectomy,* an oophorectomy performed for preventive measures. Before agreeing to a prophylactic oophorectomy, you should know what you're losing. When you lose your ovaries to surgery, you'll enter *surgical menopause.* Surgical menopause is a little more drastic than natural menopause, but consists of the same symptoms. In short, you'll experience the same symptoms caused by natural menopause, but more intensely. In addition, an oophorectomy performed before menopause also raises your risks of developing osteoporosis and heart disease if you don't take hormonal replacement therapy. Finally, it may interfere with your sexual lifestyle and contribute to vaginal dryness and loss of libido (see chapter 13).

This brings us to another hidden reason why doctors remove healthy ovaries: *the belief that a woman won't be needing them since she can't have children.* Oophorectomy has a rich medical history. There was a time when nymphomania was considered a serious disease and doctors would display removed ovaries on a silver platter at medical conventions. In reality, ovaries serve important hormonal functions that contribute to your overall health and sexual enjoyment. They secrete progesterone, three types of estrogen, and *androgen,* a male hormone responsible for libido. Essentially, the estrogen hormones trigger your vaginal lubrication, and the loss of this estrogen can cause your vaginal walls to thin, which is why sex can be uncomfortable. Meanwhile, without a libido, your sexual desire diminishes, and your sex life can change drastically. Although these hormones can be replaced with estrogen replacement therapy (ERT), they may be preserved naturally by sparing the ovaries.

Try to save your ovaries. Sometimes, only one ovary is removed, but when a *bilateral oophorectomy* is performed, both ovaries are removed. An oophorectomy *is* necessary when the ovaries are cancerous, or are badly infected as a result of PID or endometriosis. Women who should consider a prophylactic oophorectomy are those who have already had a bout with uterine, breast, or colon cancer, or those in a high-risk group for ovarian cancer (discussed in chapter 8).

Other Complications of a Hysterectomy

As many as half the women who undergo a hysterectomy will experience some of the following complications:

Hemorrhaging.

One in 10 women will require a blood transfusion as a result of hemorrhaging (blood loss) after or during the procedure. Often, a preexisting condition of anemia is the cause. You may want to consider banking some of your own blood prior to the procedure, or any elective surgery for that matter. This is called *autologous blood donation.* In the event of heavy blood loss during your surgery, *you are transfused with your own blood.*

Eventual ovarian failure.

If your ovaries are left intact, the unfortunate truth is that you may still go into surgical menopause. Women are often told that their hormone levels will not be affected if their ovaries are left intact. This is not true. Even when your ovaries are not removed, there's a chance that they will stop producing hormones. A rich network of blood vessels lies between the uterus and the ovaries and can be disturbed by removal of the uterus. Between 25 and 50% of all women who have intact ovaries after a hysterectomy will experience ovarian failure and go into surgical menopause. In addition, premenopausal women who lose their uterus but still have their ovaries go into menopause five years earlier than women who don't have hysterectomies. The hormonal side effects of hysterectomy are discussed in chapter 13.

Blood clots.

Blood clots can develop up to one week following the operation.

Depression.

Post-operative depression after a hysterectomy sets in three times more often than in other major surgical procedures. Whether you're prone to this depends on why your hysterectomy was done, your psychological state before your surgery, and whether you want to bear (more) children. Many women mourn the loss of the uterus, and some women feel as though their femininity has been stripped from them. In addition, surgical menopausal symptoms can aggravate some of these natural emotions. Hormonal replacement therapy can help.

Infections.

Fifty percent of all hysterectomy patients will suffer from various bacterial infections, which can be controlled with antibiotics. These infections include UTIs, discussed in chapter 6.

Loss of bladder function.

Aside from UTIs, sensory nerves may be cut and women can lose both the sensation of having to urinate and control over bladder functions.

Bowel problems.

If there is damage to the intestines during surgery, scar tissue can form and complicate your bowel function. This occurs in about 2% of all hysterectomy patients.

Urinary incontinence.

The uterus and its surrounding ligaments support the rest of your pelvic contents, allowing the bladder and rectum to maintain their correct positions. After a hysterectomy, you can become constipated and bloated, but also find that you can't hold in your urine.

Narrowing of the vagina.

If a vaginal repair was performed in the event of prolapse, scar tissue can form from improper healing, which will narrow your vaginal opening, making intercourse painful.

Nerve damage.

Nerves are severed during the surgery, which could cause numbness in your thigh, leg, or other parts of your body below your pelvic region. However, severed nerves can occur in any surgery and are not exclusive to hysterectomies.

Decreased pleasure during orgasm.

Orgasm can result from stimulation of the clitoris, uterus, or both. Pressure on the cervix, uterus, and its surrounding ligaments and membranes can heighten an orgasm.

Residual ovary syndrome.

Following hysterectomy with conservation of the ovaries, scar tissue forms around the ovaries and cysts tend to form, resulting in pain. This condition is difficult to treat medically and may require removal of the ovaries.

The good news about hysterectomies is that more women are taking an active role in the decision to have one—whether it is a necessary procedure or not. One study reveals that the more education a woman has, the lower her chances are of undergoing a hysterectomy. An interesting Swiss study revealed that *female gynecologists performed 50% fewer hysterectomies than male gynecologists.* This suggests that there is a gender difference when it comes to gynecological surgery.

The next chapter discusses other kinds of tumors to which your breasts and reproductive organs are prone. But again, hysterectomies need not be performed because of benign tumors. There are all kinds of microsurgery procedures that can be done to remove tumors and preserve your uterus and ovaries. Remember, 90% of all tumors are not cancerous and hence do not warrant hysterectomies.

What does all this have to do with fibroids? That's the problem. Hysterectomies shouldn't really have that much to do with fibroids anymore. So, if you should fall prey to fibroids in the future, make friends with them *first.* It could save your uterus.

CHAPTER 8

The Tumor Journey

The word *tumor* comes from the Latin meaning "to swell." A tumor is a clump of cells that are growing and reproducing, forming a lump of some sort. Whether or not the lump is visible depends on where the cells are growing. These cells are divided into two categories, *benign* (noncancerous) and *malignant* (cancerous). Benign cells are harmless; they exist without serving any particular purpose. However, there can be complications with benign tumors, which is why you'll need to get them removed. They are peaceful in nature and pose no threat to your health. Benign tumors generally stay where they are and don't bother nearby or distant organs. Fibroids (uterine muscle tumors, discussed in chapter 7) are good examples of benign tumors.

When the cells are malignant, it means they are "willful" and, if left "unsupervised," would invade nearby tissue and *metastasize* (meaning "travel") into distant organs, take over, and cause a lot of damage. They are militant or warlike in nature. Malignant cells mean cancer.

If there were any way doctors could automatically decipher a malignant lump from a benign lump, much of the anxiety over lumps in general would be alleviated. Unfortunately, there isn't any way of knowing instantly what the lump's "intentions" are. *All* suspicious lumps need to be investigated through various diagnostic procedures that can include needle biopsies, tissue biopsies via *lumpectomies* (surgically removing the lump altogether), and imaging procedures in which the lump can be photographed and studied more closely. When you feel a lump on your breasts, under your arms, or around your neck, for example, it's important to get it investigated as soon as possible.

But when it comes to the female reproductive organs, with the exception of breast lumps, tumors are very difficult to find because you normally can't feel or see them. That's why the Pap test, discussed in chapter 3, is so valuable. It's designed as a screening procedure to check up on the cervical cells once a year (although some doctors believe every two years is adequate) and make sure they haven't become abnormal and formed tumors. As a result of the Pap test, a new term has come into vogue: *precancerous.* This term means neither benign nor malignant but *potentially* malignant.

What about the ovaries, uterus, and fallopian tubes? Having regular pelvic exams and immediately reporting *any* kind of unusual symptoms, however trivial, are the *only* tools women have for keeping an eye out for pelvic tumors. In short, suspicion is still the best reason to launch a pelvic investigation. (Suspicious pelvic symptoms are discussed below.)

The *outcome* of these tumor investigations will tell you whether you have cancer. The purpose of this chapter is to describe the investigation process itself and discuss benign tumors in detail. This chapter points out high-risk groups for various cancers, as well as prevention/early detection techniques so you can stay alert. Everything you need to know about the "tumor journey" is in the following pages.

Women have a higher concentration of fat in their bodies than men do. Because of this, all kinds of lumps and bumps will form in fatty areas, but these lumps usually are *not* cancer. Potentially cancerous lumps tend to be found on the breasts, under the arms, or around the neck.

Lumps around the neck area usually don't signify a gynecological problem, and lumps around the neck are often benign. They need to be investigated, though, and *can* be signs of leukemia or Hodgkin's disease or can indicate malignancies in the throat, thyroid gland, or even lungs. If an advanced case of breast cancer developed, lumps in the neck could form as well around the collar bone. However, early detection of breast cancer is easier today, and an advanced case of breast cancer could develop only if you were neglecting other obvious signs. Because this is a gynecological sourcebook, lumps in the neck won't be discussed.

Lumps in the Breast

Breast lumps are frightening, but most of the time they're not cancerous. In addition, most breasts feel lumpy because of what they're made of: fatty, glandular tissue. The problem is, most women don't know the difference between a normal lump and a suspicious lump. A normal lump is one that's there for a good reason. A suspicious lump is one that needs to be investigated further because it has characteristics of *potential* malignant cells. Most suspicious breast lumps aren't cancerous either.

Enlarged Lymph Modes that Disappear [never suspicious]

Breasts are made up of fat, milk glands, and fibrous supporting tissue. There are also *lymph nodes* scattered throughout that extend under the arms. Lymph nodes are like small POW camps set up in the fatty, fleshy areas of your body. They work in partnership with the immune system and are designed to capture any kind of suspicious cell that roams near their "camp." A virus will make these camps active; when you're healthy, the camps will shut down. When foreign cells are captured, they're "held" in the camp for "questioning" and are then destroyed. An enlarged or swollen lymph node simply indicates that the nodes have "prisoners" and are filled up. (Anytime you have a cold, for example, the lymph nodes will swell.)

When you can't feel your lymph nodes at all, it's because there aren't any foreign cells around to keep them open for the moment. Does this mean you need to have a virus or cold in order for a lymph node to swell? No. Our bodies are constantly being invaded with viruses that we're not even aware of. Lymph nodes can fill up with prisoners all the time and then destroy them without our knowledge. These nodes will feel very small and hard, but after a menstrual cycle or two, they'll just disappear. Sometimes these little nodes might even feel tender to the touch. The bottom line is this: Small lumps that go away after two or three cycles are never cancerous. They are normal and healthy lymph nodes doing their jobs.

Enlarged Lymph Nodes that Don't *Disappear*

These are usually found on the neck area or under the arm, but they can be in the breast as well. When your lymph nodes are invaded by malignant cells, the cancer would be in a later stage and would have been around for a long time in order to have progressed to the lymph nodes. Here, the lymph nodes try to question and destroy the cells, but since the cells are so primitive, the lymph nodes are confused and hold the cells indefinitely. Therefore, the lymph nodes don't shrink and remain enlarged. It's unlikely that you'll feel these kinds of nodes in your breast; you'll probably feel them under your arm, but the malignant cells would have *originated* from your breast. If you feel an enlarged lymph node under your arm or on your breast, you'll need to get it investigated. Generally, if it disappears after one or two cycles, it's nothing to worry about. If it *doesn't* go away, this is a concern that will warrant further tests and biopsies. If you feel the enlarged node around your collar bone, get it checked immediately; it's far enough away from your breast that it won't be affected by menstrual cycle changes.

Investigating Suspicious Breast Lumps

A suspicious lump is usually hard and painless, but cancerous lumps have been known to be painful as well. The most important characteristic of a suspicious lump is that it is usually at least half an inch in size and tends to remain unchanged at your next cycle if you're menstruating. Breasts can change drastically from one cycle to the next, and sometimes even these lumps disappear. "Unchanged" means that the lump stays in the same place in your breast and doesn't move around, doesn't hurt suddenly, and doesn't shrink. (If it grows, you should continue to be suspicious.) If you're past menopause, the lump won't be affected by cycle changes. Moreover, women past menopause are in a higher risk group for breast cancer. Get your lump looked at as soon as you notice it.

If the lump is painful, it may signify one of the benign breast conditions described below. If the lump shrinks or disappears during one cycle, then magically reappears during the next, it may just be part of normal breast lumpiness and is probably not cancerous. If the lump is smaller than half an inch, is painless, and remains unchanged, it may be an enlarged lymph node, which you should have investigated.

If your lump meets these criteria, don't panic. It is probably *not* cancer and is more likely one of these: a *cyst* (a benign lump filled with fluid), a *fibroadenoma* (lazy benign cells living in a harmless clump), a *pseudolump* (suspicious at first but found to be there for a good reason when investigated), or a normal lymph node that has enlarged for harmless reasons.

Here are two questions women often ask:

1. *If I feel a lump, shouldn't I wait one cycle to see if it disappears?*
   No. Waiting will just create more anxiety. Although breast cancer grows pretty slowly, it's important to be aggressive about diagnosing or ruling out a malignancy. At the same time, it's important not to panic. In order for the lump to have formed in the first place, the cancer must have been growing for *at least* several years. Early breast cancer detected on a mammogram has generally been growing for about 9 years; by the time a lump develops that you can *feel*, the cancer has been growing for about 11 years—even then, it is considered in an early stage!
2. *Why do breasts sprout "normal" lumps to begin with?*
   All women will find lumps in their breasts from time to time. Just like any part of the body, breasts will change in size and shape as you age, diet, gain weight, and go from cycle to cycle. Some women may be plagued by lumpiness, or *nodules* (small knots of usually benign cells).

When you first discover a lump, don't wait to see if it disappears on its own. See your primary care physician. Your doctor may refer you to a breast surgeon or oncologist simply because he or she may not feel experienced enough to investigate it further. Ultimately, whoever handles the investigation will do either a needle aspiration or an ultrasound test. A needle aspiration is a simple in-office procedure performed under a local anesthetic. A long needle is used to suck out possible fluid from the lump. This will immediately tell the doctor whether the lump is a cyst, which is usually harmless. An ultrasound test can also be performed, which will tell your doctor whether the lump in your breast is solid or hollow. If it's hollow, it means the lump is not filled with mass but with fluid of some sort, which means it's a cyst. At this point, you may also need to get a mammogram, which is also useful in diagnosis.

Cysts.

Usually, a lump filled with fluid of any kind (sometimes even milk), is only a *cyst* and is not cancerous at all. Most cysts are benign. If your cyst is discovered via an ultrasound, your doctor may choose not to bother sucking out the fluid unless the cyst is bothering you. If he or she is performing a needle aspiration, the cyst will collapse or deflate when the fluid is sucked out. No more lump. If blood comes out with the fluid, the cells will be sent to a pathologist.

There is a 1% chance that your cyst may contain cancerous cells called *intracystic papillary carcinoma.* Similar to the papillary carcinoma discussed in the next chapter, this is when the cancer is restricted only to the cyst (hence the word *intraCYSTic*) and does not spread beyond it. If this is the case, the cyst will also be removed, but it's a harmless condition even though it is technically cancer.

After the cyst collapses, it can sometimes come back. If this happens, you may want to have a lumpectomy. If the lump doesn't go down after the fluid is removed from the cyst, your doctor may want to do a cellular biopsy procedure known as a *fine-needle aspiration.* This is similar to the needle aspiration procedure, but this time *cells* are sucked out of the-lump-that-won't-go-down. The cells are then sent to a laboratory for further investigation. Sometimes no fluid will come out of the cyst your doctor is trying to *aspirate* (suck out). At this point, a cellular biopsy may also be done just to double-check. (Indeed, sometimes doctors can miss the fluid if they aspirate from a bad angle.) Cysts are most common in women approaching menopause (women in their 50s), but can occur when you're in your 30s and 40s or younger. It is also common for women to develop numerous cysts or recurring cysts, a condition that may be mistakenly diagnosed as "fibrocystic breast disease," a diagnostic farce exposed below.

Fibroadenomas.

A fibroadenoma is a common, solid benign lump. It's what you get when you cross an *adenoma,* a clump of benign glandular cells (your breast has lots of glands within it), with a *fibroma,* a clump of benign cells made out of connective tissue (which your breast is also made from). If your lump isn't a cyst, chances are it's one of these.

A fibroadenoma feels like a marble inside your breast and is often very close to the nipple. It can vary from the size of a marble to the size of an egg. When it's large, it's known as a giant fibroadenoma. Actually, a fibroadenoma is a kind of breast fibroid, harmless overgrowth of normal breast tissue. (No, you don't have to have a uterine fibroid to have one of these or vice versa, nor does either kind of fibroid predispose you to the other!)

Fibroadenomas are suspected when the lump turns out to be solid via an ultrasound or when no fluid comes out during a needle aspiration. It's confirmed by *two* biopsy procedures. The first is a fine-needle aspiration, described above. If the cellular examination comes back negative, it means that no cancer is suspected, but the doctor will proceed with a surgical biopsy, which is really a lumpectomy. You'll report to the hospital, where the lump is surgically removed under either a local or general anesthetic.

Doctors may suspect a fibroadenoma just by feeling it with their fingers. Technically, if you do have a fibroadenoma, it *can* be left alone, but your doctor will probably take the lump out anyway to rule out cancer and prevent you from confusing future new lumps with *this* one. The biopsy will also give the doctor an opportunity to examine every part of the lump to ensure that he or she hasn't missed anything. Fibroadenomas are most common in younger women in their teens and 20s, but they're seen in older women, too. Like cysts, it's common to develop recurring (or even several) fibroadenomas.

Pseudolumps.

Pseudolumps fall into the "oops—I didn't realize this is *supposed* to be here" category. They look and feel like lumps but are found to be "extra lumpy" breast tissue that has every right to be there. This includes dead fat tissue lying around from a previous biopsy, hardened scar tissue from past breast surgery, hardened silicone from an implant, or the kind of lump that forms in fibrocystic breast disease.

The problem with pseudolumps is that they can scare you and confuse the doctors for a while. Usually, your doctor will try to aspirate it. When that doesn't work, a fine-needle aspiration might be done, which will come back negative, and then a lumpectomy. At this point, the pseudolump is discovered and will be removed. Pseudolumps are harmless and are never cancerous.

Enlarged lymph nodes.

Enlarged lymph nodes *that don't go away* (see above) are treated like other lumps: needle aspiration, followed by fine-needle aspiration, followed by lumpectomy. These are usually found under your arm and will be investigated for evidence of *metastasis*, the spreading of malignant cells. Often the lymph node is enlarged for unknown reasons and isn't cancerous. (A nasty virus can render a lymph node permanently enlarged, for example.)

If the doctor is going to remove a solid lump anyway, why bother with a fine-needle aspiration at all? A fine-needle aspiration always tells the doctor whether the cells inside the lump are cancerous. In fact, this biopsy is more accurate in detecting a malignant condition than a benign one. It's done more as a "ruling out" procedure than anything else. If your cells come back positive, it means the lump is malignant and you may require major surgery. In this case, having a lumpectomy performed when you're going to have (part of) the breast removed anyway is illogical. Even if the doctor suspects the lump is benign, he or she still may not know for sure. Furthermore, taking the lump out now avoids future lump "confusion." Breast cancer is discussed in the next chapter.

The Big Joke: Fibrocystic Breast Disease

Millions of women are diagnosed with *fibrocystic breast disease (FCBD).*

You may have read a lot of magazine articles on FCBD, or perhaps you've been "diagnosed" with this condition. The truth is, *there is no such thing as fibrocystic breast disease.* It is a confusing term that refers to separate and distinct breast conditions that have *nothing* to do with each other. These conditions range from normal breast tenderness that develops before your period to fibroadenomas and cysts, and are listed below.

While we're on the subject of tumors, it's crucial that this breast condition is exposed *here,* because it's a trendy diagnosis that's been erroneously linked to breast tumors and breast cancer, or even referred to as a "precancerous" condition, often treated with placebo therapies. FCBD does not cause cancer. In 1986, even the American College of Pathologists was forced to admit that this absurd label "does not increase the risk of cancer."

In fact, fibrocystic breast disease is similar to *premenstrual syndrome (PMS),* which again lumps together a hodgepodge of different symptoms into one confusing term. Like PMS, 10 different doctors will give you 10 different interpretations of fibrocystic breast disease, while 10 different women diagnosed with this mythical disease will describe 10 completely different sets of symptoms. When you hear this diagnosis, don't panic, *laugh*—because it's really just a big joke. Many times this condition refers to breasts that are lumpy and fibrous, and perhaps the term fibrocystic breast *condition* would be more appropriate than "disease."

The 'Six Conditions' Under FCBD

The term *FCBD* originated the same way *PMS* did: through sweeping generalizations, inconclusive studies, hundreds of articles all based on the *same* inconclusive study, doctors seeking diagnostic fame, illogical conclusions ("Hmm . . . these 10 women all have breast cancer. These 10 women also have nipples. Therefore, nipples must *cause* breast cancer."), and media pouncing on the latest in-vogue disease. If you suffer from any of the following breast conditions, you may be diagnosed with FCBD. It's important to remember *not* to take this diagnosis too seriously. None of the conditions below *causes* breast cancer, although on rare occasions some of the symptoms below are signs of certain breast cancers.

1. Tender breasts.

Normal physiological changes in the breast that develop during or before your period include swelling, tenderness, and lumpiness (water retention can create a lumpy feeling). If you suffer from premenstrual "tender boobs," check out chapter 2 and don't worry about it.

However, a Canadian professor of surgery made a disturbing remark about premenstrual breast pain. "Premenstrual breast pain and tenderness is not normal. If it's painful premenstrually, it's sick. I am sure that males would not accept sore testicles for 7–10 days of each month as normal." Translation: How can women just *live* with tender breasts every month? Well, it *is* normal, and all part of the *healthy* discomforts that accompany the menstrual cycle. While it's *also* true that men would not tolerate sore testicles, *would they tolerate* any *of the discomforts of a menstrual period at all?* In fact, it is *exactly* this kind of statement that reveals a troubling "reverse misogynism" at work in women's health care. On the surface, this remark seems to indicate that this doctor "cares" about our aches and pains. But underneath, it is the type of remark that *maligns* the healthy female body; it causes women to needlessly question whether they are indeed normal. In other words, instead of comforting and reassuring women about what *is* physiologically normal, some male doctors seem to be manufacturing illnesses around normal and healthy occurrences in the female body.

2. Mastalgia (or mastodynia).

Mastalgia (breast pain) can come and go or be constant. The pain varies from minor irritation a couple of times a month (often a PMS symptom) to debilitating pain. Many women diagnosed with FCBD really have mastalgia. Mastalgia is broken down into *cyclical pain,* which is the same as #1 above, *non-cyclical pain* (i.e., chronic), and *non-breast-origin pain* (a pain that has nothing to do with your breasts).

Cyclical pain (when the pain occurs only once in a while) is usually hormonal, and the PMS section in chapter 2 covers this type of breast pain. This is *never* a sign of breast cancer. For this pain, vitamin E and no-caffeine therapies, also recommended to relieve PMS symptoms, have been hailed as the ultimate panaceas for FCBD. You'll also find that this kind of breast pain "magically" disappears after menopause. (In short, hormonal breast pain *is* a PMS symptom!)

Noncyclical breast pain is trickier. This is *anatomical* (something inside the breast *itself* is causing the pain) rather than hormonal, so it does not necessarily disappear with menopause like hormonal breast pain. Often, this pain is caused by a large cyst. In fact, many women are simply prone to painful cysts. Because of this, women have come to believe that FCBD equals painful, lumpy breasts. *This is not true at all.* But women who have this particular breast problem and are told they have FCBD, may be put on an iodine treatment, which has proved helpful.

Iodine is a crucial element for thyroid gland function; too much or too little iodine can lead to thyroid problems, while *radioactive* iodine is used to treat and diagnose a variety of thyroid conditions. But studies now show that the ovaries and breasts also need iodine. (One researcher has called the breast a "big thyroid gland.") Women with painful cysts in their breasts *have* shown tremendous improvement with this kind of iodine treatment. However, if you have iodine treatment for breast pain caused by cysts, your thyroid gland can become overactive. Or, if you're on thyroid medication, the iodine can interfere with it. Just make sure your thyroid condition and breast condition are managed by the same doctor. In addition, this iodine treatment for breast pain has been heralded as *the* definitive treatment for FCBD in the past. It's not. It's only helpful for *noncyclical breast pain caused by cysts.* Period. Today, iodine treatment is rarely used.

Noncyclical breast pain can also be a bruise, and *very, very rarely,* it can indicate cancer. This type of pain should be checked out by your gynecologist or primary care physician. If you're over 35, you should get a mammogram done to screen for any kind of unusual source of the pain. The cure is either finding the source of the pain and relieving it (like aspirating a cyst, for example), or being reassured that you don't have cancer by a negative mammogram (these are 85% accurate).

Finally, non-breast-origin pain can be a form of arthritis called *costochondritis.* Men get this, too, and they think they're having a heart attack, while women think they have breast cancer. You'll need to be treated for *arthritic pain.* A pinched nerve in the neck can also cause breast pain, as well as a type of *phlebitis* (inflamed vein) in the breast. These cure themselves in time.

3. Infections and inflammations.

Breasts and nipples are like any other part of the body and can get infected, too! Antibiotics will fix this. The most common infection is called *lactational mastitis,* an inflammation of the breast due to bacteria trapped in the milk. This happens during breastfeeding. It works on the same principle as urinary tract infections (UTIs). Bacteria get inside the nipple and block a milk duct. The milk doesn't empty out of the duct completely, backs up and provides a home for the bacteria. The breast gets red and inflamed. Treatment: antibiotics. Ten percent of the time, an abscess will form that can be drained via a needle, or a tiny incision is made in the breast to drain it.

Nonlactational mastitis is a bacterial breast infection in a woman who is not nursing. Bacteria get deeper inside the breast via lumpectomy, immune deficiency, and so on. Diabetic women are prone to this for the same reasons they are prone to yeast infections. The breast can develop skin boils, and you can also have flulike symptoms. Antibiotics take care of this.

Chronic subareolar abscess is an infection of the sebaceous glands around the nipples. Bacteria are the culprit again, getting inside the glands via breastfeeding or lovemaking. The glands get blocked, and your breasts get red and form painful boils. This is an unsettling and ugly sight, but quite treatable. The gland needs to be surgically opened or the infection will keep coming back. Antibiotics and minor breast surgery are the treatments.

4. Discharge and other nipple problems.

Discharge is pretty common. One study found that 83% of women of all ages and "lactation histories" had discharge when their breasts were gently suctioned. Chapter 1 discusses how suction is an important part of milk production. Well, discharge can be caused by suction as well, even if you're not lactating. Basically, *prolactin* gets activated and tells the brain to send down fluid in a confused instinct. Although some BSE (Breast Self-Examination) pamphlets will tell you to squeeze the nipple for discharge, and some doctors will routinely squeeze the nipple during a pelvic exam, this discharge is usually normal fluid caused by the squeezing. The only time you should worry about nipple discharge is when it comes out by itself and comes out of one breast only. This is usually caused by infection, but it can be a sign of cancer about 4% of the time. See your doctor if this happens.

Finally, nipples can get itchy. This is caused by rashes, dry skin, or eczema. Rarely, a kind of "breast skin cancer" known as *Paget's disease* can occur. You'll know what it is if your rash doesn't respond to anti-itch medication. Paget's disease responds well to treatment and is discussed briefly in chapter 9.

5. General breast lumpiness ("nodularity").

Generalized lumpiness is not a concern. What you're looking for in this case is a lump that clearly stands out from other "normal lumps" and is distinct in size and shape.

6. Suspicious lumps.

Suspicious lumps are discussed above.

A final note on FCBD.

If you're diagnosed with this pseudocondition, ask your doctor what *specific* breast symptoms have led him or her to this conclusion, and ask about the "treatment." Then, refer to the list above and *calm down*. There is still an ongoing debate over whether dense breast tissue, characterized by lumpy breasts, is a risk for breast cancer. For what it's worth, the American College of Pathologists declared in 1986 that FCBD does not put you at a higher risk for cancer.

Screening for Breast Cancer and Suspicious Breast Lumps

Of all suspicious breast lumps, 85–90% are *not* cancerous. Still, approximately 1 in 10 women develop breast cancer at some point in their lives. Although knowing your family history and your age risk, as well as practicing good nutritional habits, is an important part of breast cancer awareness, it's also important to note that 75–80% of all breast cancer occurs in women with *none* of the known risk factors I've cited below. But for now, breast cancer can be detected only from a suspicious lump in the breast. There are two screening methods designed to "catch" the lump and find any possible cancer. Other nonradiation-emitting methods have been explored, but nothing has come close to being as effective as mammography combined with BSE. Some of the methods explored in the past were thermal screenings (using heat sensors) and ultrasound. Ultrasound is helpful only as a diagnostic tool, as it examines a lump that has already been *found*, rather than looking for new ones.

For the moment, mammography combined with monthly BSE is still the most reliable screening method for breast cancer. In 1993 an Israeli researcher reported that she had obtained the same screening results with magnetic resonance imaging (MRI) as she had with mammography. MRI does not use radiation, which is promising, but needs to be researched further before North American hospitals will consider it more accurate than mammography. Moreover, MRI is not useful in finding calcification, which is often an initial finding of breast cancer on a mammogram. And MRI is expensive, costing about $1500 per patient; a mammogram and biopsy costs only $300 per patient.

Finally, a better screening method is being explored through *genetic screening*: blood tests that can detect the breast cancer gene itself. This is a far more promising and feasible screening method and may be available before the next century.

There is one blood test known as the *CA-15-3*, which detects tiny, sloughed-off cells produced by malignant tumors (basically, "tumor poop") in the bloodstream. This is used only to detect breast cancer *recurrence*, however, and its effectiveness as a screening method for even *that* is still being debated.

Breast Self-Examination

BSE should be called "get to know your breasts." It involves specific steps of feeling your breasts at the same time each month and distinguishing suspicious lumps from enlarged lymph nodes. In addition, you can't know if a lump has remained unchanged unless you've been checking your breasts monthly. You should begin BSE by the age of 20. That way, you will know what your breast normally feels like, should something abnormal develop down the road.

While you're menstruating, you'll need to do a BSE after your period ends, when your breasts are least tender and lumpy. If you're past menopause, do BSE at the same time each month. The steps to BSE are outlined below, but make sure your doctor actually *shows* you how to do it as well.

1. *Visually inspect your breasts.* Stand in front of the mirror and look closely at your breasts. You're looking for dimpling, puckering (like an orange peel in appearance), or noticeable lumps. Do you see any discharge that dribbles out on its own or bleeding from the nipple? Any dry patches on the nipple (which may be Paget's disease)?
2. *Visually inspect your breasts with your arms raised.* Still standing in front of the mirror, raise your arms over your head and look for the same things. Raising your arms smooths out the breast a little more and makes these changes more obvious.
3. *Palpation (feeling your breast).* Lie down on your bed with a pillow under your left shoulder. Place your left hand under your head. With the flat part of the fingertips of your right hand, examine your left breast for a lump, using a gentle circular motion. Imagine that the breast is a clock, and make sure you feel each "hour," as well as the nipple area and armpit area.
4. *Repeat step 3, but reverse sides, examining your right breast with your left hand.*
5. *If you find a lump,* see if it has any of the characteristics of a *suspicious lump* described earlier. If it does, note the size, shape, and how painless it is. You can either get it looked at as soon as you can, or if you're comfortable doing so, wait for the next cycle. If the lump changes in the next cycle by shrinking or *becoming* painful, it's not cancerous but should be looked at anyway. If the suspicious lump stays the same, definitely get it looked at as soon as possible.
6. *If discharge oozes out of your nipple on its own, or if blood comes out,* see your doctor immediately. Don't wait.
7. *If your nipple is dry and patchy,* see your doctor immediately.

Ninety percent of all breast cancers are picked up by women themselves, either accidentally or through BSE.

Mammography

A mammogram is a breast X ray. It's used as both a screening procedure for breast cancer and a diagnostic tool in investigating suspicious lumps. Ultrasound is usually done to follow up a mammogram abnormality. A mammogram is similar to a chest X ray except it's limited to just the breast and does not display the lungs. You place your breast inside a machine that looks like a photocopier. One side of the breast is placed on a metal or plastic plate that is covered with another metal plate. Then, a picture is taken of the breast.

The risk of breast cancer increases with age (70–80% of all breast cancer is found in women over 50). For this reason the American College of Physicians, the American College of Obstetricians and Gynecologists, the American College of Radiologists, and their Canadian, British, Swedish, Dutch, and Italian counterparts recommend mammographies every two years for women age 50 or older. Meanwhile, the American Medical Association, the National Cancer Institute, and the American Cancer Society recommend screenings once a year or every other year for women 40 years and older. Deciding on a mammogram annually or every other year is currently your decision. Furthermore, the American Medical Association recommends that all women should go for a "baseline mammogram" sometime between 35 and 39 so they'll have a normal mammogram on file that can be compared to future mammograms. (Sometimes abnormalities are picked up on the baseline, too.) Then, they should have a mammogram every two years until they're 49, and *annual* mammograms afterward. Evidence suggests mammographies on women under 50 is helpful. Further research will prove whether this is correct.

Why is age such a factor? Breast cancer, as mentioned earlier, grows very slowly. By the time a mammogram can pick up what's known as early breast cancer the cancer has been growing for about *nine years!* A 50-year-old woman who has a positive mammogram would have been 41 years old when her first breast cancer cell reproduced for the first time. One breast cancer cell takes about 100 days to reproduce and become *two* breast cancer cells, and so on. In order for a mammogram to find early breast cancer in a 35-year-old woman, the first cancer cell would need to be present at the age of 26. Basically, it's highly unlikely for breast cancer to start growing in a woman this young. Furthermore, the amount of radiation exposure in a mammogram is definitely a factor to consider. Critics of mammography for women under 50 feel the amount of radiation they are exposed to would do more damage than just waiting until they turn 50. It's important to realize, though, that the radiation levels in upgraded mammogram equipment is far lower today than five years ago. In fact, mammograms now deliver less radiation than a chest X ray. Although many doctors feel that the radiation risk regarding mammography is being blown out of proportion, nobody disputes the fact that annual mammograms expose you to more radiation than no mammogram. The risk of getting cancer from an upgraded mammogram is now equal to the lifetime risk of smoking half a cigarette once. Ultimately, you need to weigh the risk of breast cancer against the lower risk of developing cancer as a result of mammogram-linked radiation.

Statistically, the age breakdown for breast cancer goes like this: 20% of all breast cancers occur in women under 50; 40% is found in women 50–65; 40% is found in women over 65.

What should *you* do? If you are under 50, are in a low-risk group (discussed below), and have no history of benign breast tumors, such as cysts or fibroadenomas, you should wait until you turn 50. If you *do* have a history of benign cysts, and you're *comfortable* waiting until 50, do so. If you're uncomfortable waiting, screening younger than 50 may reassure you and lessen your anxiety, which, in turn, will make you healthier and better able to combat breast cancer, should the time ever come. Regardless of your age, you should be doing BSE and familiarizing yourself with your breasts so you'll be prepared to notice anything unusual. You should also make sure that a manual breast exam is performed by your doctor each year with your Pap smears.

Here's how to get the most out of your mammogram:

1. Go to a reliable screening center, one that specializes in mammograms and does at least 20 mammograms a day.
2. The image of the breast on the X ray must be of the highest quality. Good equipment used only for mammography and purchased no later than three years ago is your best bet. Cheap or older equipment used by a cut-rate center will be of no value to you and could deliver false positives.
3. A dedicated, experienced technician specially trained in mammography must perform the screening, and an experienced *radiologist* must read and interpret mammogram results. (If the technician is reading the results, he or she won't be as skilled as a physician who specializes in reading X rays.) Similarly, an X-ray technician student is not a suitable person to perform the mammography.
4. For the mammogram to be as accurate as possible, there must be maximum compression on the breast during the procedure. That means it will probably hurt a little bit, but rest assured you will get a more accurate reading. Compression also reduces the amount of radiation required. (As to whether compression triggers a dormant breast cancer to grow is, to date, not proven and highly debatable.)

5. The center should have a strict quality-control program in place. Ask what they do to ensure quality before you go for the procedure. If they don't have such a program, find another center.
6. A physical examination of the breasts by a trained nurse or qualified physician *must* accompany the mammogram. Before you go, however, you'll need to see your doctor, who will indicate any concerns he or she has on your mammogram requisition.
7. Don't put any talcum powder, deodorant, or lotion on your upper body the day you're scheduled. Little flecks can get on the plates and interfere with the results.

High-Risk Groups for Breast Cancer

Every day it seems as though something else is revealed to be "linked" to breast cancer. Because researchers still don't know what causes breast cancer, much of this "new evidence" is unsubstantiated. The following list contains *established* characteristics of women who developed breast cancer in the past. Women who have one or more of the following characteristics are considered to be in a high-risk group for breast cancer. All this means is that more breast cancer was found in women *with* one or more of these characteristics than in women *without* them. However, none of these characteristics definitively "causes" breast cancer. In the list below, characteristics currently in debate are preceded by the word *may.* Remember, 75–80% of breast cancer patients do *not* fall into any of these catogories.

Women who are at higher risk:
- have had breast cancer before;
- have been exposed to high levels of radiation in the past;
- are 50 years of age or older;
- have a mother, aunt, sister, or two first-degree relatives who had breast cancer before menopause;
- have had two or more benign breast biopsies;
- *may* never have had any children;
- *may* have had their first child after the age of 30;
- *may* have had their first menstrual period before age 12 (called "early menarche");
- *may* have started menopause after age 50;
- *may* consume large quantities of animal fats and dairy products;
- *may* take synthetic estrogen hormones;
- *may* live in North America or Western Europe;

- *may* consume moderate quantities of alcohol (one to two drinks per day); and
- *may* have dense breasts.

Abnormal Bleeding and Benign Pelvic Conditions

Experiencing abnormal bleeding from the uterus, vagina, or cervix is the pelvic equivalent of finding a lump in the breast. Many women panic and jump to conclusions, fearing they have some horrible kind of cancer. Usually, abnormal bleeding is caused by a *benign* condition, which is often hormonal.

It's a signal that something is wrong and gives you the *opportunity* to fix it. In fact, it is the pelvic cancers that *don't* cause bleeding, such as ovarian cancer, that are far more destructive. Abnormal bleeding usually indicates either a benign or treatable condition. Other signs of pelvic problems are less obvious: unusual discharge (which we're not often aware of), abdominal pain, lower back pain and cramping, bowel problems, and bladder problems.

What are the Odds of Developing a Pelvic Tumor?

Millions of women will be diagnosed each year with either a benign pelvic tumor, such as a fibroid (see chapter 7) or ovarian cyst (see below), or a benign but possibly precancerous condition known as *hyperplasia* (also discussed below). Pelvic inflammatory disease (PID) (see chapter 6) and endometriosis (see chapter 2) are extremely common causes of abnormal bleeding and are often the culprits behind all kinds of symptoms, but they may be suspected as cancer until they are diagnosed.

When cancer of the reproductive organs *does* strike, it most often involves the uterus, which is usually treatable. Uterine, or *endometrial cancer*, as it's called, has a 85–92% survival rate, and about 33,000 U.S. women develop uterine cancer each year. Ovarian cancer is rarer (about 20,000 U.S. women develop this each year). Although ovarian cancer *is* dangerous and difficult to detect, the majority of women are *not* in a high-risk group for this kind of cancer. Ovarian cancer has an average survival rate of 38%, but *when it's detected in its early stages, it has an 85% survival rate.*

Cancer almost never originates from the fallopian tubes or vagina (less than 1,000 U.S. women each year develop cancer of the vagina or fallopian tubes; only five in one million women develop vaginal cancer). Less than 3,000 women develop cancer of the vulva. The only exception to the vaginal and vulvar cancer statistics is among DES daughters, who do tend to develop these kinds of cancers more frequently at young ages (at about age 19). (See chapter 3 for more information on DES daughters.) The only reason a woman dies from vaginal or vulvar cancer is usually because she is not having routine pelvic exams. As discussed below, the signs of these kinds of cancers are obvious and treatable and are now known to be almost 100% preventable through safe sex and good hygiene. For the most part, however, when the vagina, vulva, and fallopian tubes *are* involved, the cancer originates from the uterus, cervix, or ovaries. Vaginal cancer nevertheless has a survival rate of 50%; cancer of the vulva has a survival rate of 80%. Cancer of the fallopian tubes has an even lower survival rate than ovarian cancer: 30%.

Cervical cancer is more common than uterine cancer. But thanks to the Pap test (discussed in chapter 3), detecting early or "embryonic" cervical cancer is so advanced it's often treated before it has a chance to progress to a life-threatening stage. Because Pap tests are so routine now, cases of advanced cervical cancer have dropped dramatically. Still, about 13,500 women in the United States develop cervical cancer each year. If it *does* advance, it will spread to the uterus and is curable via hysterectomy. But unlike uterine cancer or ovarian cancer, cervical cancer can be prevented through safe sex (see chapter 4).

A Look at the Suspicious Symptoms

If you're bleeding or cramping when you're not having your period, these symptoms are considered *abnormal.* Any change in your normal menstrual flow (heavier or lighter flow, consistency, duration, or timing) is also abnormal. Unless you are expecting these symptoms as either post-operative side effects (following a D & C procedure or cryotherapy, for example) or as a side effect to a particular hormone or therapy (as in hormone replacement therapy [HRT] or OCs), you need to report these symptoms. Remember, though, that there are usually *noncancerous* reasons why you may be experiencing suspicious pelvic symptoms. Other suspicious symptoms that may be signs of pelvic cancer include the following:

1. *Any unusual growths or sores on or near your vulva.* Cervical cancer is now believed to be the result of human papillomavirus (HPV) infec-

tion. This virus can cause the cells that line the cervix to change, which, if left untreated, can lead to cancer. It can spread beyond your cervix toward the uterus or vagina. Cauliflower-type, flesh-toned lesions near your vagina and vulva, known as condyloma, meaning "raised wart," are often found early during a Pap smear and treated long before the virus triggers precancerous cell changes.

Vulvar cancers are basically pelvic skin cancer. Therefore, any raised sores or ulcers that are painful, ooze pus or bleed, that *won't* heal, are suspicious. (Herpes sores always heal, however.)

2. *Unusual vaginal discharge.* Watery, bloody discharge after menopause is especially suspect; unusual vaginal discharge is usually a sign of a vaginal infection (see chapter 6) but may indicate something is up elsewhere. Always report this symptom. When it's fishy-smelling, it's likely a bacterial infection or a sexually transmitted disease (STD); herpes sores sometimes wind up on your cervix and can ooze pus that imitate vaginal discharge as well. If the discharge has a sweeter odor, like baking bread or even beer, and is cottage-cheesy and white, you've most likely got yeast. However, unusual discharge could also be a sign of cervical or endometrial cancer. See your doctor if you notice unusual discharge.
3. *Pelvic pain.* Pelvic pain could indicate endometriosis (see chapter 2), PID (see chapter 6), symptomatic fibroids (see chapter 7), or may be a symptom of a pelvic cancer.
4. *Spotting after intercourse.* Unless you're a virgin and are bleeding as a result of a ruptured hymen, spotting after intercourse indicates that you may be bleeding in your upper pelvic region. This is not normal; get this looked at.
5. *Any lumps that you can feel in your abdomen, or a noticeable bloating or increase in abdominal width.* Bloating is a common PMS symptom, so you'll have to decide what constitutes "abnormal" bloating. If you're still bloated right after your period and have noticed that belts or pants don't seem to fit when you haven't put on weight elsewhere, this is generally a sign that something's up. It is often a symptom of PID, fibroids, or hyperplasia, but it could also mean uterine or ovarian cancer.
6. *Swollen glands in the groin area.* These are lymph glands that may show signs of metastasis. See the above section on enlarged lymph nodes that don't disappear. These glands will be enlarged for the same reasons but will not be affected by the menstrual cycle the way

glands around the breasts are. These should be treated as swollen lymph nodes in the neck and investigated *immediately.*

7. *Abdominal pain, nausea, vomiting, gas, constipation, weight loss, or loss of appetite.* This is a long list of miscellaneous ill-health symptoms. If any of these symptoms continues, it's a sign you're not well. Abdominal pain is also a classic symptom of endometriosis or PID. Although these symptoms could be linked to almost anything, they can also be signs of ovarian, fallopian tube, or uterine cancers.
8. *Painful, frequent, or difficult urination.* Most often, this is a sign of UTI, interstitial cystitis (see chapter 6), or a fibroid pressing against the bladder (see chapter 7). This could also mean other problems such as *metastasis* (a cancerous "invasion"). Check it out.

Pelvic cancers can be divided into two categories: estrogen-dependent cancers and disease-dependent cancers. Cervical, vaginal, and vulvar cancers tend to be associated with the presence of an STD. *That's why hesitating to report symptoms of obvious STDs is particularly dangerous.* Curing the diseases early may prevent them from developing into certain cancers.

Estrogen-dependent cancers are stimulated by estrogen. One theory about how these cancers begin is that estrogen flourishes in women who have large amounts of fat stores. The fat cells turn into estrogen factories, increasing the amount of estrogen produced by the body. Breast cancer, endometrial cancer, and ovarian cancer all fall into these categories and are more common in women who are more than 25 pounds overweight. This is why high-fiber and low-fat diets are encouraged; they seem to help prevent estrogen-dependent cancers from developing. There are also numerous other reasons, as well as external factors, for estrogen surplus in the body. Oral contraceptives may protect against ovarian cancer.

Investigating Abnormal Uterine Bleeding

The first steps in investigating abnormal bleeding is a thorough physical exam, a pelvic exam, and a Pap smear to rule out various commonplace sources: bladder infections, STDs, hemorrhoids, and so on. If the bleeding is an isolated event, your doctor may choose to do nothing and see if the episode recurs. Depending on other symptoms accompanying your bleeding, you may be required to undergo a transvaginal ultrasound procedure, a laparoscopy (discussed in chapter 2), or a D & C (Dilation and curettage). Another important procedure is an *endometrial biopsy*. This is an in-office procedure that involves placing a small plastic cylinder inside the cervix. The cylinder contains a suction device that sucks up only a small portion of the endometrial lining. The lining is then sent to a lab and analyzed. The procedure is an excellent diagnostic tool, takes only about 30 seconds to do, and is far less invasive than either a D & C (which removes the entire lining) or a laparoscopy procedure. This procedure would be done after a transvaginal ultrasound in the event of abnormal uterine bleeding. However, since it biopsies only one area, some doctors may still prefer to do a D & C. (Neither a transvaginal ultrasound or endometrial biopsy is recommended as a *routine* procedure. They should be done only when there's a problem.)

D & C is one of the most common operations performed on women of all ages. It is a short surgical procedure that can be done under a general or local anesthetic. The cervix is dilated to the size of a thumb, and the lining of your uterus is then scooped out with a spoon-like instrument called a *curette*. A D & C is most commonly done to find the cause of irregular uterine bleeding. A D & C might be recommended when an endometrial biopsy cannot be performed. This would be the case if the cervical opening was too small. This procedure can pinpoint a whole batch of problems: fibroids, uterine cancer, cervical polyps and so on. D & Cs are also done to "clean out" the uterus. (D & C also stands for "dusting and cleaning.") Women who have had miscarriages or have not delivered the placenta in childbirth are classic D & C candidates. D & Cs are also used to perform abortions.

You'll need to be admitted into the hospital. Just before the operation, your doctor will perform a pelvic exam. Then he or she will place a metal speculum into your vagina and wash off the vagina and cervix with an antiseptic solution. The doctor puts a clamp on the cervix and passes an instrument through the cervix that measures the depth of the uterus. This will tell the doctor how large your uterus is. Your cervix is gradually opened up using a series of metal rods or dilators, starting with straw-size rods and ending with thumb-size rods. The lining of your uterus is then carefully removed using curettes. The curette has a long handle and sharp edges that can scrape the inner walls of the uterus. These scrapings are then sent to the lab for analysis. Finally, the doctor removes the speculum and puts a sanitary napkin in place to soak up the blood. The whole procedure takes about 15 minutes, and you can usually go home the same day (unless there were complications indicating an infection). In the United States, D & Cs are often done on an outpatient basis, meaning that you can go home the same day.

You'll feel cramping and soreness for about a day and will continue to spot for a few weeks. If you continue to bleed heavily for more than a week, see your doctor. Since your cervix is dilated, make sure you avoid getting bacteria into your uterus, which can cause PID. Review the precautions mentioned in chapter 6. Your periods will also be interrupted (since the lining was removed) but will return to normal after about six weeks.

Endometrial Hyperplasia: It's Not *Cancer*

Abnormal uterine bleeding is often a hormonal problem that has to do with *anovulatory bleeding*. This is responsible for abnormal bleeding about 70% of the time and is particularly common in women approaching menopause. For some reason, you're not ovulating properly, and the lining of your uterus is thickening without shedding. When this happens, a condition known as *endometrial hyperplasia* can develop. *Hyperplasia* means "overgrowth," so *endometrial hyperplasia* means "overgrowth of, or too much, endometrium." Unless the lining of the uterus sheds regularly, tissues and glands will build up and may later become a breeding ground for abnormal cells. In essence, hyperplasia *can* lead to uterine cancer, but it is *not yet* cancer. It is, instead, a precancerous condition, meaning potentially cancerous.

Remember in chapter 2, where I discussed the "need to bleed?" The chapter recommended that any woman of childbearing age who has missed more than two consecutive periods—but was *not* pregnant—would need to investigate it and possibly have her period induced. Preventing the development of hyperplasia is the reason. (Preventing hyperplasia is also a concern for postmenopausal women on unopposed estrogen therapy, discussed in chapter 13.)

Depending on how long your lining has been growing, some stages of hyperplasia are more advanced than others. *Cystic glandular hyperplasia* (also called *cystic endometrial hyperplasia,* or *mild hyperplasia)* means that you have too much lining but your endometrial cells are still *normal,* which is good news. This kind of hyperplasia is always caused by too much estrogen (see below) and rarely develops into cancer.

Adenomatous hyperplasia without atypical cells is a mouthful to say, but is still good news. *Adenomatous* is an adjective that refers to harmless glandular cells. (An adenoma is, therefore, a benign tumor made up of harmless glandular cells.) When mild hyperplasia isn't treated, you get adenomatous hyperplasia, which means that the glandular endometrial cells are growing but are still benign. Again, this kind of hyperplasia rarely develops into cancer. If left untreated, 15–30% of all women with this condition would go on to develop endometrial cancer within five years.

*Atypical adenomatous hyperplasia (*also called *severe hyperplasia* or even *carcinoma in situ—CIS)* is not great news but isn't *bad* news either. This means that either a small area on your endometrium or sometimes the entire lining consists of cells that are abnormal and not necessarily benign. The cells seem to be more aggressive but may still be harmless. The worst thing you can say about this condition is that it's *suspicious.* It still isn't cancer, even though the horrible word *carcinoma* is used. What is certain, though, is that more women with severe hyperplasia go on to *develop* uterine cancer.

If you've been diagnosed with any kind of hyperplasia, the next crucial step is getting *rid* of that lining. Potent progesterone supplements are often the route; if these don't work, a D & C might be the next logical step.

Warning: For any kind of hyperplasia, many doctors still suggest a hysterectomy, which is totally unnecessary for both mild hyperplasia and hyperplasia *without* atypical cells. *Although you might be more inclined to accept a recommendation of a hysterectomy for severe hyperplasia, this procedure is not necessary unless the hyperplasia persists after the lining is removed via progesterone supplements or D & C.* In younger women particularly, severe hyperplasia can be reversed with hormonal therapy. The bottom line is that if your doctor suggests an immediate hysterectomy for any stage of hyperplasia, see another doctor! Even severe hyperplasia is still a *precancerous,* often treatable, condition. (Make sure you ask what *kind* of hyperplasia it is.)

Once the lining is shed, you'll need to get your hormones checked via a simple blood test. In fact, hyperplasia almost *always* develops because of a hormonal imbalance (too much or not enough progesterone). When this is the case, *hormone* therapy is the cure. For an estrogen surplus, progesterone will counteract it; for a progesterone deficiency, progesterone supplements are also the therapy. The menstrual cycle will often "right" itself after several "assisted" cycles.

After your lining has been shedding more regularly, you'll need a second endometrial biopsy or even D & C to see if the lining is normal again.

If you're premenopausal, you might produce too much estrogen because of excess body fat (see above). Women who are 25–50 pounds overweight are three times as likely to develop hyperplasia than women who are at normal weights. Women who are more than 50 pounds overweight are nine times as likely to develop hyperplasia.

Your ovaries may be the culprit and simply produce too much estrogen for a variety of reasons. Sometimes excess estrogen production is a genetic trait, seen in women who have long family histories of estrogen-dependent cancers (see above).

If you've always had irregular periods, you're a classic hyperplasia candidate. Diabetic women, for unknown reasons, seem to be more at risk for hyperplasia.

There is also a long list of external factors responsible for excess estrogen in the body. This includes certain herbs such as ginseng; hormone-fed meats and poultry; certain cosmetics made from estrogen; and hormonal contraceptives that contain estrogen. If you've been given estrogen therapy for another reason, discuss alternative therapies with your doctor and see if going off the therapy helps put your menstrual cycles back on track.

If you're postmenopausal and still have your uterus, unopposed estrogen replacement therapy (ERT) can predispose you to hyperplasia too. Balancing the therapy with the right amount of progesterone is all you need to do (this is known as HRT). *An estrogen/progesterone combination therapy can reverse as much as 96.8% of all postmenopausal hyperplasia cases.*

If severe hyperplasia persists and keeps redeveloping despite HRT and a repeat D & C, then a hysterectomy *is* the next logical step. This means that you've continued to bleed despite therapy and that repeat endometrial biopsy or D & C *after* the lining has shed still shows suspicious cells. If you're an older woman, you are also at a higher risk of progressing to uterine cancer and should be particularly open to a hysterectomy at this point.

Who's at Risk for Endometrial Cancer?

Although a large portion of women are diagnosed with hyperplasia and not endometrial cancer, it's important to be aware of the risk factors for both. About 99% of all uterine cancer is really endometrial cancer and might be prevented through better nutrition and balancing irregular menstrual cycles early. Like breast cancer, the following characteristics are more prevalent in women who have had endometrial cancer, but they are *not* definitive *causes* of this kind of cancer.

Women who are more at risk for endometrial cancer:

- are at least 25 pounds overweight;
- have diabetes or high blood pressure (which may be related to weight);
- have a history of irregular menstrual cycles and irregular bleeding;
- experienced menopause after 50 (late menopause);

- have a family history of endometrial cancer; and
- eat a high-fat, high-cholesterol diet (this may be the same as being overweight).

Ovarian Cysts: They're *Not* Ovarian Cancer

Abnormal bleeding and irregular periods can also be caused by an ovarian cyst. This is a scary diagnosis, but ovarian cysts are very common and are *not* cancerous conditions. Just like a breast cyst, which is a fluid-filled lump, these cysts form on the ovary. Often, ovarian cysts don't even require surgery and just need to monitored. An ultrasound can tell your doctor whether the cysts are benign.

Follicular Cysts

During normal ovulation, the follicle spits out the egg. When the follicle fails to do this, fluid, hormones, and other "guck" build up inside the unruptured follicle until a cyst develops. This kind of ovarian cyst is most common in women who are between the ages of 20 and 40. Some women are plagued by follicular cysts, which may keep forming. The symptoms of follicular cysts are different from symptoms of ovarian cancer. They include delayed periods, bleeding between periods, pelvic pain (constant dull ache or sharp jabbing), and cramping, but often there are no symptoms. As mentioned above, a full pelvic exam is done first in investigating abnormal bleeding. Often, follicular cysts are found in a bimanual exam. If your ovary is enlarged by more than two inches, it will immediately be investigated. Your doctor will order a blood test to see how well your ovary is producing hormones. Then he or she will perform an ultrasound scan to see the size and composition of the ovary. Just like an ultrasound can determine fluid-filled lumps in breasts, it can also determine fluid-filled lumps on the ovaries. In the United States, sometimes a CAT scan or MRI is done as well. Follicular cysts are always benign.

The next step in treating follicular cysts depends on your age and the size of the cyst. If you're younger and the cyst is small, waiting it out may be the best course of action. However, since most follicular cysts resolve within one menstrual cycle, the first step is simply observation, eliminating the need for expensive tests and treatment. Most go away without rupturing, but these cysts may also rupture on their own. In either case, your menstrual cycle will get back in sync and return to normal. You'll then need to be re-evaluated. If you're under 30, you can be re-evaluated in about two cycles (8–10 weeks). If you're between the ages of 30 and 40, you should be re-evaluated after only one cycle (about 4–6 weeks).

If you are experiencing a lot of pain, are over 40, or have a solid enlargement of the ovary, you'll need to be treated immediately. If the cyst persists after a second evaluation, you'll also need to be treated.

Treatment involves a laparoscopy procedure, which will tell the doctor more about the texture and size of your cyst. Depending on what he or she finds, the cyst might be aspirated on the spot, at which point it will simply collapse and you'll be cured. But if the ovary is unusually large, the cyst is removed and your ovary biopsied via fine-needle aspiration. If no cancerous cells are found, once the cyst is removed, you'll also be cured.

Sometimes a condition known as *polycystic ovary disease* can occur where a woman has numerous follicular cysts, which can be treated. This is also a major cause of infertility (see chapter 12).

Corpus Luteum Cysts

After your egg is spat out by the follicle, which then turns yellow and becomes the corpus luteum (an empty shell that produces progesterone; see chapters 1 and 2), the follicle doesn't shrink like it's supposed to. Instead, the little blood vessels that feed the follicular sac and bleed during ovulation continue to bleed into the empty sac and form a blood-filled cyst. This sounds dangerous, but it isn't. Corpus luteum cysts will often rupture and resolve on their own. If not, the diagnosis and treatment route is the same as above, the blood is aspirated during laparoscopy, and the ovary biopsied. Sometimes, though, the ovary may be too large or the bleeding too severe. At this point, some doctors may opt to remove the ovary, but this is premature. The bleeding is caused by a stubborn blood vessel that can be tied off, which will stop the bleeding, allowing the cyst to be aspirated and the ovary to remain intact.

Dermoid Tumors

These are not cysts but common benign tumors (making up about 10% of benign ovarian tumors). Dermoid tumors are more common in young women but can occur throughout the reproductive years. Prepare yourself—these are *really* disgusting! What happens here is the egg begins developing without being *fertilized*. So these growths develop hair, teeth, cartilage, and fat. Even surgeons are shocked by their appearance. The symptoms and diagnosis process for these tumors are the same as above, and an ultrasound test or even X ray can pinpoint dermoid tumors. *Teeth* (!) often show up in the scans or X rays.

Many surgeons will do laparoscopic surgery to remove the tumor and leave the ovary intact. Unfortunately, some doctors will just remove the ovary altogether. Because dermoid tumors *can* be removed, leaving the ovaries intact, your best bet is to seek out a doctor who will not remove the ovary. If you can't find one, call HERS (see chapter 7), an organization that has lists of surgeons who perform alternative surgery to hysterectomy and oophorectomy.

Preventing Ovarian Cancer

It would be comforting to hear that ovarian cysts are precancerous conditions that, when caught, prevent ovarian cancer. But this is not the case. Ovarian cysts really don't have anything to do with ovarian cancer at all. If you have a history of ovarian cysts and other problems, however, you are considered to be at a higher risk for ovarian cancer. But as you'll see in the next chapter, the symptoms of ovarian cancer are very different than they are for ovarian cysts, comprising more general signs of ill health, such as gas, bloating, and flulike symptoms. Occasionally, vaginal bleeding or even masculine hair growth might be a sign, but these are rare. Sharp abdominal pain or a continuous dull ache could be a symptom of ovarian cancer but usually points to a cyst. Menstrual irregularities are also not a common symptom. The following is a list of established characteristics that are more common in women who develop ovarian cancer than in those who don't.

Women who are at risk for ovarian cancer:

- have a family history of ovarian, uterine, breast, or colon cancer;
- are between 55 and 64 years of age;
- have never been pregnant;
- are exposed to environmental toxins (including in the workplace);
- experience irregular or no menstrual cycles, ovarian malfunctions, ovarian tumors, ovarian cysts, or have polycystic ovary disease or Turner's syndrome (a genetic disorder);
- consume a high-fat diet, low in vitamin A;
- have hypertension or diabetes;
- are Caucasian or of northern European descent; and
- are living in an industrialized country.

Ultrasound Screening for Women at Risk: The Ovarian "Mammogram"

No, there isn't any such thing as an ovarian "mammogram," but I've used this term to describe a screening process high-risk women can adopt to catch early ovarian cancer, in the same way a mammogram is designed to catch early breast cancer. If you are in a high-risk category for ovarian cancer, once you reach 50, you should request an initial pelvic ultrasound to measure the size of your ovaries even if you've already had a hysterectomy. Have blood tests done to obtain a baseline reading of your hormone levels. Then go back once a year for a comparative ultrasound and blood test. Any readings or results that veer too far from your first baseline readings can be investigated before it's too late.

Unfortunately, ultrasound is not an effective screening method for women who are not in a high-risk group. The gastrointestinal-like symptoms of ovarian cancer are simply too vague for mass ultrasound screening to be feasible or even yield any significant benefits. However, keep in mind that ultrasound or CA-125 can produce false positive or false negative results.

A Final Word

Waiting out the investigation process for cysts, tumors, and other suspicious symptoms is often more difficult than dealing with the outcome. I liken these investigations to a train ride. You board the train when you first discover the lump or suspicious symptom. The first stop is your doctor, who will start the investigation process with a manual exam. An obvious cause of your symptom or lump might be found at this first stop: swollen glands, hemorrhoids, a bacterial infection, and so on. If not, you'll proceed to the next diagnostic stop: ultrasound, endometrial biopsy, and so forth. You may be able to get off the train here, or you might continue on to the next stop: lumpectomy, laparoscopy, D & C, hormonal therapies. Many women are lucky enough to get off the train here, but many will have to take the train to the end of the line and ride through the diagnosis and treatment of a malignant condition, otherwise known as cancer. Breast cancer and cancer of the reproductive organs are discussed in the next chapter.

CHAPTER 9

When They Tell You It's Cancer

I'm in a unique position to write this chapter, because I, myself, am a cancer survivor. *Cancer* is an emotionally charged word that conjures up terrible images and fears. Contrary to what women are programmed to think, cancer is *not* a death sentence and is usually treatable. For example, cervical and endometrial cancers are almost always successfully treated, even if they are caught in a later stage. And thanks to the Pap test (see chapter 3), few women will *ever* develop advanced cervical cancer.

As for breast cancer, when it's caught early enough, it can also be successfully treated. That's why there are techniques in place to catch breast cancer *early*. Breast self examination (BSE), combined with mammography (discussed in chapter 8), are very successful screening methods. Since these screening methods have been in place, five-year survival rates of women with cancer *confined* to the breast (that is, early breast cancer) have risen from 78% in the 1940s (which was still high) to *93% today.*

Unfortunately, despite routine screenings, not all breast cancers *are* caught early, which is why breast cancer continues to be a life-threatening illness. But there are many women who survive later-stage breast cancer and go on to have normal life spans. It's also important to remember that *more women survive breast cancer than not.* For example, about 1 in 10 women will get breast cancer at some point in their lives. Of these women, three out of four will survive and live out a normal life span. Translation: *75% of all breast cancer patients* overall *survive.* So the odds are *with* you, not against you.

Bear in mind that in some cases it can take 20 years for breast cancer to recur. A 65-year-old woman whose breast cancer goes into remission for 20 years, recurs when she's 85 years old, and ultimately kills her, is *included* as a breast cancer mortality statistic.

On the downside, ovarian cancer does not carry very high survival rates (under 40%) because it is rarely *caught* in an early stage. It is treatable 80% of the time when it *is* caught early. Baseline ultrasounds, followed by regular ultrasound screenings, may become valuable diagnostic tools in finding early ovarian cancer (see chapter 8). Once these screening techniques are more widely practiced, they may do for ovarian cancer statistics what the Pap test has done for cervical cancer statistics. Thankfully, ovarian cancer is still considered rare and only accounts for about 4% of all gynecological cancers.

Cancer of the fallopian tubes has fairly dismal statistics as well, carrying a survival rate below 40%. Again, this is because it's rarely caught early. However, fewer than 3,000 women each year develop it, and ultrasound screening may also assist in finding abnormalities around or on the fallopian tubes. Vaginal cancer and vulvar cancer are also quite rare, both affecting fewer than 1,000 women each year. Vulvar cancer is very curable and carries an overall 80% survival rate; vaginal cancer is considerably lower, at 50%, but this is because it is not often caught early enough. It's crucial to note, though, that these cancers are associated with a *pre-existing* sexually transmitted disease (STD), and are preventable with regular health maintenance and good hygiene.

Whether you're diagnosed with pelvic cancer or breast cancer, there are many aspects to the diagnostic and treatment route. In addition, cancers share similar patterns of behavior regardless of where they are growing. The purpose of this chapter is to provide you with a general understanding of breast and gynecological cancer, the treatments you'll experience, the side effects of each treatment, and the post-treatment follow-up process. I'll also discuss coping with cancer and suggest some techniques that work. Finally, for those of you facing a life-threatening situation, this chapter includes a discussion of *palliative* care, which refers to treatment of symptoms rather than the disease itself.

Each cancer scenario is unique. Treatment and survival rates depend on all kinds of factors: age, overall health, genetics, history, weight, what stage the cancer is in (metastasis), what kind of cancer *cell* is involved (see below), and so on. Think of this chapter, then, as providing everything you need to know to get *acquainted* with your cancer. For those of you simply concerned with the possibility of cancer, this chapter will give you the fundamentals you'll need to know, should you face it down the road.

Cancer 101: An Introduction

Cancer is the general term for abnormal growth of cells—a cluster of cells that go out of control and multiply. When the abnormal cell reproduces, it has the ability to invade, or metastasize to, other parts of the body. The actual word *cancer* means "crab." The characteristics of the crab—slow-moving, persistent, roundish, with multiple legs that can reach out—represent the "spirit" of a cancer cell but really isn't an accurate description of what a malignant cell looks or acts like.

Unlike bacteria or viruses, the cancer cell itself is not dangerous, but its impact on the rest of your organs is. As it spreads into various parts of your body, it interferes with regular cells, confuses other organs, and can wreak havoc on your body. It's basically a "terrorist" cell that hijacks organs and other cells. Cancer cells use the lymph system to get into the bloodstream and travel throughout the body. These cells love organs that have multiple blood vessels and nutrients, such as the bones, lungs, and brain.

Cancer cells are classified in two groups: *carcinoma* and *sarcoma*. A carcinoma refers to cancerous cells made of epithelial cells, which line various tissues. You'll find carcinomas in organs that secrete milk, mucus, digestive juices, and so on. Common sites for carcinomas are the breasts, lungs, skin, and colon; common gynecological sites are the breasts, ovaries, cervix, and endometrium. Carcinomas account for 80–90% of all human cancers, are generally slow-growing, and tend to spread through the nerve endings.

The word *carcinoma* means the cells are malignant. A prefix attached to the word *carcinoma* will tell you where the carcinoma is growing and the kinds of cells that are involved. An *adenocarcinoma,* for example, is a carcinoma made of *glandular* cells. When you see the word *oma* by itself, it means "benign." An aden*oma* refers to a clump of *benign* glandular cells; a fibr*oma* refers to a clump of benign fibrous cells, and so on. If you were diagnosed with breast cancer and found out that you had an adenocarcinoma, you would know that your cancer originated in glandular tissue. It gets even more specific. You'll need to know where the adenocarcinoma *itself* originated, and may be told, for example, that you have either a *ductal* carcinoma or *lobular* carcinoma, which means that your adenocarcinoma originated in either the breast ducts or lobes. Since both ducts and lobes are *glands,* malignant cells that develop here will always be adenocarcinomas. Think of it like this: "carcinoma" used by itself is as descriptive as saying "sweater." "Adenocarcinoma" is like saying "wool sweater." A more specific description, such as "ductal carcinoma," is like saying "lambswool sweater" or "angora sweater." And there can be other prefixes that are synonymous with saying "blue angora sweater." *Papillary* ductal carcinoma describes the shape of the cancer cell, and would be like saying "V-*necked,* angora sweater," and so on. The point being that you need not worry about a lengthy, unpronounceable name that may be attached to your cancer; if a long prefix is attached to the word "carcinoma" it's just describing it more accurately. There are literally hundreds of carcinomas, all described by a different combination of prefixes, identifying the parts of the bodies that are involved, the shape of the carcinomas, and so on.

Sarcomas are cancerous cells made up of supporting connective tissue, such as the uterus. Sarcomas are rare and account for only 2% of all human cancers but tend to be more aggressive than carcinomas. Again, the prefixes before the word tell you where the sarcoma is located, what it's made of, what shape it is, and so forth. A leiomyo*sarcoma* would be a malignant tumor.

The difference between a carcinoma and a sarcoma is equal to the difference between a sweater and a boot; both are different but related. They have different physical properties and are made of different material. (You can also have a carcinosarcoma—a carcinoma and sarcoma all in one.)

The words *in situ* and *invasive* are used in conjunction with a carcinoma or a sarcoma. *In situ* means "in one place." A carcinoma in situ is cancer that is confined to a specific area and has not spread. *This is good news and means your cancer is in a very early stage.* Invasive carcinoma is cancer that has spread to surrounding tissue, the lymph nodes or other organs. *This is not good news and means your cancer is in a later stage.*

Gynecological cancers and breast cancer can involve a *lymphoma,* which refers to malignant cells that originate in the lymph nodes, seen in Hodgkin's disease, for example. Here, malignant cells spread to other parts of your body, such as the breast or reproductive organs through the lymph nodes. Lymphomas involve white blood cells that go astray and attack functioning organs. Although lymphomas may involve the reproductive organs and breasts, this kind of cancer rarely originates in these areas.

Cancer cells fall into two behavioral categories: *differentiated* and *undif-*

ferentiated. These terms refer to the sophistication of the cancer cells. Differentiated cancer cells resemble the cells of their origin. A differentiated cancer cell that originates in the breast ducts looks more like a normal ductal cell than an undifferentiated cancer cell in the breast ducts. For this reason, differentiated cancer is more treatable and carries higher survival rates. Often, you won't find a purely differentiated cell. It may look just moderately abnormal. Because of this, there are subclassifications: mildly differentiated, moderately differentiated, well differentiated, or poorly differentiated. These classifications refer to the cell's *grading*. A high grade means that the cell is immature, poorly differentiated, and fast-growing; a low-grade cancer cell is mature, well differentiated, slow-growing, and less aggressive.

Undifferentiated cancer is made up of very primitive cells that look "wild" and untamed, bearing little or no resemblance to the cells of origin. They don't assist the body at all and are therefore able to spend all of their time reproducing. This is more dangerous because the cells may then spread faster. There are times, though, where undifferentiated cancer is not very aggressive, despite the fact that it's a more primitive cell. This is often the case in breast cancers.

There are also mixes of these different cells, which affects the aggressiveness of the disease. For example, you can have mostly differentiated cells mixed in with a few undifferentiated cells, or vice versa. Whatever you have the most of will affect the behavior of the cancer; differentiated cells will slow down whatever undifferentiated cells exist, while undifferentiated cells will speed up whatever differentiated cells exist.

Dozens of other cancer cell traits have a direct bearing on how well the cells respond to treatment. In breast cancer, many cells respond to either estrogen or progesterone and hence can be treated with hormone therapy in addition to other traditional treatments. Pathologists can pinpoint where your cancer cells have invaded surrounding tissue, and then break down the metastasis into *vascular invasion* (cancer within a blood vessel) or *lymphatic invasion* (cancer within a lymph node). Pathologists can also determine how fast the cell is reproducing and whether any dead cancer cells are present, which means the cells are growing so fast they've cut off their own blood supply and are leaving a dead cell trail (called *necrosis*). All of these factors are important and will affect your treatment and prognosis. Where the cancer is growing determines the kind of cancer cell you have. For example, breast cancer will spread as breast cancer cells. They won't suddenly turn into liver cancer cells as soon as they reach your liver, or into lymphoma as soon as they reach your lymph nodes.

What Causes Cancer?

When it comes to determining the causes of cancer, it's now known that genetics plays a huge role. Breast cancer and ovarian cancer run in families. Researchers have isolated various *oncogenes* within our genetic makeup. The word *onco* means "tumor"; the field of oncology therefore means "tumorology." One theory is that every individual has certain oncogenes that remain dormant in the body until an external agent turns them on like a switch. Once turned on, the oncogene is responsible for transforming normal cells into abnormal cells. The oncogene responsible for colon cancer was recently isolated. People carrying these oncogenes would find that once activated, their colon cells would begin to transform into abnormal cells. In other cases, women carrying *ovarian* oncogenes (not yet isolated) would find that their *ovary* cells would transform when their oncogenes were activated. However, it's believed that external or environmental factors are responsible for turning on these oncogenes. These outside forces include tobacco, X rays, excess estrogen, sunlight, radioactive fallout, and industrial agents. While one cigarette may irritate your lung cells, 20 years of smoking may provide multiple "hits" to these cells that trip the lung cancer switch. One sunburn probably won't give you skin cancer, but 10 years of sun worshiping could trip the skin cancer switch.

Therefore, understanding your family history is a crucial factor in cancer prevention. This is particularly apparent when it comes to ovarian cancer: *Women who do not have a family history of ovarian cancer are not considered at high risk for the disease.* Breast cancer seems to be trickier because a long list of other factors are linked to it, chiefly estrogen. Chapter 8 outlines the differences between estrogen-dependent cancers and disease-dependent cancers. Breast cancer, uterine/endometrial cancer, and ovarian cancer are all estrogen-dependent in that an increased amount of estrogen is linked to them. Is the capacity to overproduce estrogen a genetic trait? Researchers currently believe this is a strong possibility. However, since women also ingest estrogen either for contraceptive purposes or for various hormone therapies, the "estrogen question" is more difficult to define.

All of these factors make the future of cancer detection very promising. Blood tests that detect various oncogenes are already being developed, and by the year 2000, screenings for a variety of oncogenes may be possible. This would mean that women can be treated or monitored long before their cancers become life-threatening.

Certain blood tests now detect cancer "trails" (sheddings from cancer cells) in the bloodstream. The *CA-125 blood test* may detect ovarian cancer cell sheddings; the *CA-15-3 blood test* detects breast cancer cell sheddings. These tests are currently being used to detect recurrences of these cancers in women who have already been treated.

STDs (see chapter 6) are also identified as a probable precursor to certain gynecologic cancers, such as cervical, vulvar, and vaginal cancer. Strains of the human papillomavirus (HPV) were found in over 90% of all cervical cancers. In short, *virgins are at very low risk for cervical cancer.* Cancer can be "caught" and prevented through safe sex (see chapter 4). Vaginal and vulvar cancers will not develop without the presence of certain strains of HPV.

Another "cause" of cancer is aging. Women are living longer and therefore "working" their reproductive organs harder. All this takes its toll and exposes the organs to more factors that can cause malignant cells to sprout. Are more women developing cancer today than 50 years ago? Yes, but women are living *twice as long* as they did 50 years ago. Breast cancer and ovarian cancer are classic "over 50" cancers.

A toxic environment can also be cited as a major cause of cancer. Increased levels of radiation in the air, countless pollutants, chemicals in our food, and decreased ozone layer protection all play a role in "tripping" our oncogene switch.

Stress, now known to trigger autoimmune diseases, is a major contributor to cancer as well. In the same way that stress can "give" you an ulcer, it may also turn on our oncogenes.

Finally, a high-fat diet in women can cause increased levels of estrogen in the body that are stored in fat cells. This can make you a more desirable host for estrogen-dependent cancer cells, which is why high-fiber and low-fat diets are encouraged.

The Stages of Breast Cancer

Four women can be diagnosed with the same kind of cancer, but each one will undergo completely different treatments and face a different *prognosis* (a prediction of how successful the treatment will be). This is because cancer is diagnosed at *different stages.* Most cancers have four or five stage classifications that help determine treatment and survival rate. To determine the stage your cancer is in, you'll need to go through diagnostic tests. These tests can involve imaging scans (CAT, MRI, ultrasound), biopsies, and specific blood tests. Staging will also mean different things to different cancers. Let's go through them one by one.

Each breast has 15–20 sections, broken down into lobes, which may have even smaller sections called lobules. The lobes and lobules are connected by thin tubes called ducts. While there are several types of breast cancers, 86% of all breast cancers start in the ducts, 12% start in the lobules, and the rest of the breast cancers start in surrounding tissues. Nearly all breast cancers are adenocarcinomas, originating in glandular tissue. There is something known as inflammatory breast cancer, which is an uncommon type, where the breast is warm, red and swollen, and Paget's disease is a form of breast cancer that manifests as itching and scaling of the nipple, which doesn't get better. (This is not to be confused with Paget's disease of the bone, a benign, chronic condition.) Sometimes, women with Paget's disease may also have cancer inside the breast tissue.

Staging, in this case, is determined by the size of your tumor, whether the cancer has spread to lymph nodes under the arms, and whether the breast cancer has spread to other tissues, involving the lungs, bones, or liver. You won't automatically know what stage the cancer is in until you have surgery to remove the initial carcinoma, where lymph nodes are taken out and biopsied. *Node negative* means that your breast cancer is confined to the breast and has not spread to the lymph nodes. Stage 0 means "carcinoma in situ"; your breast tumor is in very early stages. This may be discovered on a mammogram. The tumor is confined to the breast and has not spread at all. This stage carries a five-year survival rate of 95%, meaning that 95% of all women with Stage 0 breast cancer live five years completely cancer-free.

Stage 1 is similar to Stage 0, but your tumor is slightly more advanced and still confined to the breast. Five-year survival rates for Stage 1 are now at 85%.

Stage 2 means a few things: a small tumor (less than 2 centimeters) *has* spread to the lymph nodes (you're *node positive*); a larger tumor (2–5 centimeters) has spread to the lymph nodes; or a large tumor of over 5 centimeters hasn't yet spread to the lymph nodes. Stage 2 carries a survival rate of 66%.

Stage 3 means that you have a large tumor with positive lymph nodes. At this stage, five-year survival rates dip to about 41%. Stage 4 means your tumor has invaded other tissues. This is when you find a lump around your collar bone, for example, or the cancer has spread to your bones, liver, or lung. Five-year survival rates for Stage 4 breast cancer hover around 10%. Most breast cancers today are found in either Stage 1 or Stage 2, which means they respond well to treatment.

In addition to the stage classification, successfully treating either Stage 2 or Stage 3 breast cancer is extremely dependent on the number of positive lymph nodes (that is, cancerous lymph nodes). If you have only one positive lymph node, you're in better shape than if you have four.

A final and very crucial note for women with Stage 3 and Stage 4 breast cancer: *These survival statistics were compiled prior to the widespread use of chemotherapy, which has been used only in the past decade.* Survivors of breast cancer need to be tracked for at least 10 years in order for new statistics, reflecting the success of chemotherapy, to be published. In other words, there are no statistical odds against you, because there are no meaningful statistics available yet.

Cervical Precancer

As discussed in chapter 3, many women who would have developed invasive cervical cancer will now be treated at the *pre*cancerous stage. The classification of Pap smears is discussed in chapter 3. It's now thought that HPV is responsible for cervical, vaginal, and vulvar cancer. Ninety-five percent of all squamous cell cervical carcinomas (which represent 90% of all cervical cancers) contain the DNA of HPV. There are more than 50 types of HPV; types 6 and 11, responsible for raised cauliflower-type genital warts (known as condyloma) are commonly seen as precursors to cervical, vaginal, and vulvar cancers, while types 16, 18, 31, and 33 are responsible for dysplasia, flat lesions associated with cervical, vaginal, and vulval cancers. A Pap test will detect genital warts or dysplasia before your cervical cells become cancerous. Most women who might have gone on to develop in situ or invasive cervical cancer 30 years ago, will be treated for cervical precancer today, identified by their Pap smear.

A Pap test can also detect carcinoma in situ, a cancerous tumor limited to the cervix. This is very easily treated with survival rates at almost 100%. Finally, a Pap test can detect invasive cervical cancer, in which the cancer has spread beyond the cervix. Although the Pap test can't tell you how *extensive* the cancer is in this case, invasive cervical cancer can mean several things. It can mean that the cancer has spread only as far as the uterus, which can be successfully treated with a hysterectomy, or it can mean your entire pelvic and abdominal cavity is involved. Usually, invasive cervical cancer means that the cancer is confined to the uterus and is therefore "removable." Survival rates are pretty high for invasive cervical cancer, ranging from 67% to 88%. In fact, out of the sheer millions of women who will develop cervical *pre*cancer, under 7,000 will die from it. This is a very low statistic considering the high diagnosis rate. In short, most of you will be fine and go on to live a normal life span.

The Stages of Invasive Cervical Cancer

If you are diagnosed with invasive cervical cancer, your cancer will then be broken down into stages, with perhaps some crossover into the class system above. Stage 0 is the same as a Class 4 Pap smear: carcinoma in situ, which carries a five-year survival rate of 100%. Thanks to the Pap smear, invasive cervical cancer is found so early that its staging system is extremely advanced. Stage 1a means that the cancer is confined to the cervix with just minimal invasion. The five-year survival rate is close to 100%. In Stage 1a2 there is slightly more invasion on the cervix, and the survival rates dip to 80–90%. Stage 1b is a slightly more advanced version of stage 1a2, also with survival rates of 80–90%.

In Stage 2 the cancer extends beyond the cervix or into the vagina, but not yet into the pelvic wall. Survival rates are still 80–90%. Stage 2b indicates that the cancer extends more into the parametrium, and survival rates dip to 65%. Stage 3 means the cancer involves other pelvic organs and the vagina; survival rates drop to 40%. Stage 4a indicates that the bladder or rectum is involved, and stage 4b denotes distant invasion into other organs. Survival rates for 4a are about 10%, while fewer than 10% of women with Stage 4b survive.

The Stages of Endometrial Cancer

There's a big difference between endometrial cancer and uterine cancer. Endometrial cancer is always a *carcinoma;* uterine cancer means uterine sarcoma, which is discussed separately below. Seventy-five percent of endometrial cancer is discovered in Stage 1. Stage 1a means that the cancer is limited to the uterine lining, but the depth of invasion, cell type, and grade of cells are also important. Treatment will involve a hysterectomy/oophorectomy/salpingectomy to remove the *possibility* of cancer's developing beyond the uterus. Survival rates are generally 90–95%. In Stage 1b the cancer has invaded the uterine wall; survival rates range between 70–80%. Stage 2 may involve the lymph nodes in the groin area, and they'll be examined individually during a hysterectomy procedure to determine the extent of metastasis. Stage 2a means that the glands that line the cervix are involved; Stage 2b indicates that the cervix itself is involved. Both 2a and 2b have survival rates of 60%. In Stage 3 the cancer has spread into the lymph nodes and beyond the uterus into the greater pelvis area. Stage 3a involves the uterine surface, tubes, and ovaries; Stage 3b involves the vagina; and Stage 3c involves the pelvic lymph nodes. Survival rates drop in all three cases to 30%. Stage 4 is rarely seen and means that the cancer is involving other organs: bowels, the abdominal cavity, bladder, whatever. Stage 4a means the bladder and rectum are affected, while Stage 4b indicates distant invasion. Survival rates in either case hover around 5%. Treatment varies and depends on what organs are involved. Few women ever experience Stage 4 endometrial cancer.

The Stages of Uterine Cancer

Uterine sarcomas are fairly rare, accounting for only 1–5% of all uterine cancers. But these cancers are very aggressive. In Stage 1a, the sarcoma is limited to the endometrium, with a survival rate of 75%. Stages 1b and 1c indicate that the sarcoma has invaded the uterine wall, with survival rates of 50%. Stage 2a means the lymph glands or the endocervical canal is involved, while Stage 2b involves the cervix. Survival rates for both these stages remain at 50%. In Stage 3a the sarcoma has gone beyond the uterus to the tubes and ovaries. Survival rates here dip to between 0 and 20%. Stages 3b and 3c are worse; Stage 3b means that the vagina is involved, while Stage 3c indicates that the pelvis and lymph nodes are involved. Survival rates range between 0 and 10%. Stage 4a means that the bladder and rectum are affected, while Stage 4b shows that there is distant invasion. Survival rates here only range from 0 to 5%.

The Stages of Ovarian Cancer

Unlike breast cancer, ovarian cancer is usually discovered beyond Stage 1. About 1 in 70 women will develop ovarian cancer, and most will be over age 40. Most ovarian cancer originates in the epithelial cells lining the ovaries. About 10% of ovarian cancer originates in the eggs and is known as *ovarian germ cell cancer.* In fact, two-thirds of all ovarian cancers are detected after the cancer has already spread. In Stage 1, the cancerous tumor is limited to the ovaries. This is treatable and has a survival rate of 60–100%.

Stage 2 means the cancer involves one or both ovaries and has spread into other areas of your pelvis. Evidence suggests the survival rate for Stage 2 ovarian cancer is now about as high as it is for Stage 1. Current statistics put it at about 60%. Prior to this study, Stage 2 ovarian cancer survival rates were believed to be significantly lower.

In Stage 3 the cancer involves one or both ovaries but has spread beyond the pelvis into the bowel and abdominal cavity. Survival rates drop to only about 20%. The most promising information I can offer here is taken from *JAMA,* which published that the five-year survival rate for women with Stage 3 ovarian cancer who underwent platinum-based chemotherapy (a specific type of chemotherapy drug) was significantly higher than that of Stage 3 ovarian cancer patients who received chemotherapy *without* platinum. However, the women who received platinum-based chemotherapy in this study were also younger than those who did not. Nobody knows if age played a role in the survival rates.

Stage 4 ovarian cancer means that the cancer has spread to the lungs or other major organs far beyond the bowels and abdominal cavity. The statistics are dismal: 10% survival rate. Ovarian cancer is not more dangerous or insidious than other kinds of cancers; it is simply more difficult to *find* and therefore has more opportunity to spread. If you are at Stage 4, outlook and attitude are important. You must believe that you are among the 10% who will survive. Someone has to, so why shouldn't it be *you?*

Ovarian germ cell cancer paints a brighter picture. Stage 1 carries statistics as high as 95%, Stage 2 is as high as 80%, while both Stage 3 and Stage 4 have survival rates of about 75%.

The Stages of Vulvar Cancer

Vulvar cancer accounts for about 3–5% of all gynecological cancers. Eighty percent of all vulvar cancers develop as a result of exposure to HPV. Other vulvar cancer develops after exposure to the following STDs: syphilis, lymphogranuloma venereum, and herpes (all discussed in chapter 6).

Eighty-six percent of all vulvar cancer is squamous cell carcinoma. Melanoma, a very aggressive type of skin cancer, represents about 6% of all vulvar cancers. Four percent of vulvar cancers originate in the Bartholin's glands, 2% are sarcomas, and 0.5% are Paget's disease (the same Paget's seen in breast cancer). However, no matter what kind of vulvar cancer you have, it's usually confined to the skin anywhere from 1 to 10 years before it spreads. Symptoms include lumps, open sores, itching, pain, burning, bleeding, and discharge. Statistics reveal that whenever vulvar cancer is diagnosed, two-thirds of the women have had symptoms for more than six months, while the remaining third have had symptoms for more than a year. In the past, vulvar cancer was normally seen only in postmenopausal women. *Today, 40% of all vulvar cancers are seen in women under 40, particularly in women with multiple partners.*

Stage 0 is vulvar carcinoma in situ, and survival rates are 100%. In Stage 1 the cancer is confined to the vulva, with survival rates at 90%. Stage 2 is similar to Stage 1, but the cancer is slightly more advanced, with survival rates of 80–90%. Stage 3 indicates that the vagina, anus, or lymph nodes are involved, with survival rates at 50%. Stage 4a means the upper urethra, bladder, rectum, or pelvic bone is involved, and survival rates plummet to about 15%. In Stage 4b there is a distant spread, and depending on where the cancer has spread, survival rates range from 5–25%. If melanoma is the cause, survival rates range from 40–80%.

The Stages of Vaginal Cancer

Vaginal cancer is a cousin to cervical cancer but accounts for less than 2% of all gynecological cancers. Like cervical cancer, the most common vaginal cancer develops on the surface of the cells that line the vagina. Called vaginal intraepithelial neoplasia (VAIN), it is caused by HPV; that is, the cells begin to grow abnormally after exposure to HPV. A Pap smear that collects cells lining the vagina will find early abnormal cell changes in the vagina, just as it finds them on the cervix. The symptoms of vaginal cancer are vaginal bleeding and a foul-smelling discharge often attributed to an infection. Women who develop advanced vaginal cancer are clearly ignoring their symptoms.

Another kind of vaginal cancer is seen in DES daughters (see chapter 3), where the cancer originates in glands within the vaginal wall. It is possible to develop melanoma in the vagina, but this accounts for a tiny portion of all vaginal cancers.

Stage 0 means vaginal carcinoma in situ and has a survival rate of 100%. In Stage 1 the cancer is limited to the vaginal wall, with survival of 70–80%. Stage 2 involves the adjacent vaginal tissue, excluding the pelvis; survival rates are about 50%. Stage 3 means that the cancer has penetrated the pelvic wall, and survival rates dip to 30%. Stage 4a indicates that the cancer involves the bladder or rectum; Stage 4b shows that there is distant metastasis. Survival rates in both cases plunge to about 10%.

Who Will Manage My Cancer Treatment?

Doctors work in teams to manage cancer therapy. This means that your primary care physician, surgeon (for breast cancer) or gynecologic oncologist (surgeon for pelvic cancers), radiation oncologist (in charge of radiation therapy), and medical oncologist (in charge of chemotherapy) will all be involved with your treatment together.

If you have a lump in your breast, you may be referred to a breast surgeon for the lump investigation process (see chapter 8). He or she will handle everything from the biopsy phases to the actual diagnosis of breast cancer. If it is your family doctor or gynecologist who makes the breast cancer diagnosis (from a positive biopsy), he or she will immediately refer you to a breast surgeon. If you're not referred to a breast surgeon, insist on it unless your gynecologist is trained in breast care. *Unless your gynecologist is trained in breast care, a gynecologist should* never *manage your breast cancer treatment.*

The breast surgeon will decide on the type of surgery, which will vary depending on the stage of cancer you have. (Breast surgery is discussed below.) After your surgery, you'll be referred to two more specialists: a medical oncologist who will look after your chemotherapy and possible hormone therapy treatments, and a radiation oncologist, who will look after the external radiation phase of your treatment. You may need to see only one of these specialists. Your breast surgeon will be the project manager, coordinating and consulting with both oncologists regarding your progress. In some cases, a family/primary care physician might be involved as an overall "coach." He or she would be continuously updated on your progress by the specialists and might be in charge of finding the specialists for you. You may wish to see this doctor regularly for question-and-answer sessions. He or she can inspire you and help you cope with all your treatments. The primary care/family physician should not be in charge of making any decisions about your treatment, however.

If you have *in situ* or *invasive cervical cancer, endometrial, ovarian,* or *other pelvic cancers,* and if your regular gynecologist also does gynecologic oncology, you may not need to see anyone else. He or she will be qualified to do colposcopies and biopsy procedures and perform the necessary scans, laser surgery, cryosurgery, or major surgery. For chemotherapy and/or radiation, you'll be referred to a medical oncologist, a radiation oncologist, or both. If your cancer was diagnosed by either a primary care physician (see chapter 3) or a gynecologist who does *not* do gynecological oncology (please ask!), you'll need to be *referred* to a gynecologic oncologist. Surgery, chemotherapy, and radiation are usually necessary only for ovarian cancer and cancer of the fallopian tubes. Invasive cervical cancer and Stage 3 endometrial cancer generally involve surgery and radiation. With the exception of ovarian cancer, chemotherapy for pelvic cancers is necessary only when other organs have been invaded. Your gynecologic oncologist will serve as the project manager in charge of your treatment.

The first thing you'll need to do after your cancer has been diagnosed is to get some answers directly from your project manager, whether he or she is a gynecologic oncologist or a breast surgeon. Schedule a separate appointment with him or her, and use the *entire* appointment time for a question-and-answer period. Write down all of your questions ahead of time, and tape record the answers so you can review them later by yourself or with a supportive spouse, partner, or friend. When we're anxious, we often don't hear correctly, and we misconstrue facts and block out what we don't want to hear. Questions will vary depending on the person and the conditions, but here are some general areas to get you started:

1. Have the doctor draw you a diagram of the cancerous organ or part and shade in where the cancer is situated or has spread. Visualizing the cancer makes it easier to understand.
2. Ask whether the cancer is differentiated or undifferentiated. Breasts and reproductive organs can be invaded by either kind of cancer cell.
3. Find out how long the cancer has been growing, where it *can* spread (or continue to spread), and what stage it's in *now.*
4. Find out what treatment is being recommended and why, and what kind of diagnostic procedures (tests, scans, and so forth) you'll need to have.
5. Find out how the treatment will help, the risks and side effects associated with it (including how all this affects your menstrual cycle), and the survival rates associated with successful treatment.
6. Find out what will happen to you if you choose *not* to undergo treatment. Say, for example, that you have an advanced stage of a particular cancer. If you are told that you will most likely *not* survive and that chemotherapy treatment is *not* considered to be significantly useful, you may choose to fight the cancer with less toxic and

unpleasant therapies. That way, you can more fully enjoy the time you *do* have left. *Many women do not regret this choice.*

7. Find out where and when the treatments will take place and how long they'll last. This will help you plan your life.
8. What if you miss one treatment? Can you "make it up?"
9. What other health problems should you be on the lookout for during treatment?
10. How can you contact your "managing doctor" between visits?
11. Can you take other medications during treatments? How will the treatments affect other medications you're taking?
12. What about alcohol? Considering what you're going through, you might want a glass of wine or a shot of hard liquor occasionally. Is this OK?
13. If you're not given a very good prognosis, find out if you can participate in new studies or clinical trials using new drugs or therapies.
14. Find out where you can go for more information, and ask to be referred to a support group or a therapist or social worker who specializes in working with patients who have your particular kind of cancer.

Treatment for Particular Types of Cancer

Once you're diagnosed, you will need to undergo various scans, blood tests, and possibly more biopsies throughout the treatment process. Depending on where your cancer is located, scans will vary from imaging scans, such as CAT scans, X rays, magnetic resonance imaging (MRI), or ultrasound, to pelvic procedures such as endometrial biopsies, examinations via hysteroscope and colposcope, and possibly D & Cs. All of these diagnostic tests and procedures may seem exhausting and time consuming but are necessary to determine the extent of your cancer, determine appropriate treatment, gauge how well you're responding to treatment, and determine whether the cancer has gone into remission. Treatment usually starts with surgery and, depending on the stage and the kind of cancer you have, is followed by chemotherapy, hormone therapy for some breast cancers, drugs to boost your immune system, and finally radiation therapy.

Breast Cancer

Treatments are divided into three categories: *local,* where only the breast is involved (surgery and external radiation); *systemic,* where the whole body is involved (chemotherapy and/or hormone therapy); and *immuno complementary,* where you're given treatments to boost the immune system. (Check out chapter 5 for a review of how a normal immune system works.) One theory of breast cancer is that each case is systemic at the time of diagnosis, which is why all women are usually referred for chemotherapy. In *adjuvant therapy,* systemic treatment is used even when there is no indication that it's necessary (because the cancer hasn't yet spread). This is often recommended as an "overkill" therapy and has been successful.

You'll need some kind of breast surgery no matter what. This will be in the form of a *partial mastectomy,* which is also known as a *lumpectomy* (not to be confused with the biopsy procedure discussed in chapter 8), a *wide excision,* a *segmental mastectomy,* or a *quadrantectomy.* A partial mastectomy removes the lump and part of the surrounding tissue and is usually followed by external radiation. The part that is removed can be anywhere from 1–50% of the breast tissue. The surgeon will also remove fat and lymph nodes from the armpit area to determine how many lymph nodes are positive.

For more advanced breast cancer, you may need a *modified radical mastectomy.* This will remove all of the breast tissue from the edge of the ribs to the collarbone, and from the breastbone to the muscle at the back of the armpit. Lymph nodes will also be removed to determine how many are positive.

There is an older mastectomy procedure called *radical mastectomy,* or *Halsted radical mastectomy.* This is rarely done and is considered a deforming, archaic surgical procedure. Here, in addition to removing the whole breast, the underlying pectoral muscles are removed, and sometimes even portions of the rib cage. Don't automatically consent to this procedure without getting a second opinion. Any breast surgeon who recommends this is pretty much in the Dark Ages.

If you're having a mastectomy, you may also have breast reconstructive surgery done at the same time. (Most surgeons feel it's wise to wait and get it done at a later time.) Because of the controversy surrounding silicone implants and "gel bleed" (in which the implant ruptures and the gel leaks out into your body, possibly causing other health problems), you'll need to do research before making a decision. Get several opinions, read up on the controversy, and look into alternative procedures, and prosthesis products. As of 1994, silicone implants have *not* been banned, and the health hazard raised by their usage is considered unproven. As a reconstructive agent, silicone may be very beneficial for your psychological health and well-being. In one study, 70% of breast cancer patients reported improved self-image, 84% viewed breast reconstruction as an important aspect of their lives, and 89% said they came to view the "new" breast as real. The procedure also involves taking tissue from your abdominal area to reconstruct the nipple and areola with the aid of a "staining" tattoo.

Reconstructive surgery is a highly individual choice, but about 20% of all mastectomy patients choose breast reconstruction at some point. If you *do* decide on it, you'll need to plan well in advance, discuss the pros and cons with your surgeon, and find out whether it is covered by your health insurance. What to expect in major surgery, chemotherapy, hormonal therapy, and radiation therapy are discussed further below. Some methods use body tissue only and no synthetic materials. In fact, there are some ingenious methods that don't involve silicone at all. For example, one procedure gives you a "tummy tuck" and a new breast in one fell swoop; tissue is taken from the tummy to form the breast mound.

Cervical Carcinoma in Situ

If you haven't yet read chapter 3, go back and read the section on positive Pap smears, which covers treatment for precancerous Pap test results. Cervical carcinoma in situ is treated with a minor surgical procedure known as *conization* or *cone biopsy*. This can now be done using a laser or a wire loop (such as LEEP, discussed in chapter 3). If your gynecologic oncologist even *suspects* carcinoma in situ, he or she will remove a cone-shaped chunk of tissue from your cervix. Your doctor will then remove all of the abnormal tissue as well as some of the healthy surrounding tissue. This procedure can completely cure cervical carcinoma in situ. You'll then need to be closely monitored and go for follow-up colposcopies and Paps *religiously*.

A procedure known as *endocervical curettage* may also need to be done. This is exactly the same procedure as a D & C (see chapter 7), except instead of cleaning out the uterine lining, the cervical canal leading to the uterus is scraped. This helps the gynecologist see the condition of your cervical cells. You may also need a D & C so your gynecologist can check the condition of the uterine lining and make sure that the cervical cancer was indeed in situ. If a hysterectomy is recommended for cervical carcinoma in situ, you may want to get a second opinion. What you decide depends on your age, childbearing status, whether the cancer is a recurrence, or whether it is likely to recur in the future.

Invasive Cervical Cancer and Endometrial Cancer

You will need a radical hysterectomy for invasive cervical cancer and a radical hysterectomy *and* oophorectomy (with possible salpingectomy) for endometrial cancer. Here, the cervix, uterus, and tissue surrounding the cervix and surrounding lymph nodes are all removed, as well as the ovaries and fallopian tubes for endometrial cancer. To date, removing cancer-free ovaries for invasive *cervical* cancer is considered premature, but many surgeons will remove them as a *preventive measure*. This is one circumstance where a prophylactic oophorectomy (see chapter 7) may *be* a good idea.

You may be required to undergo either pre- or post-operative radiation treatment, discussed below. For extremely advanced endometrial or cervical cancer, you may also need chemotherapy. Chapter 7 discusses hysterectomy surgery in detail. You may need to have an abdominal procedure done in the case of cancer. Review the post-operative side effects of hysterectomy in chapter 7; you will not suffer all of these side effects, but will go into surgical menopause after an oophorectomy. Chapter 13 discusses both natural and surgical menopause in detail.

Ovarian Cancer

A radical hysterectomy, bilateral oophorectomy (removing both ovaries), and bilateral salpingectomy (removing both fallopian tubes) should be done if you have ovarian cancer in *any* stage. Anything *beyond* Stage 1 will need to be treated with chemotherapy and radiation therapy. When your treatment is completed, you may need to undergo follow-up laparoscopies (see chapter 2) and/or laparotomies (see chapter 6). See chapter 7 on the side effects of hysterectomy and chapter 13 on surgical menopause.

Cancer of the Vulva

In the past, a disfiguring surgical procedure known as a vulvectomy (removal of the vulva) was a traditional treatment for this kind of cancer. Today, treatment can include laser surgery, cryosurgery, radiation, or topical chemotherapy drugs. Surgery is usually confined to a local excision of a particular cluster of tumors. Advanced invasive cancer may still require a vulvectomy.

Vaginal Cancer

For early stages of vaginal cancer, a vaginectomy, laser therapy, intravaginal chemotherapy, and radiation are used. For later stages, treatment can include a vaginectomy, hysterectomy, and removal of lymph nodes, while late stage vaginal cancer involves chemotherapy with any combination of the above procedures.

Cancer of the Fallopian Tubes

This cancer is so rare that most gynecologists will never see one case in their lifetimes. It is as hard to detect as ovarian cancer because of the murky symptoms. There are also no real statistical data on who's at risk, the stages of this kind of cancer, or survival rates for each stage. It's suspected that inflammation of the fallopian tubes may be one precursor. The treatment scenario is identical to that of ovarian cancer.

Chemotherapy

Whether you're having chemotherapy for ovarian cancer, leukemia, or breast cancer, your experience will be similar to that of other chemotherapy patients. Of all treatments, chemotherapy is by far the most miserable. For many women, it makes the notion of having cancer a *reality*.

Chemotherapy involves treating a medical condition with drugs. Technically, taking aspirin for a migraine headache, an antifungal suppository for a yeast infection, and an antibiotic for a bacterial infection are all forms of chemotherapy. When it comes to cancer, you are taking *anticancer drugs*. These drugs are designed to kill cancer cells. They interfere with the process of cell division or reproduction so that the cells can't divide and therefore die. But the drugs are not very selective and kill *healthy* cells that are also dividing, including hair cells and bone marrow cells. There is a fine line between a therapeutic dosage and a toxic dosage and for this reason only a highly experienced medical oncologist is qualified to manage your chemotherapy. (In some cases, certain gynecologic oncologists or surgeons are trained in administering chemotherapy.)

Chemotherapy drugs can be administered orally or intravenously. You might be given one kind of drug or a combination of drugs. Each anticancer drug has the ability to destroy one kind of cancer cell; however, cancer is made up of more than one kind of cell. That's why combination drug therapy is often done because it destroys more cancer cells. In the past, chemotherapy was reserved for cases where surgery failed to treat the cancer. Today, even when there is no sign of cancer after surgery, chemotherapy is used as a preventative or prophylactic therapy; this is known as adjuvant chemotherapy and is common for early-stage breast cancer that responds well to surgery.

No matter how balanced your chemotherapy dosage is, your healthy cells will be affected. The side effects to chemo are frightening and unpleasant, but the reactions *do* vary from person to person. Some of the more common reactions include tiredness, weakness, body aches, bloating and weight gain, night sweats, nausea, and changes in your sense of taste and smell. Chemo can also cause a chemically induced depression and dramatic mood swings. If you're menstruating, your periods may become irregular, or they may just stop altogether. This is because your ovaries begin to fail, which causes you to go into surgical menopause, discussed in chapter 13. In some cases, periods may return to normal after the treatment is over.

Now for the most disturbing side effect: hair loss. It's important to be prepared for this, but there is also a possibility that your hair may *not* fall out. For most women, the idea of hair loss is worse than the reality of it; it is a stripping away of femininity and an announcement to the world that you have cancer. Talking to a counselor and sharing your feelings with other chemo patients will help put this side effect into perspective. Your hair may thin gradually, or you may lose it all very suddenly. It may come out in clumps; this happens about three or four weeks after your first chemo treatment. Scarves, hats, or turbans, and *good* wigs (do *not* have someone else pick one out for you) will come in handy.

Other side effects include a decrease in your blood *platelets*, which are responsible for blood clotting. You might find that you bleed more or suddenly. This will improve after your treatment.

Drugs you may come across in your treatment include *cyclophosphamide* (Cytoxan), used for breast and ovarian cancer; *amethopterin* (Methotrexate), *mitomycin-C* (Mutamycin), *vincristine* (Oncovin), used for breast cancer; and *cisplatin* (Platinol), a drug with platinum used to treat ovarian, cervical, and uterine cancers. *Note: A drug known as 5 fluorouracil (5-FU) is also a chemotherapy drug used for a variety of cancers. This contains the same active ingredients as the*

5-FU discussed in chapter 3. There is an excellent antinausea drug called Zofran you can inquire about that may relieve much of the discomfort. As well, a newer drug known as GCSF can also be added to your therapy. GCSF stimulates the production of healthy, infection-fighting white blood cells, which reduces your risks of contracting any infections while you're undergoing chemotherapy.

Whether you lose your hair or not, you should look for a wig—before your hair starts falling out—that matches your hair color. Get a longer wig and then have your own hairstylist cut and style the wig to match your current hairstyle. That way, the wig will be far less obvious.

Three months or so into your chemo, you'll feel completely drained. You'll feel depressed, tired, scared, fat, ugly, and cursed with this terrible "cancer thing." You'll cry a lot, feel completely isolated, and may be continually amazed at how rude other people can be. People will either openly pity you: "If it were *me* going through it, I couldn't handle it—you know, being *bald*!" One woman told me that when she confided to a friend that she needed to have chemo, her friend casually said, "Why don't you just shave your head *now?* Your hair's going to fall out *anyway.*" Cancer is like a wedding: It brings out the worst in people. Talk to other chemo patients and share your experiences; surround yourself with supportive people; write; watch funny films; get incredibly selfish and let yourself *feel bad* without feeling guilty.

After your treatment is over, you'll start to feel better. You'll gradually regain your usual energy and the depression will lift. *Your hair will grow back!* You'll shed the bloat and your complexion will return to normal. Food will taste right again, and you may crave foods you never have in the past. You *will* be yourself once more.

Radiation Therapy

In some instances your surgeon will want you to have radiation therapy. This is the last stop on the treatment train, but it is not as unpleasant as chemotherapy. If you haven't had chemotherapy, this *will* be the worst part of your treatment. It's an overkill type of treatment.

Radiation therapy involves high-energy X rays or gamma rays (also referred to as cobalt). X rays use photons (an electron with a different "dosage" of energy) to penetrate the skin; gamma rays use electrons. It is *not* chemotherapy. Therefore, your hair will not fall out unless your scalp is being radiated. Radiation treatment is very exact and directs radiation only at the areas where the cancer has spread. For breast cancer, you'll most likely have *external radiation*; for ovarian and endometrial cancers, you'll be given *internal radiation*, where small amounts of radioactive materials are placed high *inside* the pelvic cavity (discussed below).

The concept of radiation is very simple. Radiation destroys the DNA (the molecules that carry genetic information) in the cancer cell's nucleus (center) in the body cells it targets, arresting the reproduction of cancer cells. The actual process, however, is a little more complex. First, you'll be referred to a radiation oncologist, one who specializes in radiation therapy (*not* to be confused with a radiologist, a doctor who specializes in reading X rays and diagnostic test results).

Radiation therapy is given over a long period of time because it involves, again, a fine balance: enough radiation to destroy cancer cells, but not enough to destroy your healthy tissue. Certain cancer cells are also more sensitive to radiation than others, in the same way that some cockroaches are killed by poison while others aren't.

External Radiation Therapy

If you're having *external radiation* (meaning a beam aimed at the outside flesh) the radiation oncologist will "tattoo you" by injecting tiny dots of special dye in precise areas he or she has marked off in red ink (these will wash off). The therapist will use the tattoo as the bull's-eye of a squared-off section predetermined by the radiation oncologist.

After you're tattooed, you'll report a few days later to a radiation clinic, located in the hospital basement. Radiation clinics are situated in the basement because hospitals want to minimize the risk of radiation exposure to healthy people. It's really just a security measure; however, reporting to a clinic in the bowels of a hospital feels very isolating and depressing. That's why it's important to bring someone along for support, so make sure you don't go alone. You'll need to have a simulation of your radiation done so the machine can be tailored to your size and shape and the proper shieldings molded to the parts of your body *not* receiving radiation.

The amount of external radiation treatments varies for each individual, depending on the severity of your cancer. For example, you might need only 30 seconds of radiation every weekday for a month, while another woman may require four minutes of radiation every day for six weeks. The average dose is about two to four minutes of radiation for five consecutive days each week for a period ranging from two to eight weeks. You'll receive a total dose of radiation, which is then referred to in terms of daily doses. This is called fractionation. The radiation clinic will have a number of radiation therapists on staff who will operate the actual machinery and administer your treatment. You'll go into a dark room and lie down on something that looks like an examination table with a device overhead. The overhead device activates the beam. Then you'll be covered in lead blankets, and only your targeted area will be exposed. The beam will then be turned on.

Although the procedure itself is painless, the aftereffects are not. Knowing this in advance may not alleviate the symptoms but may make them more understandable and more bearable. Although radiation therapy delivers far less radiation to your tissues today than five years ago, you'll still have side effects from the treatment. For the first week of treatment, you probably won't feel much. By week two, the squared-off area that the beam targets will look and feel like a bad sunburn. If you're fair-skinned, you'll have a worse reaction than people with darker pigments. A small raw area might develop in places where your skin rubs together—under the arms, in the folds between your thighs and buttocks, or under your breasts. Not all patients will experience skin changes because equipment is more refined now than it was even a few years ago. But if you do have a problem, you'll need to treat your skin as though it *were* sunburned: avoid sun, cover up exposed skin, don't use any deodorants or perfumes, and use lotions safe for sunburned skin. To help with the sunburn symptoms, use either over-the-counter sunburn creams or ask the radiation oncologist or radiation therapist on staff to recommend something. Generally, diaper rash creams or sunburn creams safe for babies are quite good. Creams that contain lanolin will soften and moisturize your burnt areas (Nivea cream, for example). If a small area of skin actually peels and is raw, a 1% cortisone cream helps. For itchiness, cornstarch in a bath or applied topically with a towel and bandage will help. If you're being treated for breast cancer, your breasts will also be very sore as a result, and you may find that going braless is best. Loose, cotton clothing is recommended. Wool can really irritate your breasts.

If your upper chest or throat area is being radiated, your throat will feel extremely sore. *Absolutely do not smoke during these treatments. This worsens the reactions in your throat and limits the effectiveness of the radiation.* Swallowing will be very painful. As the treatment progresses, your throat will become so tender you'd be better off spitting out your saliva than even attempting to swallow it. To relieve throat symptoms, the best suggestion is to chew Aspergum continuously. Some clinics will prescribe a topical anesthetic to gargle with such as Xylocaine, which numbs all feeling in your throat. It tastes pretty bad, so it may not always work. Eating soft and cold foods may help. If you have no appetite, you could survive on a meal supplement drink (such as Ensure) sold in drugstores or hospital pharmacies. These drinks are like a sweet milkshake and taste like the meal replacement drink from various diet programs.

You may also experience a dry cough or sputum if the radiation is in your lung region. Cough suppressants shouldn't be used because you need to cough up the sputum. A humidifier will help to loosen the sputum so you can get rid of it.

You'll also feel tired by the third or fourth week of treatment; the procedure is mentally as well as physically draining. You may experience some nausea or just loss of appetite. As soon as the treatments are finished, you'll start to feel much better and regain your strength. You'll then need to undergo an imaging scan (CAT or MRI) to see how well the treatment worked.

For certain stages of endometrial or uterine cancer, you may have external radiation directed at the abdominal/pelvic region. Skin reactions will be the same as above, but you'll experience tenderness in the abdominal area, nausea, and usually diarrhea. In a standard, five-to-six-week regimen for the abdominal/pelvic area, the beam begins to affect the bowels after about two weeks. There are medications available that can control your diarrhea, such as atropine and diphenoxylate (Lomotil) and Imodium A-D. If your rectal area is being radiated, your anal opening will be irritated. This can be soothed with cortisone cream. Finally, if your bladder area is being targeted, you'll experience bladder problems such as urinary stress or urge incontinence (discussed in chapter 13) and bladder infections (discussed in chapter 6). Phenazopyridine (Pyridium), oxybutinin (Ditropan), or terazosin (Hytrin) may help with urinary incontinence or frequency.

"Internal" Radiation Therapy: Intercavitary Radiation

For pelvic cancers, radiation therapy in the pelvic/abdominal area is usually administered by placing a radioactive solution into the pelvis and abdomen through a thin tube, coating the organs and total abdominal contents. Specially designed hollow applicators are placed in the uterus under a general anesthetic. After you wake up, a small plastic tube containing the appropriate radioactive isotope (an unstable element) is inserted into the applicators. The isotope is left in place for 48–72 hours, and you'll be required to stay in bed during this time. You'll also be required to stay in isolation because some radioactivity leaks out. Some hospitals developed a way to do this on an outpatient basis, giving a more potent dose of radioactivity with a shorter half-life. Sometimes the applicator is placed in the vagina. This can cause scarring of the vaginal walls, redness, and vaginal dryness. If the applicator is placed in the abdomen, you'll also experience skin irritations in the treated areas, and sometimes bowel and bladder problems (which can be corrected via surgery). Loss of energy and appetite, nausea, and vomiting may also occur, but again, you'll begin to feel better after treatment.

Preventing Surgical Menopause: The Oophoropexy

Any woman receiving radiation to the pelvic region will lose ovarian function either temporarily or permanently after about two weeks of treatment. This will cause surgical menopause. There is a surgical procedure called an *oophoropexy* that literally *moves* the ovaries out of the way of the radiation beam. After your treatment is over, the ovaries are repositioned correctly. This procedure will preserve ovarian function. Request the procedure if it's possible. Unfortunately, if you're also receiving chemotherapy either alone or in conjunction with radiation therapy, this procedure will do you no good.

Hormone Therapy and Immunotherapy

Hormone therapy is used only to treat breast cancer. After your surgery, if your lymph nodes are positive, your doctor may recommend this treatment. It is an estrogen-blocking drug that changes the body's own output of hormones in order to affect the growth of hormonally sensitive tumors. The side effects of this treatment are minimal, but the purpose is the same as chemotherapy: to kill cancer cells.

The most common drug used is called tamoxifen (Nolvadex), but there are many other estrogen-blocking drugs available. Tamoxifen interferes with protein synthesis and prevents an estrogen-responsive cancer cell from extracting estrogen from the body. The drug blocks the estrogen from the cancer cell. This will stop the estrogen cancer cell from growing. The treatment is administered orally and the only side effects reported are hot flashes and possible nausea for the first month or so. It's a tea party compared to chemo or radiation. If you have this treatment (which not all breast cancer patients do) you'll be on the drug for about two years. There is one catch to tamoxifen, however. Because it has an estrogenic effect, women on it who have not already been treated for endometrial cancer will need to be monitored for signs of endometrial hyperplasia, which can develop into endometrial cancer.

In immunotherapy, you may be given interferons and interleukins to boost your immune system. The drug involved here is called *levamisole* (Ergamisol).

A Word About Diet

During your cancer therapy, diet is crucial. An appropriate diet will help you get through all your treatments. Many well-intentioned family members and friends tend to force food on the cancer patient, who is usually nauseous or suffering from poor appetite and/or chronic diarrhea. Don't eat to please; this will do you no good. What you need to do is see your oncology unit's hospital dietitian, or an independent dietitian who specializes in working with oncology patients. Together with the dietitian, you can design a food plan that is realistic and palatable to you during each stage of your treatment.

Follow-up Treatment

Follow-up treatment involves regular visits to all of your cancer doctors: medical and radiation oncologists, breast surgeon, and gynecologic oncologist. Each specialist will see you about every three months for the first two years, then every six months for the next four or five years, and annually thereafter. Each visit will entail various diagnostic tests: blood tests, chest X rays, bone scans, CAT scans, mammograms (for breast cancer follow-up), full pelvic exams and Paps for pelvic cancers (especially cervical cancer), a "second look" laparoscopy or laparotomy for endometrial or ovarian cancers, and endometrial biopsies and ultrasound. The ultimate question is: *Are you cured after all of these treatments?* The answer depends on the stage your cancer was in to begin with (see the section on staging). Statistically, the answer is "usually."

Cancer goes into *remission,* meaning that the cells stop growing and what *was* there was removed or effectively killed. But cancer cells *can* start up again and begin to grow at some future point. Endometrial cancer and cervical cancer rarely come back. Both breast and ovarian cancer may recur, but these can be detected with the CA-125 blood test for ovarian cancer and the CA-15 blood test for breast cancer. If you have a recurrence, you'll need to repeat some or all of your treatments. The longer you go cancer-free, the greater your chances are of being permanently cured. If you've had a mastectomy or lumpectomy, it's crucial to have a mammogram done regularly on the opposite breast.

Palliative Care

If you're not responding to treatment *and* your cancer is in an advanced stage (or has come back in a more advanced stage), your specialists may decide to treat you with *palliative measures.* This means that your pain will be alleviated with strong painkillers or narcotics, such as morphine. Your symptoms will be treated, but you will not be required to undergo any further chemo, surgery, or radiation therapy. (Morphine addiction is really not a concern here. When you're on morphine for pain, the pain is *real,* and the drug's effects are beneficial.) There comes a point in advanced and, inevitably, terminal cases of cancer where you and your doctor decide that enough is enough. After an exhausted regimen of various treatments, you and your doctor will at this stage feel that you tried your best but are unable to reverse your fate. When you get to this stage, your "prognosis" will come as no surprise. You'll be tired and ready to resume as normal a life as you can, and will *look forward* to your dignity. When you're undergoing palliative treatment, it's important to seek out counseling and therapy that will help you accept and *live* with terminal cancer. Never give up, and remember that there are no rules and statistics to follow at this point. Spiritual therapies have been known to work; the mind's ability to heal the body is significant and well beyond the scope and power of the medical community. *I have met women who are living proof.*

Speaking from my own experience, people who have survived cancer have the unusual opportunity to see all angles of the health picture. They experience a variety of diagnostic procedures and treatments, but the subsequent *balancing* of different specialists, medications, and treatments makes cancer patients particularly wise. In a sense, it prepares them for any future health scenario. The experience also provides many patients with coping skills for future crises (health or otherwise) that may arise. Cancer is often what we fear most; after having dealt with it in a treatable version, we are less fearful of other potentially threatening situations.

Surviving invasive gynecological cancer that results in a hysterectomy, oophorectomy, or salpingectomy will bring up for some women the painful reality of infertility and surgical menopause. Keep in mind that women without some of their reproductive parts *can* have children through techniques known as *assisted conception,* discussed in chapter 12. Women without any reproductive organs can still have children through surrogacy or can adopt children. Survivors of breast cancer or cervical carcinoma in situ can go on to get pregnant and give birth. Women with one breast can even breastfeed. All of the reproductive consequences in store for cancer patients are addressed in chapters 10, 12, and 13.

CHAPTER 10

Pregnancy in the 1990s

Pregnancy and childbirth are wonderful and fulfilling experiences for most women. To make the most of a pregnancy and to prepare for a safe delivery, it's crucial that you know what your options are and anticipate potential problems in advance. Living in the 1990s, we are in the midst of a second baby boom; the birthrate hasn't been this high since the 1950s and early 1960s. The new baby boom began around 1980 and is predicted to continue steadily into the early 2000s. *This* baby boom is very different from the last one, however, for many mothers are older, wiser, more highly educated, and often professionals. As a result, the obstetrics "industry" has undergone radical changes. These new mothers are better informed about health and nutrition than their predecessors; they are more concerned about maternal and fetal health; they are questioning procedures, medications, and challenging the old pregnancy myths. But they are also under far more personal and financial stress than the pregnant women of 30 years ago, and are bearing children at a much older age than their forebears. All this has led to a completely different picture for North American women giving birth in the mid-1990s and beyond.

Obviously, the subject of pregnancy cannot be done justice within the scope of a single chapter. The following pages will address everything you need to know about pregnancy in the 1990s. In addition, a list of alternative sources and organizations you can go to for more information is listed at the back of this book. For an expansive look at pregnancy and postpartum health, please consult my book, *The Pregnancy Sourcebook*, which was originally inspired by this chapter. The subject of getting pregnant and preparing for conception is covered in chapter 12, "Fertility Awareness and Infertility."

Everything you need to know about terminating unwanted pregnancies is covered in chapter 11.

The Pregnant Consumer

Because, as you've no doubt heard, no two pregnancies are alike, you'll need to understand how to tailor your prenatal care to your own unique needs, prepare for possible complications, and plan ahead to obtain the most comfortable and appropriate labor and delivery conditions. Since most first-time pregnant women have a more colorful gynecological or medical history than the generation before them, it's important to keep your own history in mind when you're pregnant.

In the 1990s, you don't need to see a doctor to confirm that you're pregnant. Instead, you just pop over to a pharmacy and spend about $20 on a home pregnancy test kit. There are a variety of kits, all of which are about 99% accurate. Most of them are easier to use than the average brand of microwave popcorn. Many pharmacies even offer a pregnancy confirmation service you can use. This entails bringing in a urine sample to the pharmacy and finding out the results within 24 hours. (The pharmacy uses a home pregnancy test kit to confirm the results!)

When the pregnancy is confirmed, women immediately assume that they need to find an *obstetrician,* a doctor who specializes in prenatal care and delivery. Not so. First, not all women *need* an obstetrician. If you're under 35 and healthy, and have never had any significant health problems, you can continue to see your primary care physician throughout your pregnancy and arrange to have him or her deliver you. If your primary care physician doesn't "do" obstetrics (see below), the normal scenario is to see your primary care doctor throughout the first trimester. Your doctor will then refer you to an obstetrician or a primary care doctor who *does* obstetrics, for the remainder of the pregnancy.

Another misconception is that *any* gynecologist will handle your pregnancy. Also not so. Although all gynecologists are initially *trained* as obstetricians (hence the term OB-Gyn, which stands for obstetrician/gynecologist), not all gynecologists *practice* obstetrics, for reasons of insurance. Because even the most routine pregnancy is "risky business," the cost of malpractice insurance significantly increases for obstetricians. These costs are more pronounced in the United States than in countries with universal health care, but the insurance issue exists regardless of where you live. What about primary care physicians? Again, the reason why some primary care physicians do obstetrics while others don't revolves around the insurance issue as well.

If you haven't read chapter 3, go back and do so. Finding good obstetrical care means finding good *primary* care first, then finding a gynecologist who *practices* obstetrics. For any woman considering children, obstetrics care should be a chief concern when you're "doctor shopping." (In fact, some gynecologists do more obstetrics than general gynecology, which is a concern to women who *don't* need the service.)

When Should You First See the Doctor?

Planned Pregnancies

When you're planning pregnancy, you should see the doctor before you conceive, as I'll discuss below. You'll need to be screened for a number of conditions and will need to establish an accurate menstrual chart (see chapter 2) so you can properly date the pregnancy when you do conceive. Many women like to see their doctor after a "positive" home pregnancy test. They often request an "official" blood or urine test to double-confirm it. With the quality kits on the market today, this really isn't necessary, but if it makes you feel better, do it. To figure out your due date, count nine months, plus one week from the first day of your last menstrual period (the first day of bleeding). For example, let's say the date of your last period was November 22. November plus nine months = August; 22 plus one calendar week = 29. Therefore, your due date will be August 29. Another way of calculating the due date is to simply *subtract* three months back and *then* add seven days: November minus three months = August, and again, 22 plus one calendar week is still 29—August 29. When you go for your first prenatal exam (discussed below), your doctor will do the same thing, calculate a little room for error, and give you a rough date. That date is never precise. Only about 5% of women actually give birth on their due dates. A normal pregnancy ranges anywhere from 254 to 294 days! A typical scenario is preparing to deliver anywhere from two weeks prior or past the due date. The *real* answer to "when should I see the doctor?" depends on the prep work you've done *before* the pregnancy. It also depends on your current health situation.

As discussed in chapter 12, when you're healthy and planning to get pregnant, there are a number of conditions, diseases, and infections you must be screened for. The list is long and includes genetic disorders, such as Tay-Sachs disease or sickle cell anemia, German measles (rubella), vaginal infections, urinary tract infections (UTIs), and the whole gamut of STDs (herpes, gonorrhea, syphilis, and chlamydia are the most important ones). You should have a Pap test done and make sure it's clear (see chapter 3). *If you have reason to suspect that you've been exposed to HIV (human immunodeficiency virus), you must take an HIV antibody test if you're either planning a pregnancy or are already pregnant.* (HIV and pregnancy are discussed in chapter 5.)

You should also have a complete physical and make sure that your blood pressure, cholesterol levels, and heart rate are all normal. You may want to be screened for some of the more common autoimmune disorders (diseases that develop because the body "attacks" itself), such as thyroid disease, if you have a family history. A typical prenatal "lab package" in the United States, for example, consists of screenings for Rh positive/negative factors and blood type, anemia, syphilis, gonorrhea, chlamydia, German measles (rubella), hepatitis B, and a urinalysis. At about 14 weeks into the pregnancy, you can expect an alphafetoprotein test (discussed in the prenatal testing section), and your HCG (hormone produced by the fetus) and estrogen levels will be checked. Depending on your history, you might also be screened for diabetes if you're in a high-risk group, but many doctors now screen *all* patients for diabetes, regardless of family history.

If you've done all of this already, you don't need to repeat these tests unless you have reason to believe you contracted an STD or have a specific infection *now.*

If none of this was done, *don't panic!* All you need to do is see your doctor, tell him or her that you are *X* amount of weeks pregnant and that you haven't been screened for anything yet. *Request a complete physical and an STD screening.* He or she will take it from there. The screenings will be done via blood test, urinalysis to check for UTIs, and swabbings taken during a pelvic exam and Pap test. Most likely, the doctor will also do another pregnancy test. If everything is negative ("all clear") you can discuss things like nutrition and diet with your doctor. He or she will probably put you on a vitamin supplement as well. Then, all you need to do is wait out the first trimester until you go for your first prenatal exam, discussed below. If you do have an STD or an infection, you'll be given antibiotics safe for pregnancy. These are discussed in chapter 6.

If you have a history of other health problems and you haven't *already* discussed your plans for pregnancy with your doctor and the health consequences of it, do it as soon as you can. For example, you might be a cancer survivor, have been treated for cervical *pre*cancer, have had major pelvic surgery, have had radioactive iodine (a standard treatment for thyroid disease), have endometriosis, have a clotting disorder, be taking certain medications, be asthmatic or highly allergic, have diabetes, have a heart problem, or have multiple sclerosis or herpes. All of these histories and/or chronic conditions mean different things in the case of pregnancy and carry special concerns and warning signs. Here are some key questions to ask:

1. How will the pregnancy affect my current condition?
2. How will the *treatments* I've had in the past (lasersurgery, chemotherapy, radiation, other surgical procedures) affect my pregnancy and fetal development?
3. How will my condition affect labor and delivery? For example, if I had treatment for cervical dysplasia five years ago, can I still expect to have a vaginal delivery?
4. What kind of symptoms am I likely to experience because of my medical history?
5. What warning signs should I be alerted to during the pregnancy?
6. How can I contact you should something go wrong?
7. What can I do during the pregnancy to avoid any of these symptoms? (bed rest? diet? vitamin supplements?)
8. Are there any activities I should refrain from to maximize my health during pregnancy? (For example, sexual intercourse may be safe for some women and not for others.)
9. What sort of prenatal testing do you plan for me and why?

Whatever your medical history, you should also contact the specialist who usually manages your condition and see him or her a few times during your pregnancy. For example, if you're diabetic or are taking thyroid hormone, it's crucial that your endocrinologist sees you when you're pregnant to balance your medication appropriately. If you've had breast cancer, it's important that your breast surgeon and medical oncologist see you during the pregnancy to make sure that all is well. If you've had cervical dysplasia, human papillomavirus (HPV), or herpes, you may need special gynecological checkups during your pregnancy. If you have certain allergies, you should see your allergist a few times during your pregnancy. The list of special health problems is too long to include here, but you get the idea! You *will* need to seek out the services of an obstetrician if you have other health problems.

"High-Risk" Pregnancies

Your pregnancy is considered high-risk if you:

- are over 35 years old (because of the risk of Down syndrome);
- are having a multiple birth;
- have a history of chronic gynecological problems, such as pelvic inflammatory disease (PID), endometriosis, large, symptomatic fibroids, and pelvic cancers (a yeast infection, treated STD, or UTI does *not* make you a high risk);
- have a history of breast cancer or cancer therapy;
- have a chronic health condition that requires ongoing care (see above), such as diabetes, blood clotting disorders, and heart problems;
- have a history of troubled pregnancies (repeated miscarriages, an ectopic pregnancy, premature births, stillbirth);
- have the potential of passing on a genetic disorder to your child, or have already had one child with a genetic disorder;
- have an untreated or undiagnosed STD;
- are pregnant as a result of assisted conception techniques (see chapter 12);
- have ever had an abortion;
- are a DES daughter (see chapter 3); or
- have an IUD still in place.

The rules for a higher risk *early* pregnancy don't change, except in this case you *will* definitely need an obstetrician, not just a primary care physician. As the pregnancy develops, you may need to take greater care than low-risk pregnant women. You will also need to undergo more prenatal testing. As a result, you'll need to ask the same questions of your doctor as women who have a complicated medical history do (see above).

Unplanned Pregnancies

If your pregnancy was an accident, it's fairly safe to assume that you will *not* have had any appropriate screenings done. These screenings should be your first priority. You should also make sure you inform your doctor about the circumstances of your pregnancy and the contraception situation, if any.

The news will affect each woman in dramatically different ways. If, for example, you're married and were using the withdrawal method combined with fertility awareness techniques, your pregnancy might be unexpected but not unwanted. If you're single and were actively trying to prevent pregnancy, that's a whole different ball game.

If you have an IUD in place and still got pregnant, if you got pregnant while on oral contraception or other hormonal contraception, the situation needs to be addressed. If you had a casual encounter with a man and the condom broke, this will warrant an HIV-antibody test for sure. If you were raped (including date rape), there are special gynecological exams that need to be conducted and can be used in trial evidence. If you don't know who the father is, tell the doctor; if you weren't using any contraception, this needs to be addressed to avoid future accidents. In many circumstances, free counseling, legal advice, and birth control or abortion counseling are available.

After all of these factors are considered, you'll need to level with your doctor about your diet and lifestyle. Are you using drugs? Do you smoke? Do you drink alcohol? Do you normally practice safe sex? What is your medical history? What other medications are you taking? The condition of your ovaries, progression of the pregnancy, and your answers will mean different things to the pregnancy, and in some cases may warrant a *therapeutic* abortion.

What About My First Prenatal Exam?

You should have an initial prenatal exam as soon as you discover you're pregnant—anywhere between 6 and 10 weeks. Here, you'll be given a full physical and perhaps be screened for some of the conditions outlined above. Most important, the date of your last menstrual period—and hence, the pregnancy, can be more accurately established at this point. Dating the pregnancy accurately to begin with can avoid all types of problems later. At this first visit, you'll also be registered as a prenatal patient. Then, should problems develop, such as bleeding, and so on, you'll have established a rapport with your doctor. From here on, you'll be seen about once a month. What to expect in a routine prenatal exam is discussed further on.

It's important to note that traditionally, the basic prenatal exam didn't take place until the end of the first trimester. Even today, many obstetricians (particularly in Canada) will not see you until you're at least 12 weeks pregnant. The high rate of pregnancy loss in the first trimester, coupled with the fact that the pregnancy was—until recently—viewed as too "early" for the doctor to really add any value to the patient, was what postponed the prenatal exam until this point.

But attitudes regarding when to have a prenatal exam are changing. Many doctors feel that the earlier you're examined, the better your pregnancy can be managed overall, preventing miscalculating your due date, poor nutrition, as well as missing the opportunity to screen for certain conditions. If your obstetrician is still using the "12 week" rule, you should be seen by your primary care physician when you discover the pregnancy. Then, at 12 weeks, you can graduate to your obstetrician if you need to.

Finding the Right Hospital

The most important decision you'll ever make as an obstetrics consumer concerns the *hospital* you choose for your delivery, *not the doctor.* For an unremarkable, routine pregnancy, the hospital will make the difference between a good labor experience and a bad one. Do bear in mind that if you live in a small town or less-populated area, you may not have much of a choice in terms of a hospital or birthing facility. The biggest misconception many women have is the belief that their hand-picked, Harvard-graduate obstetrician who looks after their prenatal care, should be the same doctor who delivers them. It doesn't work that way. Most doctors will *try* to be available for your delivery, warn you that they may not be, and ultimately are often *not* available on the "big day." The reason is simple: Labor is unpredictable, and most obstetricians' schedules are jam-packed. They are available for deliveries on a first-come, first-served basis. The exception to this rule is when you've prearranged a cesarean section or are being induced (see below).

Primary care physicians are a little more likely to be available because they're not as booked up and are not exclusively seeing pregnant women.

If your doctor doesn't guarantee delivery, who *does* deliver you? In a teaching hospital, whoever is on call in the OB-Gyn unit of the hospital when you go into labor. Actually, many women are rudely awakened to the fact that, after all is said and done, an OB-Gyn resident (a recently licensed general practitioner who is studying for a particular specialty, in this case, OB-Gyn) may wind up delivering them. In a community hospital, you'll be delivered by any physician or midwife on staff (not necessarily a resident). In some communities (particularly in Canada) if you go into sudden labor and need to be rushed to the hospital, whoever is on call in Emergency may deliver you if the hospital is short-staffed. In this case, you should be more concerned about finding a great hospital than finding a great doctor. But if you're seeing a private physician in a group practice, either your own doctor or another doctor in the group will attend to your labor. If you're seeing a doctor in solo practice, you may be delivered by one of the doctors who backs him or her up when he or she is unavailable.

Choosing a Birthing Facility

You'll naturally want a hospital that has top-notch facilities, such as a neonatal intensive care unit and state-of-the-art fetal monitoring equipment. You should also *expect* to find a 1990s' maternity facility that offers you choices without having to do a long, arduous search. For example, there are very few hospitals left in North America that *don't* offer the following:

- *Birthing rooms* (a one-stop room where you labor, deliver, and bond with the newborn, after which you'll be moved to another room to recover). This is preferable to a separate labor room followed by a separate delivery room. It's also much homier. These rooms are usually nicely decorated to mimic a home environment. Some U.S. hospitals now offer LDR (labor delivery recovery) or LDRP (labor delivery recovery postpartum). Today, U.S. hospitals are under pressure to discharge patients earlier and earlier. Women may give birth, recover and return home in 24 hours or less. So you may either labor, deliver, and recover in one room, then transfer to a traditional hospital room for the remainder of your stay, or you may do everything in the same room until you check out.
- *Birthing beds.* These are adjustable, comfortable beds that allow you a variety of labor and delivery positions. The flat, 1950s' gynecological exam-style beds with stirrups are not used anymore in a modern hospital.
- *Birthing chairs.* Ideal for the squatting-style delivery. Squatting deliveries, discussed below, are *really* popular now.
- *"Leboyer births."* Frederick Leboyer was a French obstetrician who advocated gentle deliveries that included warm baths for the newborns after delivery, immediate bonding with mom, soothing lights, and so on. Essentially, the days of whisking the baby away, immediately severing the um-

bilical cord, and spanking the baby to start his/her breathing are over! Most hospitals incorporate some aspects of this method; not too many go the whole 9 yards, however.

- *"Rooming in" privileges.* Your baby stays in your room and nurses are available round-the-clock to assist you in breastfeeding, bathing, and so forth. It's sort of like an "instant nanny" service at your disposal. You also have the option of *not* doing this.
- *Total father involvement.* No hospital will prevent the baby's father from *complete participation* in labor and vaginal delivery. In fact, this is encouraged. Some hospitals may have a problem with his presence during cesarean sections. Just ask.
- *Total midwife involvement.* Some hospitals today offer midwife services, acknowledge midwifery as professional training, and welcome midwives into the birthing process. They're helpful, knowledgeable, and comforting. (Midwives are discussed below.)
- *Breastfeeding lessons.* There is currently a worldwide effort, led by UNICEF and WHO (World Health Organization), to make hospitals "baby friendly." This means doing away with and adopting practices that support breastfeeding in the hospital. In other words, a hospital in this decade should not only show you how to breastfeed properly but ensure rooming in, end the distribution of free or low-cost formula to new mothers in hospitals, not provide the baby with artificial nipples (which discourages breastfeeding), and so on. For more details consult my book, *The Breastfeeding Sourcebook.*
- *Baby bathing lessons and baby changing lessons.* Someone will show you how to change and bathe your baby.

  Note: Canadian women may need to shop around more for certain facilities, simply because American hospitals are usually better equipped.

When choosing a birthing facility, some women may be concerned about certain archaic hospital practices they read about in various pregnancy books. Many of the things they warn you about aren't done anymore, including:

- *Shaving the pubic area before delivery.* Hospitals now realize that pubic hair is perfectly sanitary and doesn't need to be shaved. In fact, nicks and cuts in the area as a result of shaving are recognized as more hazardous.
- *Enemas before delivery.* First of all, you'll be given a choice regarding an enema if your doctor feels you need one for any reason. But it's now an accepted fact that the mother will most likely "go" on her own because of

a kind of watery diarrhea that precipitates labor. This is much like the kind of diarrhea that often accompanies heavy menstrual cramps.

- *Stirrups during standard labor.* Old-style stirrups are not used anymore, in the sense that you're involuntarily "tied down," but there are certainly foot supports available to help you bear down during labor. In cases where forceps are needed for difficult deliveries, these foot supports are necessary as well.
- *Synthetic hormone.* Bromocriptine (in pill form) was once used to inhibit the production of prolactin, a hormone necessary for the production of breastmilk. The benefits of breastfeeding have been recognized for a long time. The hospital will assume that you'll want to breastfeed unless you state otherwise. If you want to bottle-feed instead, or need to for medical reasons, speak to your doctor sometime before your due date about it. (Lactation supression is still available for moms who want it.)

You *might* want to know the following about the facility:

1. Is the maternity unit well staffed at all hours?
2. What credentials does the on-call staff have, in case one of them does the delivery?
3. What is the hospital's philosophy regarding cesarean sections? When are they done? Who does them? Are they open to vaginal births after a cesarean birth?
4. As a reference, can you contact a new mother who recently had her baby there?
5. What is the hospital's philosophy on *underwater birth?* This is a new process in which a baby is born in a kind of large Jacuzzi-style bathtub. Some women really like this! Some hospitals have these facilities, others are concerned that the newborn might drown in the process—which is considered *a very small* risk by underwater-birth advocates. Although to date, Jacuzzi births don't add any proven benefits to the baby, it's helpful during labor and is soothing for mom.
6. Does the hospital have midwives on staff or should you "bring your own"?
7. What is the hospital's philosophy on *episiotomies* (a procedure in which the vagina is slit open a little to allow room for the head to come out) or *epidurals* (a painkiller that numbs the pelvic region but doesn't interfere with labor). Both of these are discussed in the labor section below.

Midwives

In North America there are two types of midwives: a *certified nurse-midwife* (CNM) and an *independent midwife,* sometimes referred to as a *certified midwife* (CM). A CNM has a professional graduate degree in midwifery, and has gone through more officially recognized medical training. A CNM always works in partnership with your managing practitioner. This means that she might manage your entire pregnancy and refer you to a doctor only if there's a problem. Or, she may work right alongside your doctor and be with you during all your prenatal exams and tests. Most hospitals have CNMs on staff. If you're American, you will have a choice of CNMs on your health plan, just like you have for a doctor. This care is covered by your insurance. For more information, call The American College of Nurse-Midwives at 202-728-9860. Canadian women can choose CNMs through their hospitals or can contact the Ontario Association of Midwives at 416-538-4389 to find out more about Ontario or Canada-wide services.

An independent midwife, or CM, has less "official" medical training but usually has combined university courses with a type of "internship" or apprenticeship. These midwives are less likely to be covered by American health plans, and would be paid for independently. For a low-risk, routine pregnancy, this midwife *is* qualified to act as the managing practitioner as well. Hospitals and primary care physicians will have lists of both kinds of midwives. If you are a first-timer or are in a high-risk group, the best scenario is going with the CNM-physician combination. Ultimately, whoever you choose will need to be interviewed (see chapter 3) and will need to be a compatible personality. In some states, a *lay midwife* is also available, but she has absolutely no medical or academic training. She has apprenticed with another lay midwife who also has had no medical or academic training. You may need to rethink this type of midwife.

Your midwife's role is to be a real friend and "constant" to you throughout your pregnancy. She will help you through the discomforts of pregnancy and may be more available for delivery when you go into labor. A midwife will also assist you in more perilous circumstances, such as miscarriage, or other complications. Throughout your pregnancy, she will come to see you at home if you require immediate care and she will also be active during the postpartum period. It's important to remember, though, that a midwife isn't qualified to manage complications during pregnancy, labor, or delivery; you'll need to be referred to an obstetrician under these circumstances.

The First Trimester

The first trimester is an exciting time in your pregnancy, but it's important to be prepared in the event of any problems, which are more common in the first trimester.

Early pregnancy is a different experience for each woman. Obviously, you won't be menstruating regularly, but you might continue to bleed scantily throughout the first trimester, which is why some women often don't realize they're pregnant until about three months into the pregnancy. About seven days after conception, you may get what's called *implantation bleeding*. This is normal vaginal spotting caused by the formation of new blood vessels, but it rarely happens.

You might also find that you're urinating more frequently. First, your uterus is enlarging and pressing down on your bladder. Second, because of all the hormonal changes you're experiencing, such as megabursts of progesterone in your body (see chapter 1), you'll be retaining and releasing more water.

Most women will feel changes in their breasts. The breasts may swell, tingle, throb, or hurt. This is because your breast is developing milk glands. There is also an increased blood supply going to your breasts, and the veins will become more pronounced. Your nipples will also enlarge and become more erect, and your areola will darken and become broader. Some women will notice early on that their nipples feel sensitive and sore. (Breast changes during pregnancy are discussed in chapter 1.)

Fatigue is another major symptom at this stage. It begins after the first missed period and persists until the 14th to 20th week of pregnancy. The remedy is simple: *Get more sleep!* If you're at home, take naps in the afternoon. If you're working, take a nap after work. Try to arrange for help around the house. About 10 hours of sleep is suggested during the first trimester.

Increased levels of progesterone will also cause you to feel faint and constipated. The faintness happens because the progesterone dilates the smooth muscle of the blood vessels and causes blood to pool in the legs. In addition, more blood begins to flow to the uterus. This can cause low blood pressure and result in fainting. Standing or sitting for long periods of time tends to trigger it. Lying flat and doing exercises that get the blood circulating again will prevent this.

As for constipation, progesterone relaxes the smooth muscles of your small and large intestines, slowing down the digestive process. To combat this, enrich your diet with more fluids (about six to eight glasses a day) and high fiber, and eliminate fatty foods such as red meat. One to two tablespoons of unsulfured blackstrap molasses in warm water once or twice a day is an old reliable remedy. Molasses is also high in iron and trace minerals. Prune juice can work miracles. Walking or mild physical exercise also helps. Finally, don't *force* your stools. If you're on the toilet and nothing's happening, get up! If you sit there, strain, and force a bowel movement, you might develop hemorrhoids. Get into the habit of waiting until the stools are almost out before you go to the toilet. (Most pregnant women get hemorrhoids anyway because of hormonal changes, as well as an enlarged uterus, which puts pressure on pelvic veins.) Stool softeners might help, which can be prescribed by your doctor. Some doctors suggest that you try sitting on the toilet for about 10 minutes after each meal. The stimulation of your stomach from eating will be transmitted right down through to your bowels, which will train your body to defecate at regular times each day. This is called the gastro-colic reflex. And finally, you can adjust your diet to include more fruit, vegetables, fiber, and fluids, and less milk, calcium, and simple sugars.

Other things that might plague you early on are *yeast infections*, discussed in chapter 6. Lower back pain occurs because your expanding uterus might put pressure on your *sciatic nerve*, which runs from your buttocks down through the backs of your legs.

Morning Sickness

Morning sickness refers to the infamous nausea and vomiting women tend to experience during early pregnancy. Between 60 and 80% of all women suffer from morning sickness in their first trimester, but be forewarned: Morning sickness may *begin* in the morning, but it often persists 24 hours a day for the first few weeks of pregnancy. Sometimes the nausea isn't bad enough to cause vomiting and is sort of an ever-present condition, warded off by dry crackers or juice.

For more severe cases, the nausea and vomiting begins 6–8 weeks after your last menstrual period, persists strongly until about 14 weeks after your last menstrual period, and then either disappears or gets much better. But it can persist well into the second trimester, too.

Numerous other symptoms that accompany morning sickness include an aversion to certain tastes or smells that never bothered you before, such as coffee, cigarette smoke, meat, and my favorite example (from a chronic dieter), *salad!* Just the sight of some of these foods may send you "heaving."

Some women find it difficult to prepare any food and may be turned off to everything except one food in particular, like grapefruit, yogurt, or crackers.

Unfortunately, skipping meals and fasting is the worst thing you can do. Childbearing practitioners suggest eating frequent, small meals or snacks. Nibbling on dry crackers throughout the day and keeping cracker stashes at the office, at your bedside, in the car, or wherever really helps. The nausea is caused by changes in hormone levels that somehow affect your stomach lining and stomach acids. So an empty stomach aggravates the nausea. Giving your stomach something to actually *digest* is a way to combat it. There is also a strong connection between nausea and low blood sugar levels. If you're diabetic, this could mean trouble, so make sure you're on top of your blood sugar levels no matter what.

The problem with nonstop nausea and vomiting is that you might become malnourished or dehydrated. Try to sip fluids such as fruit juices and keep drinking water. (You don't have to worry about drinking milk just yet.) Cheese, yogurt, or calcium supplements are just fine. If you're vomiting more than three times a day, see your doctor and make sure you're not dehydrated. Most women have enough "reserves" in their body to nourish the fetus regardless of how nauseated they are. A most ironic statistic shows that the presence of morning sickness is associated with more favorable pregnancies than the absence of it. Perhaps this fact will give you comfort as you face the "Tidy Bowl" man every morning.

A final word: Just because you're in early pregnancy doesn't mean you don't have a stomach flu or another ailment causing the nausea. Be sure to check it out if it persists beyond what's tolerable.

Concerns about Nutrition and Weight Gain

Eating well is extra important during your pregnancy. The best thing to do is request a referral to a *nutritionist* and work out your daily nutritional needs with him or her. Or, book a separate appointment with either your doctor or midwife to design an appropriate diet that's right for you. You might ask, "Why not just consult a general pregnancy book and follow a *standard* diet?" The answer is simple: Not every pregnancy is "standard." Each woman experiences different symptoms, has a different medical history, and lives a different lifestyle, and therefore *needs to eat different things.* Some women need to have a vitamin supplement; some women need to go *off* vitamin supplements they're taking to relieve or prevent other symptoms.

One of the major problems with the current nutritional information on pregnancy is that *there's too much of it.* It's too overwhelming and puritanical for the average, working, nauseous, stressed-out pregnant woman to follow. One woman I interviewed was relieved to discover that she could have one cup of real coffee each morning. She had "read" that caffeine in any amount would cause fetal abnormalities. Her doctor felt that, in light of the fact that this woman was working, battling traffic jams, and fighting off fatigue, one cup of coffee each morning was appropriate for *her.* Someone else, on the other hand, who is more sensitive to caffeine may not be able to have coffee. Another woman I spoke to was reassured that one glass of wine, *once in a while* during her pregnancy, was fine. Nevertheless, most of us *will* want to avoid alcohol, but under certain circumstances, it may be difficult. The lower limit of safe alcoholic use during pregnancy hasn't yet been determined.

Other concerns include the "no junk food" rule. Pregnant women in the 1990s are *only human.* A Big Mac once in a while, a chocolate bar, or a bag of potato chips *is not* going to cause fetal abnormalities. If you're caught in a horrendous traffic jam, eating *something*—even if it's *not* a sandwich made with all-natural, free-range chicken—is better than nothing. Furthermore, many workplaces aren't exactly pregnant-friendly. You might be busy all day and have time only for fast food, which you can adjust to your needs. (Even McDonald's has salads!)

And as for all that *milk,* what if you have a lactose intolerance problem, can't handle any dairy products, and don't want to take Lactaid? Other unique dietary problems during pregnancy revolve around being vegetarian (many vegetarians eat neither dairy nor eggs). What if you have other food allergies? What if you're diabetic? What if you are anemic or are on certain medications that interfere with certain foods? Weight gain is also highly individualized. What if you're already battling a weight problem? What if you have a history of eating disorders?

The bottom line is that nutrition during pregnancy is *too important* to get out of a book or magazine article. Your age, weight, history, and pregnancy symptoms will *all* affect your diet and vitamin supplementation during pregnancy. And, the diet may need to change throughout your pregnancy. So forget the cookbooks and see a qualified nutritionist, your own doctor, or a midwife. And *relax!*

As far as weight is concerned, yes, you're technically "eating for two," but remember that what's growing inside you will weigh only about 10 pounds at the very most. (Although infants over 10 pounds have been known to be born, it's rare!) You'll need to work out a realistic food plan and weight-gain strategy with your nutritionist. What is important is to increase your calcium intake to prevent premature bone loss. This is discussed more in chapter 13. Don't look at your pregnancy as a food bingeing "free for all." Gaining too much weight will make it more difficult for you to take it off after the delivery, could put you at risk for other problems such as hypertension or gestational diabetes, and might also aggravate other problems down the road that result from water retention.

Both fitness and exercise are important, but in moderation. Your doctor or midwife is the best judge of what kinds of activities are appropriate. Some women will need to speed up their activities and become more fit, while others will need to slow down. There are several good aerobics classes designed for pregnant women that work the right muscles and prevent you from overdoing it. Another benefit to getting in shape during pregnancy is that you'll be more prepared for the physical work involved with labor. Whatever you decide, it's best to exercise under the supervision of a trained aerobics or fitness instructor who can guide you toward the right exercises and prevent you from damaging yourself.

Things that Can Go Wrong

When something goes wrong during the first trimester, it has to do with the pregnancy's not "taking." This usually means two things: a miscarriage (bleeding and cramping are the main symptoms) or an ectopic pregnancy (sharp, abdominal cramping or searing pain on one side, depending on the tube). Often, women don't even *realize* they're pregnant until they experience a first-trimester problem like this. But these problems are common.

Ectopic pregnancies were considered less common until about five years ago, when the results of untreated STDs, PID, and assisted reproductive technology started to factor into the childbearing population. If you've had PID, discussed in chapter 6, you are at a higher risk of suffering an ectopic pregnancy. If you're walking around with *undiagnosed* chlamydia or gonorrhea, you're also at risk. *Fifty percent of all women between the ages of 18 and 30 have chlamydia and don't know it.* This is why it's important to be regularly screened for STDs and to be particularly prudent about screening if you're planning a pregnancy.

As for miscarriage, one in six pregnancies ends in miscarriage, *and 75% of these miscarriages occur before 12 weeks.* The risk of a miscarriage also increases with age, which is discussed further below. This is why it's crucial to have your birthing team and birthing facility in place *now.* You'll need these professionals if you *do* miscarry.

After carefully reviewing many of the pregnancy books out there, I've concluded that miscarriage is very much *downplayed* in most of the pregnancy books. Information about it is listed as a kind of afterthought in the "first trimester" sections when it should be a major focus. This is a pity considering how common it is. And while the majority of you *will* carry full-term, the women who *don't* typically need more information.

Again, it's important to understand that normal, low-risk pregnancies are *risky business*. There are several reasons why a miscarriage occurs. Some studies indicate that about 60% of all first-time, first-trimester miscarriages occur because of genetic abnormalities. It's your body's way of doing its own "genetic engineering," expelling malformed fetuses. More than 90% of women who miscarry once will go on to have successful pregnancies.

But women who experience miscarriages today are sort of left "hanging" when they refer to their pregnancy books. They scramble to the index, look up *miscarriage*, and if they're lucky, find a couple of pages on it at the back of the book. They feel like failures, they're in a kind of "no-man's land" information-wise. Then they suddenly "graduate" to an *infertility* book or a book on pregnancy loss. As far as I'm concerned, a first-trimester miscarriage is very much a *pregnancy* issue, not an infertility issue. It's important for all women in their first trimester to learn about miscarriage so they don't panic needlessly and can be prepared in the event that it happens. This is why information on miscarriage is a very central part of *this* section. Few women have repeated miscarriages; when you miscarry once, usually the next pregnancy is successful.

You may *not* have had an official prenatal exam at this point, and you may not have realized you were pregnant. If you do have your team and birthing facility in place, call your doctor (obstetrician or primary care physician) as well as your midwife. Midwives are wonderful during these kinds of crises and will give you marvelous support and advice. The right way to handle emergency symptoms depends on the severity of your symptoms, your health care system/coverage, and the kind of birthing facility and health care team you've chosen. In the United States, if you're under the care of a private physician, you will usually have a chance to consult with your doctor about your symptoms over the phone (most of them are on 24-hour pagers). Depending on your situation, your doctor may be able to evaluate what's going on just by what you describe over the phone; ask you to come into his/her office for an ultrasound, which can determine the status of the pregnancy; or ask you to meet him/her at the hospital. If you *are* miscarrying, a D & C can be scheduled at a convenient time for you rather than done as an emergency procedure. In fact, many doctors in private practice can actually do a better job of evaluating the problem in their offices than a hospital Emergency room, which, of course, wouldn't be as familiar with your case as your own doctor.

For American women in less exclusive health care plans as well as Canadian women (whose physicians do not have appropriate ultrasound equipment in their offices) you will need to inform your doctors' offices (via receptionist or answering machine) of your symptoms and go directly to the birthing facility. For severe symptoms, ask your midwife, your doctor, or both to meet you there. Someone will take care of you when you get to the birthing facility. (Even if it's not a hospital, all birthing centers are staffed for emergencies.)

If you're taken by surprise by any of the symptoms discussed below, and feel they are severe (heavy bleeding, onset labor, severe pain, or loss of consciousness), immediately call either your regular gynecologist or primary care physician's office. If it's during business hours, ask the receptionist or answering service what hospital he or she practices at (each will be affiliated with a hospital). Have the receptionist inform the doctor that you will meet him or her there and that you're leaving now! *Then, get yourself to an Emergency unit of that hospital ASAP.* If you can't drive yourself or find someone to take you, by all means *call 911 and request an ambulance.* If it's after hours, there should be a recorded message at your doctor's office that gives out an emergency number and the address of the hospital he or she is affiliated with. If you're well enough to go to Emergency on your own, have someone (friend, mother, spouse, neighbor) call that emergency number and arrange for the doctor to meet you at the hospital. If you're going by ambulance, the ambulance staff will call for you. If for some reason you can't get hold of any doctor, and he or she does not have prerecorded emergency instructions, get yourself to the Emergency unit of *any* hospital ASAP, either on your own or by ambulance. Once you're there and being looked after, the hospital will sort everything out and find the doctor and appropriate hospital for you. Never *wait* for the doctor to call you back. Just get moving!

Bleeding.

It's important to remember that not all bleeding means that a miscarriage is imminent. Nevertheless, although some bleeding during early pregnancy is fairly *common,* it is still not "normal."

Heavy bleeding that requires heavy-duty pads that need to be *frequently* changed should be reported immediately. You'll also have other symptoms: cramps, pain in the abdomen, fever, weakness, and possible vomiting. The blood may have clumps of tissue in it. You may also notice an unusual odor. Another kind of bleeding is brown, intermittent, or continuous vaginal spotting or light bleeding accompanied by severe abdominal or shoulder pain. Finally, when light bleeding continues for more than three days, this is not a good sign.

Miscarriage.

Heavy bleeding and cramping anywhere between the end of the second month to the end of the third month are classic signs that you're in the process of miscarrying. Cramps without any bleeding are also a danger sign that you're miscarrying. The bleeding can be heavy enough to soak several pads in an hour, or may be "manageable" and more like a heavy period. You may also be experiencing *unbearable* cramping that incapacitates you. Sometimes you can *pass clots,* which are dark red clumps that look like small pieces of raw beef liver. Sometimes you may pass grayish or pinkish tissue. A miscarriage can also be taking place if you have persistent, light bleeding and more mild cramping at this stage.

Once you're in the hospital, your doctor will be able to tell whether you're indeed miscarrying, and if so, what stage the miscarriage is in. He or she will do a gentle pelvic exam and/or ultrasound. You might be sent home with a list of instructions and told to wait it out, which is often the only thing to do. Sometimes it takes several hours for a miscarriage to run its course. Or, depending on what's going on, you might need to stay and have an emergency D & C procedure (D & Cs are discussed in chapter 8).

When you miscarry before 20 weeks, it's actually called a *spontaneous abortion.* Staying in the hospital or going home will depend on what kind of miscarriage you're experiencing, what stage it's in, and so on. There are several kinds of spontaneous abortions:

- *Threatened abortion:* Your cervix is still closed and holding everything in securely, but you are having cramps, bleeding, or staining. Your doctor will do a physical exam and check the fetal heartbeat. You may also need an ultrasound. Then you'll be ordered to bed. In some cases, the bleeding will stop and the pregnancy will continue normally. Sometimes you might miscarry anyway because of unsalvageable problems, such as severe genetic deformities.
- *Inevitable abortion:* In this case, nature has already taken its course and the process of miscarriage has started. Bleeding is heavy, cramps increase, and

the cervix begins to dilate. You may wind up expelling everything while it's still intact: the fetus, amniotic sac, and placenta, accompanied by a lot of blood. This is the most traumatic kind of first-trimester miscarriage because you'll need to *save* what you've just expelled. Sometimes you'll have to dig these things out of the toilet. If you're going through this, try not to be alone. Call a friend or make sure your partner is with you. If your doctor suspects an inevitable abortion, abnormal bleeding is usually heavy enough to warrant a D & C before any tissue passes out on its own. However, if a D & C is not done, the pregnancy tissue would come out on its own eventually. Save what you expelled, in case your doctor wants to do tests. In general, it's difficult to determine the cause of a miscarriage by examining or testing expelled tissue.

- *Incomplete abortion:* This is when you're not naturally expelling all of the uterine contents. Some, but not all pregnancy tissue has been spontaneously expelled. Usually, what remains is fragments of the placenta. Only half of the fetus is expelled; the other half remains. This needs to be corrected with a D & C procedure, which will clean out the uterus and help it to heal. You'll still need to save part of what comes out, but it will look like just clumpy pieces of blood. You may be sent home from Emergency, only to have to go back into the hospital a couple of days later for the D & C.
- *Complete abortion:* This is when all pregnancy tissue is passsed spontaneously. You will be sent home and will *slowly* expel everything by steadily bleeding. This will feel like a miserable period, and the bleeding can actually go on for days, but everything will come out in time. You still may need a D & C anyway just to clean out any bits of tissue left behind but this usually isn't necessary. In this case, save anything that looks like pregnancy tissue, and give it to your doctor when it's all over.
- *Missed abortion:* This is also very traumatic. The fetus dies in the uterus but doesn't come out. You may not have symptoms that anything's wrong for quite some time. This is when you just lightly spot. In this situation, all of your pregnancy symptoms will gradually disappear and you obviously won't progress at all. This condition is frequently diagnosed during a routine exam, and the fetal heartbeat can no longer be heard. Treatment depends on the duration of the pregnancy.

The risk of miscarriage increases with age. The risk is about 10% for women in their 20s, and skyrockets to 50% for women in their mid-40s. This means that a significant portion of thirtysomething pregnancies will end this way. There are all kinds of reasons why you might be miscarrying, but 90% of all women who miscarry either once or twice, do go on to have normal pregnancies and deliveries. Usually, the reason has to do with a fetus "self-terminating" because it wasn't developing properly. You'll need to wait anywhere from three to six months after a miscarriage before you try again. Review chapter 4 and choose an appropriate barrier method to prevent conception during this period.

After two miscarriages, you should *stop* trying and go for diagnostic tests to see *why* you're miscarrying. Often, the reasons are unknown and you'll go on to have a successful third pregnancy. In fact, even after two miscarriages, there's a 70% chance that your third pregnancy will be fine. But if a reason does turn up, it may be easy to fix, and finding the cause at this point will prevent further trauma to you. Possible causes of miscarriage at this stage involve hormonal deficiencies that interfere with fetal development, uterine structural problems, genetic error, and blood incompatibility.

When miscarriages keep repeating (three or more in a row), this is considered an *infertility* problem (see chapter 12). *However, one or two miscarriages do not make you infertile and are generally* not *precursors to future problems.* Seek out other women who have gone through pregnancy loss as well. There are several support groups for women who have miscarried once or twice. For more information on pregnancy loss and miscarriage, review the resources at the back of this book, organized alphabetically by subject.

Ectopic pregnancy.

An ectopic pregnancy occurs when the fetus fails to implant itself in the uterus and starts to develop in the fallopian tube. This is very dangerous. If your tube ruptures, it could be a life-threatening situation. The classic symptoms of ectopic pregnancy are sharp abdominal cramps or pains on one side. The pains may start out as a dull ache that gets more severe. Neck pains and shoulder pains are also common. You may also have a menstrual type of bleeding along with the pain, but the pain is the most *obvious* sign.

The problem with ectopic pregnancies is that often women don't realize they're pregnant until they have one. So if you're trying to get pregnant or are not practicing birth control, and notice any kind of unexplained abdominal pain, get yourself to a doctor as soon as you can.

Women in high-risk groups for ectopic pregnancies generally

- have intrauterine devices (IUDs);
- have a history of PID;
- have a history of pelvic surgery (scarring may block the tube and prevent the egg from leaving);
- have a history of ectopic pregnancy; or

- were pregnant as a result of assisted contraception techniques, where gametes or embryos have been injected into the fallopian tubes.

If you have symptoms of ectopic pregnancy and suspect it, follow the same instructions outlined above in the "bleeding" section. Your doctor will check the human chorionic gonadotropin (hCG) hormone levels in your blood to see if they're elevated (a pregnancy test). An ultrasound will be done to investigate the condition of the uterus and fallopian tubes. Once an ectopic pregnancy is confirmed, you will need *emergency surgery (laparotomy, laparoscopy, or open abdominal surgery) and a skilled surgeon.* The surgery involves removing the embryo from your fallopian tube. This is delicate surgery, and you'll want someone who is capable of saving your fallopian tube *if possible.* Sometimes this isn't possible, and your fallopian tube will need to be removed (salpingectomy). Depending on the progression of the pregnancy, you may need one ovary removed as well. You'll then need to recuperate for at least a week from surgery. After surgery, you'll need to have another blood test to make sure no embryonic tissue is left. Usually, women go on to have normal pregnancies. You'll need to have at least two periods before you try again. If you have only one fallopian tube, the remaining tube will pick up the slack and you'll ovulate regularly.

The Second Trimester

Once your pregnancy has progressed to the fourth month, the risk of complications decreases considerably; miscarriages at this stage, known as late miscarriage, account for less than 25% of *all* miscarriages. Meanwhile, ectopic pregnancy occurs usually in the first trimester, but it can go to term. This is known as an "abdominal pregnancy." It is at this stage that you'll begin to look pregnant, rather than just be mistaken for "chubby." Most women will begin to feel a little less nauseated at this point, too, but morning sickness occasionally persists well into the second trimester or even throughout the third trimester. You'll also be watched for signs of hypertension or diabetes, common in women who come from high-risk families. Begin having "official" prenatal exams, which will include regular testing of your blood sugar levels because of the frequency of gestational diabetes developing at this stage. Also, begin to go for various prenatal tests depending on your age and risk group.

How Does It Feel?

When there *is* an end to morning sickness, you'll begin to feel better in some ways but decidedly more "pregnant" in others. By now, your waist will have expanded considerably and you won't be able to fit into many of your prepregnancy clothes. You'll begin to feel fetal movement, sometimes called quickening, in the early part of the second trimester. This date is important to note because it will help your doctor date the pregnancy more accurately.

At this point, your entire circulatory system is changing. Your total blood volume increases, your bone marrow produces more blood corpuscles, and your heart will be changing position and increasing slightly in size. You may notice that you're salivating more frequently, which is sometimes associated with nausea or is more pronounced if you're nauseous. You may sweat more as well. At this stage, the weight of your uterus increases 20 times, *while the bulk of your weight gain will take place after the 20th week.* As your abdominal area stretches, you may notice stretch marks, lines with pinkish or reddish streaks that appear across your stomach. Your skin may also be drier. There are other symptoms that might creep up, such as iron-deficient anemia and a host of other problems that vary from woman to woman.

By midpoint in your pregnancy, your breasts will have become fully functional, ready for breastfeeding. Around the 19th to 20th week, your nipples will secrete a yellowish liquid known as *colostrum,* a crucial premilk substance that nourishes the baby until your mature breastmilk comes in.

Constipation gets worse as the pregnancy progresses. A good high-fiber diet (discussed with your doctor and/or nutritionist) will help this. Even so, hemorrhoids may become unavoidable at this point because of pressure on your pelvic organs and the dilation of veins in your rectum. Another tip is to prop your feet up on a stool when you move your bowels. For remedies, Preparation H, petroleum jelly, or vitamin E oil work fine.

Women can experience heartburn all through the pregnancy. It is most common in the last trimester, but it can also start at some point in the second trimester and continue until the end. Heartburn is a burning sensation in the middle of your chest or upper digestive tract. It's caused by progesterone, which relaxes the muscle that controls the opening at the top of the stomach. Progesterone also causes the stomach, which is pressed upward by the growing fetus, to empty more slowly. The bottom line is that the stomach doesn't work as well as it should. Here are some tips that might help:

1. Avoid fatty and greasy foods, carbonated drinks, processed meats, and junk foods. Ask your nutritionist to recommend a heartburn-friendly diet.
2. Eat slowly and chew your food well before you swallow. This will give the enzymes in your saliva a chance to work better and help to break down the food, which will relieve some of the digestive "workload" from your stomach.
3. Try not to eat later in the evening (after 8 p.m.) when you're less active.
4. Try not to drink with your meals. If you don't wash down the soilds with liquid, you're likely to eat slower and swallow less air.
5. Avoid coffee, tea, smoking, and antacids that contain bicarbonate.

Because your blood volume has increased by about 40% and your hormonal levels have increased, you might notice an occasional nosebleed. This is nothing to worry about. Keep a little petroleum jelly in each nostril, which will help prevent dryness, which can, in turn, trigger a nosebleed.

A thin, milky, painless, inoffensive-smelling vaginal discharge will develop around now and get heavier as the pregnancy progresses. This is known as *leukorrhea,* caused by an increase in hormonal activity. You may need to wear lightday pads for this. You should also review vaginal hygiene rules, outlined in chapter 6 in the yeast infection section. Yeast infections may persist throughout your pregnancy, however.

Edema means "water retention" and can cause swollen ankles, swollen fingers (to the point where you might need to take off your rings), and general all-around puffiness. Depending upon the severity of the edema, a number of other problems can develop. *Carpal tunnel syndrome* is one of them. This is when the increased fluid in your wrists cuts off the nerve in the wrist responsible for feeling in the fingers and hands. Women who develop this may feel tingling or burning sensations in their fingers. This usually corrects itself in time or can be corrected with a splint. If the problem persists after delivery, minor surgery can correct the problem. Other edema-related problems also tend to correct themselves in time as the fluid levels in the body drop. When you are pregnant, the increase in estrogen causes you to retain more fluid, essential for nourishing the placenta and maintaining adequate milk flow.

The Venous Chronicles

Your veins may change drastically, but this is a normal part of pregnancy.

Venous changes range from unsettling blue lines under the skin around the breasts or abdomen to bonafide varicose veins. These blue lines are just more prominent and expanded veins. They've expanded because your blood supply has increased, which is necessary to nourish the fetus.

Some women get spidery, purplish lines up and down their thighs, known as "superficial varicosities." "Spider nevi," or *telangiectases* may develop too, which are similar lines on the chest. Both result from hormonal changes. These lines might fade or disappear after pregnancy. If they don't, they can be remedied through minor cosmetic procedures.

As for varicose veins, these tend to run in families. The veins carry blood back from all your extremities and your heart. The veins are designed with valves to prevent the blood from flowing backward in the veins. The valves need to work against gravity when they're carrying blood up the leg. Sometimes the vein valves are faulty or missing, which causes the blood to collect in areas where the gravity is most pronounced: the legs, rectum, or even vulva. These blood "pools" in the legs are noticeable, clumpy, and painful. Unfortunately, an expanded blood volume and an increase in progesterone just makes the condition more pronounced or will initially trigger it in women who haven't yet suffered from varicose veins but who are vulnerable to them.

Sometimes the only sign of varicose veins is the appearance of faint bluish lines in the areas where the blood pools. A bulging can crop up anywhere from the ankles to the vulva. In more severe cases, *thrombophlebitis* can develop, which means "inflammation of the vein due to blood clot." When a clot develops in a vein, this is known as *venous thrombosis.*

Clotting usually occurs in the postpartum period, but varicose veins can develop at any point in the pregnancy. The treatment revolves around prevention: maintaining a healthy pregnancy weight (overdoing it can worsen varicose veins); raising your legs while lying down (stick a pillow under them to get the blood flow moving); wearing support pantyhose (this keeps the blood circulating); avoiding restrictive clothing, such as tight belts, snug shoes, garters, girdles, and so on; and daily walks (about 20–30 minutes a day).

Things that Can Go Wrong

When something goes wrong during the second trimester of your pregnancy, it usually has to do with your health (gynecological or otherwise), premature labor, or a problem with the *placenta.* Space does not allow me to list *everything* that can go wrong, but the following are among the most common problems affecting average and high-risk pregnancies.

Bleeding.

In the second trimester, light or spotty bleeding is often caused by either an increasingly sensitive cervix, which may be irritated during an internal exam, or by sexual intercourse. Notify your doctor immediately.

Late Miscarriage.

Between the third month and 20th week of pregnancy, a spontaneous abortion is known as a late miscarriage. The symptoms are similar to the first trimester miscarriage variations. In many cases, a condition known as an "incompetent cervix" is responsible. This is when the cervix dilates prematurely and can't hold in the fetus. If an incompetent cervix is caught early enough, the cervix can be stitched up and the pregnancy can be resumed. Then, at labor, the stitches can be removed and a normal vaginal birth can take place. Some stitching techniques are permanent, however, and a cesarean section is required.

If the miscarriage is inevitable and can't be prevented, a D & C can be performed up until the 20th week. A miscarriage after 20 weeks is no longer a miscarriage. It graduates to either a premature birth or, in unfortunate cases, a stillbirth, discussed further below. You'll also need to follow emergency instructions outlined above.

Premature labor.

Premature labor is characterized by contractions accompanied by bloody discharge, anywhere from the 20th week to the 37th week. Other symptoms of premature labor are menstrual-like cramps, with possible diarrhea, nausea or indigestion, lower back pain, and all the other symptoms of labor discussed below. This is an emergency situation and can be treated with medications that postpone the labor. In the worst-case scenario, the baby is delivered prematurely and treated in a neonatal intensive care unit.

The Prenatal Exam and Prenatal Testing

Before we go on to the third trimester, let's discuss the prenatal exam. You'll need to be screened for a whole batch of STDs, genetic disorders, and other diseases, as well as have a complete physical. This can be done either just before you plan to get pregnant or right after you first discover the pregnancy. Once all these things are in order, you don't technically need to have a prenatal exam until at least 12 weeks into the pregnancy. As discussed earlier, depending on your health care system or plan, many obstetricians won't even schedule your appointment until this point. However, if you're seeing a private physician, he/she may encourage a prenatal exam in the first trimester. This is always a good idea because the sooner you see the doctor, the more accurately your pregnancy can be dated.

Whether you have your first prenatal exam at three months or four months, you'll begin to see the doctor every month thereafter, and sometimes more often if your pregnancy is a difficult one. A prenatal exam usually lasts about 10–15 minutes and consists of the following:

- Weight and blood pressure check (via scale and blood pressure instrument). This is a good time to bring up dietary questions and request an appointment with a nutritionist, if you haven't already.
- Urinalysis for sugar and protein levels.
- Fetal heartbeat check (by putting a stethoscope to the outside of your uterus).
- Size of your uterus. (Your doctor can do this just by feeling the outside of your uterus. If there's a question regarding your due date, an ultrasound may be necessary.
- Checking the height of the *top* of your uterus (also called the fundus).
- A visual inspection for edema and vein changes.
- Questions about your symptoms.
- Suggested remedies or safe medications for your symptoms, and possible follow-up visits in between your monthly checkups.
- Possible blood tests for certain conditions depending on your age, weight, and symptoms.

You shouldn't need an internal exam during a prenatal exam (unless your doctor suspects a problem and needs to check your cervix for some reason), nor will the exam change very much from month to month.

Contrary to what you might think, ultrasound testing is not necessary in a normal, routine pregnancy. However, most women will have it anyway for the reasons discussed below. For women older than 35 and for certain high-risk pregnancies, amniocentesis will be recommended but is also *not* imperative. Women do have a right to refuse amniocentesis for a variety of reasons, also outlined below. Some newer tests have been developed, however, that can screen for some of the same things as amniocentesis.

Ultrasound

In prenatal testing, ultrasound is also called *ultrasonography*. It is the use of an echo sounder to produce a picture of the baby *inside* the uterus. The way it works is that high-frequency, low-energy sound waves are used to scan your abdomen, reflecting the fetus's outline on an electronic screen through a series of bright dots. Most pregnant women can expect to have at least one ultrasound anywhere from the fourth month on. You will need to have a full bladder for the procedure. This entails drinking copious amounts of water about an hour before the procedure, which takes place either at the doctor's office (more likely in the United States) or at the birthing facility you chose (more likely in Canada). Jelly is rubbed all over your abdomen, and a probe is placed on the jellied area and moved around. The procedure takes about 30 minutes, and you may be uncomfortable because of your full bladder. In early pregnancy, scanning may be done with a vaginal probe and an empty bladder.

Although many women assume that ultrasound is completely safe and harmless, we still don't know if ultrasound carries risks that have not yet been published. Obviously, many women will want the experience of ultrasound because they can actually see the child in the womb and want to be reassured that everything is healthy. Ultrasounds are important if you have a high-risk pregnancy or have encountered a problem. Certainly, in these circumstances, the diagnostic benefits of ultrasound far outweigh any *possible, not-yet-published* risks affiliated with ultrasound. However, if you're having a routine, low-risk pregnancy, and you don't require an ultrasound other than for "curiosity" purposes, you may want to research the process more and rethink it. It's always crucial to ask your physician why he or she wants to perform an ultrasound and how frequently he or she will do one.

Here are some legitimate reasons for an ultrasound:

- To date the pregnancy when the dates of the last menstrual period are in question or unknown. This is done between 15 and 18 weeks of pregnancy or earlier. Ultrasound for this purpose could be easily eliminated by more careful charting of menstrual periods. (In early pregnancy, a vaginal scan would be better for this, however.)
- Your doctor may suspect developmental problems.
- As a diagnostic tool to help pin down abnormal bleeding, pains, or other suspicious symptoms at any time during the pregnancy.
- Your doctor may suspect a multiple birth.
- You are in a "high-risk pregnancy" category.

- Your doctor may suspect a structural problem with the uterus or other part that may cause problems during delivery.
- *You're* concerned and worried about the baby's development.

Depending on why the ultrasound is initially performed, you may need to have it repeated between 32 and 34 weeks.

Amniocentesis

Amniocentesis is always recommended to mothers who are over 35 or who are at high risk of giving birth to a baby with genetic or chromosomal disorders. The procedure involves using ultrasound to locate a pocket of fluid around the fetus. Then, a long needle is inserted through the abdomen into the amniotic sac, and amniotic fluid is withdrawn. Most of the time a small amount of local anesthetic is used. You will also need a full bladder for the procedure. The cells in the fluid are then grown in a laboratory and tested for chromosomal abnormalities. The sex of the baby can also be determined through amniocentesis. The results can take anywhere between three and four weeks. The procedure is done at 16 weeks to ensure the results are back by 20 weeks. That way, if there *is* a problem, you have time to terminate the pregnancy if you wish. Some research centers are performing amniocentesis as early as 14 weeks.

There are risks involved in amniocentesis. One in 100 normal fetuses is miscarried as a direct result of the procedure. Other reports indicate that the risk of miscarriage is as low as 1 in 500. The risk needs to be weighed against the general risk *overall* of a baby born with a deformity: about 4 in 100. Other uncommon side effects include a puncture of the placenta, the baby, or the mother's bladder, or an infection or leakage of the amniotic fluid.

Amniocentesis may make no sense under certain circumstances. For example, if you are adamantly opposed to abortion for any reason, or believe that your child deserves to live regardless of what kind of genetic disorders are found, there is no reason to have amniocentesis done except to prepare parents and family ahead of time and to make a decision not to do a cesarean section if the fetus goes into distress during labor. In this case the risks outweigh the benefits. However, even if you won't abort, you may wish to *prepare* for the outcome of the birth.

The following are legitimate candidates for amniocentesis:

- Women who are clearly at risk of having a child with a genetic disorder or birth defect. These problems include spinal chord defects, missing brain tissue, exposed spinal column, Tay-Sachs disease, and sickle cell anemia.

- Women who are over 35 or who are at risk for giving birth to a child with a chromosomal disorder, known as Down syndrome, a form of retardation. (Down syndrome children are now shown to have a much higher capacity to learn and develop than was once believed. You may need to research your decision to abort a Down syndrome child.) Ninety-five percent of all Down syndrome cases are age-related. At 30, your chances of having a Down syndrome child are 1 in 885 births; at 35, your chances are 1 in 365; at age 40, the chance goes way up to 1 in 109. This test also picks up other chromosomal abnormalities and would be recommended to someone with a previously affected infant or when either parent has a known chromosome disorder.
- Women known to be carriers of diseases linked with the female X chromosome, such as one type of muscular dystrophy and hemophilia. These diseases are passed on only to a male child, who in 50% of the cases will develop serious illnesses.
- Women who are diabetic. In the past, amniocentesis was done in the last months of pregnancy to determine the maturity of the baby's lungs. The information was used to determine whether inducing labor was necessary. Yet the tendency these days is to use ultrasound to date pregnancy and then simply monitor the fetus, allowing the labor to occur naturally. There is much less use of amniocentesis in diabetics unless some other condition makes early delivery likely.
- Women who are Rh negative and have produced antibodies that pose a danger to their babies. This is now an uncommon problem. If the baby has been affected, he or she may need an intravenous transfusion or early delivery, frequently by cesarean section with a transfusion after birth.

The following are legitimate reasons to refuse amniocentesis:

- You oppose abortion for ethical, moral, or religious reasons.
- You do not wish to risk miscarrying a normal fetus.
- You are comfortable accepting whatever fate is in store for you, and are not able to handle the emotional stress involved with the procedure, regardless of the outcome.

Alpha Fetoprotein Screening

Alpha fetoprotein (AFP) is a voluntary blood test you can request. It can be performed anywhere between the 14th and 20th week of pregnancy. AFP is a compound normally manufactured in the liver of the fetus, and it is an important carrier of molecules in the fetus's bloodstream. This protein is known as a *glycoprotein* that can be measured in both amniotic fluid and maternal serum. This test is often referred to as the "triple screen" because in many clinics it involves three separate tests for AFP, hCG levels, and a serum estrogen called estriol. From this triple screen, a calculation can be performed that will identify whether you're at risk for a Down syndrome pregnancy. It can also pick up Down syndrome in women under 35. If the alpha fetoprotein is elevated, it's possible that there may be neural tube defects. An ultrasound is then done to examine the anatomy of the fetus, and in some cases amniocentesis is recommended. If the level is low, this could indicate Down syndrome. A follow-up amniocentesis would then be done to confirm Down syndrome. However, there are a number of false positives and false negatives associated with this blood test, which make it necessary to follow up results with further testing. The test is not considered "conclusive" in any way; it merely identifies whether your pregnancy is at a higher risk for certain defects, and encourages you to seek other tests to confirm such suspicions. Elevated AFP sometimes is due to incorrect dating of the pregnancy or a multiple pregnancy—both of which can be determined with an ultrasound.

Chorionic Villus Sampling: The Amnio Alternative

If the idea of amniocentesis bothers you, chorionic villus sampling (CVS) is considered the amnio alternative. This is one of the newest prenatal tests around (developed in the late 1980s), and it's actually performed in the *first* trimester, between 10 and 12 weeks of pregnancy. With the help of ultrasound, a piece of placenta can actually be sampled. This is done by inserting a catheter through the vagina and into the uterus. In some cases, due to the location of the placenta, a needle is inserted into the uterus through the abdominal wall.

CVS can detect the same chromosomal defects as amniocentesis, but it cannot diagnose open neural tube defects. Depending on the type of analysis you need, results may be available within 24 hours or can take up to two weeks. Some doctors report that results can take as long as four weeks. However, you will need to have a serum AFP done again at 15–16 weeks if you go the CVS route.

There are risks. First, CVS carries a slightly higher risk of miscarriage than amniocentesis. *Your risk for miscarriage with CVS increases 2–4% over the natural risk for miscarriage during this trimester: one in six pregnancies.* Studies suggest that if the test is performed before 10 weeks, there can be an increased risk of fetal limb development problems.

It is also more difficult to interpret the results of CVS. Occasionally, chromosome variants, or mixtures of cell types, make interpretation difficult. A blood sample might be needed from both parents to see if there really is a problem.

Cordocentesis

Cordocentesis is a test that can sample some of the fetus's blood. This test is done in the second half of the pregnancy *usually when a fetal abnormality has already been detected via ultrasound.* Genetic studies are done to confirm or even pinpoint a problem. You also can get the results very quickly, in about 48 hours, so that you can make the proper decision about whether to terminate the pregnancy. This test is done by using ultrasound to identify the area where the umbilical cord inserts into the placenta. You'll receive a local anesthetic, and a small amount of fetal blood is withdrawn with a long, fine needle. After the procedure, the fetal heart rate will need to be observed for several minutes.

The risk is considered higher than that of amniocentesis. There may be signs of immediate fetal distress or premature labor. Again, this test is done only if a problem has already been identified. The procedure can also be used for intravenous transfusion in pregnancies affected by Rh incompatibility.

Terminating the Pregnancy

The purpose of prenatal testing is to tell you whether your baby will be "normal." Obviously, most women will be anxious about the results and will want to be comforted by the good news that all is well. However, bear in mind that there are countless *physical* deformities that are correctable with surgery; these options should be discussed with a neonatal specialist and factored into your decision.

If amniocentesis confirms Down syndrome or another chromosomal abnormality, you'll need to discuss with your doctor *exactly* how your baby will be affected. Attitudes toward persons with Down syndrome are changing, and many families choose to welcome these children with their special needs, which can include mild to moderate retardation and physical and medical problems. For other families, abortion might be the best choice. Other chromosomal abnormalities cause conditions that are not salvageable. Being aware of the problem ahead of time can prepare you for the likelihood of stillbirth or neonatal death. In these cases, many parents consider pregnancy termination (even though they would not in other circumstances). It's also important to note that if the decision is made to allow the pregnancy to continue, a futile cesarean for distress of the fetus during labor may be avoided. Whatever you decide, remember that the decision to abort or *not* to abort is a personal and private choice that has more to do with your civil rights as an individual than it does with your health.

The Third Trimester

Once you've made it into the "home stretch," the risks of complications go up again. This time most of the problems that occur are related to labor complications: premature labor and delivery, delivery complications, cesarean sections, and so on. Other problems revolve around your baby's oxygen supply; if it's interrupted in any way via cord complications, for example, a normal, uneventful pregnancy can result in a stillbirth. Hypertension is also a common problem at this stage. This is why a technologically advanced birthing facility is so important. Many of these problems are expertly and speedily dealt with when they come up, to ensure both your own and your baby's health.

How Does It Feel?

By this stage your uterus has become very large. The baby's movements are visible, and you'll begin to experience what are known as *Braxton Hicks contractions*. You'll feel periodic tightening in the uterus that makes it feel like a kind of drum. There will also be an increase in urinary pressure, and you'll need to urinate more frequently, as you did in the first trimester.

You'll also experience more shortness of breath because the baby is pressing on your diaphragm. Once the baby moves down more into your pelvis in the last month or so, this will ease off. This is known as *lightening* because some women report that they actually *feel* much lighter as a result—but don't count on it!

You'll also have more difficulty sleeping. First, depending on your size, you may not be able to find a comfortable sleeping position. As a result, you'll be tossing and turning all night. Second, you'll become more anxious and excited about the baby and may not be able stop your mind from racing in a hundred different directions. All this boils down to one word: *fatigue.* Some women find adjustable beds helpful, which you can rent for this last period.

Because you'll gain an additional 10–15 pounds in this trimester alone, you'll become uncoordinated, feel awkward, and may experience backaches and leg pains. You may also experience a type of joint looseness caused by progesterone, which relaxes certain muscles (preparing your body for labor).

Finally, all the second-trimester health problems you may have developed will persist: edema, venous changes, autoimmune disorders, and so on. Believe it or not, some women *still* suffer from morning sickness at this stage! By now you'll have learned to live with these changes, but you may need to consult with your doctor if symptoms become really uncomfortable.

Things That Can Go Wrong

Bleeding.

Heavier bleeding at this stage is usually caused by a *low-lying placenta* or *placenta previa.* In this case, the placenta is a little too close to the mouth of the uterus and may cover the cervix. The bleeding is bright red and painless. It starts out of the blue and can be triggered by coughing, straining, or sex. This condition is diagnosed via ultrasound. If it happens in the second trimester, the placenta may "move" away from the cervix by this point and can correct itself. A combination of bed rest, a variety of vitamin or dietary supplements, hospitalization for bed rest and monitoring, and even transfusions may be required. Sometimes the pregnancy is kept going until about the 36th week, and you're then delivered by cesarean. The baby will be kept in a neonatal wing until it is strong enough to survive at home. In the worst-case scenario, a very premature delivery may be necessary.

One in four cases of mid-to-late pregnancy bleeding is caused by *premature separation of the placenta* or *abruptio placenta,* in which the placenta separates itself prematurely from the uterus. In 90% of the cases, mother and baby are fine. The bleeding is like a light or even heavy menstrual flow and may contain clots. You may experience cramping or mild cramps or pain in the abdomen. In more severe cases, bleeding is heavy, which could cause fetal death and maternal blood problems. Cocaine use during pregnancy can cause this. The remedy is bed rest, careful monitoring, and, in the worst-case scenario, induced labor and premature delivery, or a cesarean section.

Warning signs at this stage are symptoms of labor as well as an absence of fetal movement. Any perceived decrease in fetal movment should be reported ASAP. Often, the fetus is just sleeping, *but do not take any chances.* You'll no doubt be wondering, *Is it alive or not?* which all mothers go through. You might want to purchase an actual stethoscope earlier on in the pregnancy and have your doctor show you and your partner how to use it and what to listen for. Remember, 30 years ago this was the only kind of prenatal "monitoring" that was done. You'll want to be able to check for the heartbeat and observe any abnormalities. Toxemia is another big problem, characterized by water retention, hypertension, and protein in the urine.

Premature labor and delivery.

There's no such thing as miscarriage at this stage. When you "miscarry" in late pregnancy, you graduate to "premature labor." This means that for a variety of reasons, your body isn't able to carry full term and begins to give birth to the baby. Reasons for this include infections, hypertension, drugs and smoking, placental problems, uterine abnormalities, and cervical incompetence, but most causes are unknown. Premature labor is no different from any *other* labor; it just happens before the baby is as physically able to exist in the outside world as it is at nine months, but it's considered one of the biggest problems for obstetricians in the U.S., where neonatal technology is very expensive. Labor is discussed below.

Stillbirth.

Stillbirth is pretty rare these days, particularly in facilities equipped with advanced fetal monitoring equipment. When a fetus dies in the womb, its oxygen supply is somehow cut off. During a normal labor and delivery, cord complications are anticipated, and the delivery staff is prepared for any number of problems. Women are monitored for this, and if it does happen, an emergency cesarean section is done.

If the amniotic environment becomes hostile for any reason, labor is induced to prevent a *potential* stillbirth. This can happen because of leakage of amniotic fluid, placental malfunctions, an overdue pregnancy, toxemia, or a variety of reasons too numerous to list.

Sometimes, a perfectly healthy baby, born alive, may have problems when the cord is cut. Its lungs or heart may fail to oxygenate its system. In a hospital setting, the baby would be given oxygen immediately and speedily resuscitated.

The first scenario *can* happen at some point in the second or third trimester, well before labor complications are even a consideration. Should you experience a stillbirth, you *will* need to give birth to that fetus. Labor is usually induced as soon as the tragedy is confirmed. You will definitely need to seek out counseling, and must expect to grieve properly for that child. You might also find it helpful to have an autopsy conducted to find out exactly what happened. Naming the child and properly burying or cremating it is the normal practice. Stillbirth is considered one of the most difficult and traumatic experiences a woman will ever go through. As a result, you will need to surround yourself with supportive people and come to terms with the loss before you try to conceive again. Clergy may be very helpful to you during these times. For more information, see the sources at the back of the book on pregnancy loss.

A Normal Labor and Delivery

Whether you experience labor prematurely, right on schedule, or well past your due date, no two labors are alike. The following *briefly* describes what you can expect in a normal, routine labor and delivery. Keep in mind that there are entire books on the subject of labor and delivery, so don't consider this section anything but incredibly *basic!*

Preparing for Labor

By the sixth or seventh month, you should consider beginning some sort of childbirth class with your partner that will explain "coaching" and labor, show films, and discuss all kinds of labor and delivery scenarios, *including what to do in emergency situations.* Childbirth classes are definitely one of the best ways to prepare yourself and your partner for labor and delivery. However, many women do find that these classes are a joke. This can happen if you have a poor instructor or if the class has a weak "curriculum" and teaches you nothing that you don't *already* know from articles, magazines, or books. Make sure that the class is teaching you the kind of childbirth method you intend to *use*. If you're against Lamaze, for instance, don't take a Lamaze *class*.

To avoid bad classes, make sure you go to one that your practitioner or midwife *personally* recommends, or that is provided at your birthing facility. Make sure the instructor is qualified and certified by the International Childbirth Education Association, not just "the mother of six." Just because the instructor has children doesn't guarantee that she can *teach*. She (or even *he)* needs to have teaching and communication skills, and some medical training (nurse, midwife, and so forth). You can also sit in on some classes before you sign up to test out various centers or instructors.

Essentially, there are three basic "methods" out there: Grantly Dick-Read, Lamaze, and Bradley, all named after the practitioners who invented various techniques, from breathing, to working with pain, to teaching fathers to be coaches and active participants in the labor process. Other classes are more health-care oriented, borrowing techniques from all three methods, tailoring your class to the newest technology and information available, and, if given by your birthing facility, tailoring information specifically to *it*.

Labor isn't a "swift" process. Unlike what sitcoms lead us to believe, most women have *time* to get to the hospital, even if they go into a "sudden labor." If you need to be induced, you'll experience all phases of labor in the hospital and report to the hospital feeling fine. Cesarean sections are discussed below. Labor is divided into three segments: pre-labor, early labor, and active. Then, you "graduate" to delivery.

Pre-labor

Pre-labor can begin anywhere in the last few weeks or last days of pregnancy. Of course, many women will experience this prematurely or past their due date. This is when you experience the "lightening" described above, and begin to feel more pressure on your bladder. You may also get diarrhea and possibly a severe backache, both precursors to early labor. The diarrhea is "nature's enema" and is your body's way of emptying everything out before actual labor begins. You'll also feel the Braxton Hicks contractions more frequently (these are painless).

Your cervix at this stage softens and may start to thin out a little, which allows it to dilate (open up) slightly. You will also get some mucusy, bloody discharge. This is charmingly referred to as "bloody show." All this means is that the mucus plug that has been sealing the cervical opening is now pink or blood-streaked and is leaking discharge.

As the baby's head presses down against the amniotic membranes containing fluid, the membranes may break. This is what's known as "breaking your water." This is the classic pre-labor symptom. Women expect this event to be like a flood of water suddenly rushing out of their vaginas and it frequently happens this way, but the fluid may also just *trickle* out. It normally will be clear, odorless, and milky. Some women think that they've wet their pants when this happens. If your water doesn't break at this point, it will probably happen during more active labor. In other words, if it doesn't break now, don't worry about it. Membranes more commonly rupture after the onset of contractions than before. If membranes rupture more than 24 hours before contractions start, this is called "premature rupture of membranes."

Now is a good time to get ready to go to the hospital! Some women may choose to stay home until active labor begins. This is an individual decision and depends on how "high risk" your pregnancy is, how anxious you are, and a hundred other things you'll have been prepared for by your practitioner. For the purposes of this chapter, I'll assume that all phases of labor take place in the hospital. If your water has broken, you'll need to follow some special, common-sense hygiene practices at this point. Showers, no baths, is an obvious one. Your practitioner and midwife will give you more instructions as well. Your doctor or midwife (or whoever is on staff at the hospital) will also want to examine you vaginally to see how much your cervix is dilating. The "real stuff" of labor, the more active phases, begin between 12 and 24 hours after your water breaks. The "bloody show" is also a sign that it's beginning.

Early Labor

Pre-labor slowly unfolds into early labor. This phase lasts about seven or eight hours. You may not even notice a "change" in the process, however. Early labor and active labor are also known as the *first stage* of labor. Early labor is characterized by contractions that cause the cervix to dilate about 3–4 centimeters. These contractions can feel sort of wavelike. They build up and then recede. They will be mildly painful and begin in the lower back. They can also feel like heavy menstrual cramps. At this point you may want to start practicing what you learned in your childbirth classes in terms of breathing, relaxing, and so on. The contractions will be anywhere from 5 to 20 minutes apart, become more intense each time they occur, last anywhere from 30 to 45 seconds, get longer each time they occur, and get closer together. (If you're not in the hospital already, you'll need to go in *for sure* when the contractions are about 5 minutes apart.) The contractions may also become more pronounced with walking. You'll be able to sleep, eat, and engage in normal activities throughout this phase.

Active Labor

Active labor is similar to early labor but is *far more pronounced.* This phase lasts from 3 to 5 hours. If you're sleeping, for example, you'll be waked up by the intensity of these contractions. Now the contractions occur every 2 to 4 minutes and last up to 60 seconds. They may be moderately or extremely painful depending on the woman. At this phase, keep emptying your bladder regularly. If you want to have an *epidural,* a painkiller that numbs you from the breasts down, take it now! You will have a choice and have the right to accept or refuse it. This will take the edge off your pain, but you may want to feel everything. With an epidural you'll also need to remain in bed because your legs will now be numb. Epidural or not, you may also get an incredible urge to push, which mirrors the urge to push out a bowel movement. You may also start to feel either very warm or even get chills. At this stage, your nurse, midwife, or practitioner will continuously check your cervical dilation and your baby's heartbeat. When an epidural is administered, an intravenous line and electronic fetal heart monitoring will be started, but this can also be done earlier. You'll also need to use a bedpan if you've had the epidural.

The Transition Phase

The transition phase takes you into delivery and lasts anywhere from 30 to 90 minutes. You may have been in active labor for approximately 3 hours now. You may be tired, abusive, and frustrated; have no clue what time it is; may be shaking, hiccupping, vomiting, or having chills; have cold feet, dry mouth, and lips; and are hyperventilating, moaning, crying, or screaming. Meanwhile, you now have a *TREMENDOUS* urge to push and you will feel rectal pressure. Your contractions are the most intense now, occurring every 30 seconds and lasting 90 seconds, and your cervix is almost fully dilated. Some women may want to go to the toilet, which will help relax them and get the pushing going.

Delivery: Bearing Down

Now you can push. Essentially, instead of holding back the urge to push, you'll actually get to do it. This is tough work. Your face will turn red and you'll be soaked with perspiration. You should only push when you feel the *urge* to push, however. Try not to force it. The uterus will contract on its own and help the baby out anyway, so waiting for the urge will make the delivery easier for you. In fact, you might be so overwhelmed by the urge to push that you'll be frightened by it and hold back.

Whatever delivery position you've chosen, you'll be in it by now although you may need to switch if the position isn't as comfortable as you planned. Your pushing may "push out" some stool (*everyone* does this—don't be embarrassed). At this phase, the hardest part is pushing out the head. As the head emerges, you may feel intense burning and stinging sensations, feeling as though you are about to "tear apart." You won't. The vagina is like a huge elastic band that stretches for this. In fact, you might be coerced at this point to consent to an *episiotomy*. Once you read the next section, you may want to resist *this* urge in particular.

The Episiotomy

An episiotomy is a minor surgical procedure where an incision is made in the *perineum*, the area between your rectum and vagina. It's done to enlarge the opening for vaginal births, making it easier for the baby's head to come out. You will probably be given a local anesthetic for this between contractions, but won't need it if you had an epidural. However, after the birth, the area is frozen via local anesthetic and you'll be sewn back together.

On the general consent form you sign when you register as a maternity patient, there is usually a space for your signature, giving your consent to an episiotomy. Before you sign it, you should discuss *alternatives* with your practitioner or midwife, and find out when the procedure is truly necessary. Some women find this an uncomfortable procedure and a hindrance to the overall childbirth experience. In addition, the procedure is only necessary about 25% of the time, even though it's almost *always* performed. Why? All doctors will tell you that they perform an episiotomy only when necessary. This is not so. First, the doctor who tells you this may not be *delivering* you. Meanwhile, the resident or intern who's on call when you go into labor may do an episiotomy for any number of reasons, usually having to do with a mistrust of natural "vaginal engineering." The real truth is, many doctors have never completely *witnessed* natural childbirth and have been taught in medical school that the vagina cannot stretch to the extent that it needs to.

This just isn't true. Most vaginas have an incredible "Lycra" quality to them. But doctors don't usually wait around in a delivery to witness this; they just make the "cut," which they consider minor.

A *routine* episiotomy cuts through skin, vagina mucosa, and three layers of muscle in an otherwise sensitive area. The side effects include pain, bleeding, a breakdown of stitches, and delayed healing. The pain afterward can be enough to keep you from sitting comfortably for several weeks, which is the last thing you need when you're nursing a newborn. One of the few studies done on the side effects of this procedure shows that 6% of women who had episiotomies suffer from persistent pain during sexual intercourse.

Remember, midwives are trained to deliver babies without the assistance of surgery. That's why a good midwife, *combined* with a good hospital, is the best system. The midwife will "watch over you" during delivery and can help gauge whether your vagina *can* make the stretch it was designed to make. Many doctors believe that a little natural tearing, which will often take place without the episiotomy, not only will heal much quicker than a surgical "tearing," but is less painful.

When *is* an episiotomy necessary? Any medical emergency during delivery can be reason for episiotomy, for example, when the baby's heartbeat becomes abnormal during pushing; to facilitate the delivery of a premature or breech baby; and whenever forceps are necessary (for instance, if the head is in an awkward position). The procedure is also necessary when the delivery of the baby's head is progressing at a rate or manner that will badly tear the perineum, or when the vagina *isn't* making the stretch. But for the majority of normal, vaginal deliveries, episiotomy is *not* necessary.

The Cesarean Birth

A Cesarean section, or C-section, is a surgical procedure that is essentially abdominal delivery. This is considered major pelvic surgery that usually involves either a spinal or epidural (only in some cases is a general anesthetic necessary). A vertical or horizontal incision is made just above your pubic hair line (you may need to be shaved for this). Then the surgeon (usually) cuts horizontally through the uterine muscle and eases the baby out. Sometimes, this second cut is vertical, known as the "classic incision." It is this *second cut,* into the uterine muscle, that will allow a VBAC (vaginal birth after cesarean). With a horizontal cut, women have gone on to have normal second vaginal births; with the classic cut, the scar is less stable and will mean that for *you,* "once a C-section, always a C-section" is a reality.

In some instances, you'll know in advance whether you need to have a cesarean section. Your pelvis may be too small; you may have irreparable scarring on your cervix from previous pelvic surgery that will prevent dilation; or an emergency situation may be detected in utero (in the womb) that requires the fetus to be taken out immediately.

Usually, the problem doesn't come up until you're in labor, which entails a dizzying array of complications too numerous to list, that will necessitate a cesarean.

There are, of course, many *unnecessary* cesarean sections performed. Most *second* cesareans are not necessary, for instance, if the uterine cut was horizontal. Another common practice is to perform a C-section when a woman fails to go into labor after being induced. Reasons for being induced usually have to do with progressing past the due date. In this case, if the fetus isn't in distress, you may want to wait or get a second opinion. In a U.S. study, situations in which a C-section was performed depended more on the doctor than on any other single factor. The rate of C-sections varied from 19 to 42%, according to the individual doctor's preference. This is a huge discrepancy. What it boils down to is the *doctor's* definition of *emergency,* which may arise in the event of prolapsed cord, fetal distress, failure to progress, placental complications, or primary genital herpes, to name just a *few* of a dozen good reasons why a C-section is performed. And, no competent doctor will delay a C-section if he or she thinks that the labor is endangering the baby's or mother's health.

To avoid an unnecessary procedure, consult with your practitioner and midwife *before* the third trimester. Find out what situations truly warrant a C-section, and whether you're a VBAC candidate. If you're experiencing a difficult or high-risk pregnancy, or will be having a multiple birth, you *may* be more likely to have the procedure than a woman with a low-risk pregnancy.

A Word About the Placenta

This is known as the "afterbirth," "birth of placenta," or just the "third stage of labor." In a vaginal delivery, episiotomy or not, after the birth of the baby, your uterus will contract enough to loosen the placenta from the uterine wall. These contractions may be painful, but they are mild in comparison to what you just went through. Besides, you'll be so busy with your newborn, you probably won't even notice them. The placenta will then slip out with one or two pushes. The uterus than continues to contract against exposed blood vessels from where the placenta used to be, as a natural way to control bleeding.

Postpartum Issues

There are a number of postpartum issues you'll need to be concerned with. Because of space restrictions, these issues are covered thoroughly in *The Pregnancy Sourcebook,* but unfortunately, not in this chapter.

Review some of the hygiene rules in chapter 6. To avoid an infection, you'll need to follow special precautions after your cervix has been dilated. You'll also need to consult with your practitioner and midwife about exercises that can help strengthen your vaginal and abdominal muscles, as well as follow some dietary precautions if you've chosen to breastfeed. Remember that breastfeeding will also cause your uterus to contract and shrink back to normal size.

If you've had either an episiotomy or a C-section, you'll need to find out about postoperative healing and hygiene and whether certain activities should be restricted.

You might have heard of the infamous "postpartum blues," which is sometimes confused with postpartum depression. First, normal fatigue and feelings of "let down," in that you've been excited and preparing for the birth, are common and normal. True postpartum psychological and emotional disturbances range from what's known as *"maternal blues"* to true *postpartum depression,* where one experiences symptoms of major depression or clinical depression, to something known as *postpartum psychosis,* the kind of diagnosis made in a situation where a woman *kills* her newborn, believing that it is evil or abnormal in some way. Postpartum psychosis occurs in 2 out of every 1,000 deliveries, not as uncommon as one is led to believe, but 80 percent of all women will suffer from maternal blues after delivery. Maternal blues are common, nothing to worry about, and transitory. It usually occurs within the first 10 days (averaging 3 to 4 days) after delivery. Symptoms are frequent crying episodes, feelings of sadness, low energy, anxiety, insomnia, restlessness, and irritability. These symptoms are seen in all classes and cultures, and there's no specific link between these symptoms and hormonal changes. Women who experience these feelings should take comfort in that these feelings are *normal* and will pass.

If you are going to breastfeed your baby, first review chapter 1 to find out how the body actually produces milk. Second, review "The Big Joke: Fibrocystic Breast Disease" in chapter 8 to find out more about nipple infections and bacterial infections you're prone to as a result of breastfeeding. Chapter 8 also discusses milk cysts, which are common.

There are numerous benefits to breastfeeding: it's more nutritious, it's cheap, it's convenient and safe, it's instant, fast food, it's available for as long as you need it, it helps your uterus shrink, it helps you lose weight, it helps you bond, and it can be done by working mothers with the aid of breast pumps. Breastfeeding has been touted as being a "natural contraceptive." *This isn't true.* It has *some* contraceptive effect in the first three or four months, but it's not 100%. You'll need to practice a barrier method or use condoms, unless you don't care whether you get pregnant so soon after delivery. Review chapter 4 for safe contraception methods. Breastfeeding is obviously a huge topic that is covered in more detail in *The Pregnancy Sourcebook* and exhaustively in *The Breastfeeding Sourcebook.*

As I've stressed throughout this chapter, pregnancy is a far-from-perfect process and is always risky. Not all pregnancies result in a child, and not all successful pregnancies result in a *perfect* child. Not all pregnancies produce only *one* child. Not all pregnancies are wanted. Not all pregnancies are achieved through *natural* means. And most important, not all mothers necessarily *experience* pregnancy. These are just some of the issues facing potential parents. To learn more, see chapter 11 and chapter 12.

CHAPTER 11

Abortion: The Right to Know

Imagine what it would be like to live in a society in which sperm is considered sacred and a potential *life*. Any kind of activity that "wastes" sperm, such as male masturbation or fellatio, is banned. In this culture, men are expected to "save" their sperm and ejaculate it into a woman's vagina only during the act of intercourse. Consequently, male masturbation, fellatio, anal sex, male homosexuality, and, certainly contraceptive use become synonymous with *murder*. Men who don't obey the rules are hunted down, tortured, and killed. As a result, underground "organizations" are formed where these forbidden practices are performed secretly. These organizations are public health disaster areas, breeding grounds for diseases and bacteria. Many men and women die from infections they contract while visiting these places; they cannot get medical treatment, fearing that they would call attention to their murderous acts of sperm wasting. (Women who participate in these activities are considered "accessories" to murder.) Over time, this society becomes hotly divided. People of both sexes stand on either side of the issue: pro–sperm waste activists and anti–sperm waste activists battle it out in the streets, on television, and in the headlines. Sperm wasting becomes a platform for politicians and is legally debated in the courts. Ultimately, the issue that emerges is whether one is entitled to *biological privacy.*

Thankfully, no man is subjected to the absurd puritanical society I just described. What he does with his sperm is his own business, and whether he chooses to waste it or not, is a *private* matter, not a political one.

Until recently, however, women did *not* enjoy the same rights to *their* biological privacy. What a woman chose to do with the contents of her uterus was . . . *legislated!* Until the late 1970s, many North American women who wanted an abortion were forced to go underground. Consequently, many women died from infections resulting from unsanitary conditions or improper procedures. Even today, although abortion is legal in North America, it remains a political issue, not a health issue. This is unfortunate indeed. As a result, women don't have enough information about abortion procedures to make an informed decision. Worse, women are not even given *choices* about which procedures are even available to them.

This chapter provides guidelines for seeking abortion counseling and choosing an abortion clinic, where to go for an abortion, who is qualified to perform the procedures, the current abortion procedures available, what the procedures entail, the risks involved with the procedures, and how to take care of yourself afterward.

The Therapeutic Abortion

Abortion is far from a dirty word. Medically, the word *abortion* simply refers to pregnancy loss before the 20th week. This may be either a *spontaneous abortion,* also known as miscarriage (which includes *complete, missed,* or *incomplete abortion,* discussed in chapter 10), or a *therapeutic abortion (TA),* a deliberate termination of pregnancy for medical or social reasons. Yet among the general lay public, there is a *huge* misconception about what a therapeutic abortion really means. Most people think that a therapeutic abortion refers only to the kind of procedure sought out, for instance, by a couple who discovers they are carrying a deformed or defected fetus. *This just isn't so.* A teenager who hasn't the financial means to support a child or the support structures to take care of the child, will also be a therapeutic abortion candidate. A woman who was impregnated during a rape will be a therapeutic abortion candidate. Finally, a woman who simply does not *desire* a child, for *any combination of reasons,* is also a candidate for a therapeutic abortion. The abortion is "therapeutic" because it *enhances* the quality of life for the mother and prevents the *inevitability* of a life of poverty, unreasonable struggle, or unreasonable trauma for both the mother and the unborn, unwanted fetus.

The surgical abortion *procedure* you undergo will depend on whether you're in your first or second trimester of pregnancy. After the pregnancy has progressed *beyond* a certain number of weeks in the second trimester (usually 24 weeks, but the limit varies in your state or province), you will *not* be able to elect to terminate the pregnancy legally. But all women in North America can expect to have a legal abortion *up until at least their 20th week of pregnancy.*

Currently, about 1.5 million abortions are performed annually in the United States alone. People who are ethically opposed to abortion may find it interesting to learn that this statistic hasn't changed much since the days when abortion was illegal. In the 1950s, about one million illegal abortions were performed. Factor in population changes over the last 40 years, and *you have roughly the same abortion statistic for 1950 as you do for 1990.* Why?

Abortion is clearly not an easy decision for any woman, but when she decides to abort, she considers the decision a *necessary* step she must take to preserve her welfare and happiness. Legalizing abortion has not made it a more appealing or easier option; it has only made it a safer and noncriminal act.

Making the Decision

Every woman will have different reasons for choosing a therapeutic abortion. Five of the most common reasons are listed below.

1. *Contraceptive failure.* Obviously, any woman who practices some form of contraception does not *intend* to get pregnant. This is reason enough for an abortion, but you'll need to review why your method failed, and consider using a better method next time around (see chapter 4 for more information on contraception).
2. *Socioeconomic concerns.* This would include the inability to support a child financially due to sudden unemployment or separation from a partner. You may have indeed planned, or not *prevented* pregnancy, but find that your personal circumstances may have changed drastically.
3. *Medical conditions where continuing the pregnancy endangers the mother's life.* You may have developed a heart condition or a severe illness

during the pregnancy, or discovered that you are HIV positive, and now have to choose between your life or that of the unborn child.
4. *The pregnancy is the result of rape or incest.*
5. *The fetus is malformed or will be born with an inevitable genetic/chromosomal deformity.* Review the prenatal exam and testing section in chapter 10.

It might surprise you to learn that, whether you've *elected* to abort or have miscarried, universal feelings of sadness and loss are natural and should be expected. There are no "good" or "bad" reasons for choosing an abortion. What *is* important, however, is that you're *clear* about why you want to abort *before* you undergo the procedure. It's difficult to predict how you will feel once the pregnancy is terminated, but studies indicate that there *are* certain groups of women who will suffer *more* emotional side effects of the procedure than others. These include:

- Women who abort for medical reasons (see above).
- Women under 20 years of age. (Many of these women are not emotionally mature enough to handle the enormity of the decision.)
- Women with poor support systems in place. (Do you feel isolated? Do you feel as though you have no supportive friends or family around you to validate your decision?)
- Women who have been pressured into making the decision. (Have you been pressured by your boyfriend or parents?)
- Women who are clearly torn between terminating and continuing the pregnancy. (Your mind says yes, your heart says no, or vice versa.)
- Women with a past history of psychiatric illness. (Do you have a history of bulimia, anorexia nervosa, or clinical or major depression? Are you taking lithium for any reason?)
- Women who are not psychologically stable. (Are you recovering from any kind of addiction? Are you currently using drugs or alcohol to escape your problems? Have you ever required therapy for any reason?)

If you fall into one of the above categories, you should *definitely* seek out counseling prior to undergoing the procedure. A qualified counselor should help you be confident in your decision, not try to convince you to either terminate or continue the pregnancy. The counselor will also help you come to terms with normal feelings of guilt but will also validate your reasons for the decision.

Finding a Counselor

Until the Clinton administration took office in 1993, it was illegal in the United States to provide abortion counseling to women who went to federally funded clinics or agencies. Privately owned clinics or doctors in private practice were free to provide or recommend counseling, however. (Canadian women have never been subjected to such insane legislation.)

This outrageous law, known as the "gag rule," has now been lifted. Today, any private or federally funded hospital in North America has counselors on staff who are experienced with abortion patients. Any abortion clinic should also have counselors on staff or at least refer you to a counselor. Any primary care physician or gynecologist has a legal and moral responsibility to discuss abortion options with you, and refer you to a qualified counselor as well.

Both Americans and Canadians can also call the National Abortion Federation in Washington, D.C. at 202-667-5881. The federation has a toll-free hotline that gives out referrals for abortion services. In the United States, the number is 1-800-772-9100. In Canada, the number is 1-800-424-2280. This organization operates a massive database that contains the names of abortion clinics throughout Canada and the United States. You can call anonymously and just tell the operator where you're calling from. You'll then be provided with a list of clinics in your area. Counseling is available at any of these clinics.

Know Your Options

Abortion is not the definitive solution for every unwanted pregnancy. That's why it's important to explore *options* to abortions first, to make sure that an abortion is what you *really* want. In general, these are the groups who may not benefit from an abortion:

- *Women who are morally or ethically opposed to abortion.* For example, even though you *know* you're carrying a child that is malformed, you may not be able to go through with terminating the pregnancy. The psychological trauma to you may be lessened by giving birth to the child and letting fate decide the outcome.

- *Women who don't feel informed enough about their options.* Have you considered adoption, or looked into social programs that might support you until you get back on your feet? Have you researched your decision to abort? Are you familiar with what the procedure entails? Have you explored all other solutions?
- *In most states, women under age who cannot obtain consent from their parents or legal guardians.* Unless you have consent, you'll be forced to get the abortion illegally, and could wind up getting an abortion from an incompetent doctor or under unsanitary conditions. That means you could suffer from serious postoperative infections. Not all states require parental consent, however.

There are viable options to an abortion, depending on who you are. In white, middle-class North America, there is currently an infertility epidemic, which is creating a great demand from childless couples for white, healthy newborns. (Some couples may sponsor you through the pregnancy, paying your medical bills, buying you the necessary groceries, and so forth; others may be willing to pay you a lump sum, *but make sure you do this legally through a legitimate agency or lawyer. Beware of the underground "baby market!")*

If the child isn't healthy or is a visible minority, it will be far more difficult to find a home for that child.

If you are concerned that you may not have the support networks in place to take care of the child, have you exhausted supportive networks in your family? How about the father's family, or the father himself? Have you looked into social programs available to you that are provided by your government or community?

If the concern is financial, have you looked into programs that will support you while you retrain, upgrade your education, or finish school? Government programs are now in place that enforce child support by deducting money from the father's wages.

You might want to call the Planned Parenthood Federation of America (or its Canadian counterpart) to request counseling regarding alternatives to abortion. Look in your local phone directory for the chapter nearest you. As a last resort, you could also visit a pro-life organization that can tell you what options *it* recommends. (Be careful, though. They might show you gruesome pictures of aborted fetuses or preach fundamentalist dogma to you.) Typically, pro-life organizations have hefty funding made available to them through private benefactors. But *that* money could be passed on to *you* in the form of financial support, while you get your life together enough to take care of a child.

Whatever the outcome, making a decision about abortion can be stressful. In general, studies on the psychological complications of abortion report that most women suffer a minimal degree of psychiatric stress. Although there *is* a natural grieving process that *all* women can expect to go through, regardless of how secure they are in their decision, there is no *permanent* trauma connected to abortion for most women.

On the flip side, some women may feel relief and experience *immediate* psychological benefits after the abortion procedure. This was the experience of one women I interviewed, who recalls that she felt "elated" after her abortion. This particular woman was about 25 at the time, middle-class, and educated. When she got pregnant after an encounter with a casual lover, she was immediately "repulsed" by the idea of the fetus within her. Having neither the desire nor the inclination to *ever* marry or become a parent, this woman recalls feeling bewildered at the sight of the frightened and almost tormented faces of the women in the waiting room of her abortion clinic. She wondered why they weren't as happy about terminating their pregnancies as she was. She recalls that the procedure *she* underwent was painless, psychologically effortless, and welcomed as a tremendous weight off her shoulders. Today, in her early 30s, this woman has *never* regretted her decision and is convinced that her abortion saved *her* life.

Who Should Perform Your Abortion?

An abortion procedure in the first trimester basically involves variations of the D & C (dilation and curettage) procedure described in chapter 7. (The specific variations are described further below.) Obviously, the *best* person to perform an abortion is a board-certified gynecologist (see chapter 3). Of all abortions done in hospitals or clinics, 75% are either performed or supervised by gynecologists. Most abortions in the United States are done in free-standing centers by gynecologists. If you're having your abortion done in the hospital, a gynecologist will either perform the procedure or supervise an intern (a licensed M.D. who's in his or her first year of practice) or an OB-Gyn resident (a general practitioner training to be a gynecologist) who is doing the procedure.

The remaining 25% of abortions are done by family practitioners or general practitioners. This is fine as long as they're *trained* to do abortions. In fact, many family or general practitioners exclusively do abortions and may even head an abortion clinic. In these cases, they may actually have *more* experience in abortions than an average gynecologist. Abortions do involve minor surgery, and as a result carry a certain degree of risk and potential complications. Any doctor experienced in abortion will be able to handle these problems. Your medical (and gynecological) history, current health, and emotional state all factor into the outcome of the procedure as well.

Depending on your reasons for the abortion, your own gynecologist or primary care physician (if he or she is trained) may be perfectly willing to perform the abortion. Be forewarned, however, that many doctors are ethically opposed to abortions and will not perform them. To find a qualified abortion practitioner, call the National Abortion Federation at 1-800-772-9100 (U.S.) or 1-800-424-2280 (Canada), or call the Planned Parenthood Federation of America (your local chapter is listed in the White Pages). Either organization can refer you to an abortion clinic, and you can then call the clinic to find out the credentials of the abortion practitioners there.

The following professionals are *not* appropriate abortionists:

- Nurses (but they can assist and help you through postoperative care)
- Physician assistants (they can assist and help you through postoperative care)
- Certified nurse-midwives or independent midwives (they can also assist and help you through postoperative care)
- A medical student or clerk (a clerk is a fourth-year medical student.)
- Any non-M.D. health practitioner (never!)

The following people are qualified to perform the abortion *under supervision*. In other words, a senior, experienced doctor must be in the room or at least in the same building to manage any complications that arise.

- A hospital intern (you'll encounter this only in a hospital)
- A hospital OB-Gyn resident (again, you'll find this only in a hospital)
- A physician assistant, *well trained* in abortion procedures (*Vermont only)*
- A certified nurse or certified nurse midwife, *well trained* in abortion procedures (*Vermont only*)

In a typical abortion scenario, unless you live in a large metropolitan center, you'll end up in an abortion clinic that is licensed by the state or province. These clinics need to follow the same guidelines as any hospital. An abortion is a simple procedure that doesn't require a genius IQ. However, it is not the procedure itself but the *complications* that can develop during or after the procedure that require the skill of an experienced M.D. In a smaller city, you are likely to find only a *handful* of doctors who *do* abortions at all. Most women do *not* have the luxury of being terribly selective. However, you *do* have the right to ask your doctor the following questions:

1. *Are you a board-certified gynecologist?* If the answer is yes, the doctor is *more* than qualified. If the answer is no, you might want to probe further.
2. *What are your credentials? Are you an M.D.?* If the individual is a board-certified family practitioner, this is fine. Proceed to question 3. If the individual is not an M.D., ask who will be supervising and *where* the supervising doctor will be during your procedure. If you're told that the doctor can "be reached by phone in an emergency," *this just won't do!* Go elsewhere. Unless the individual is an M.D., he or she is not qualified to "manage" the abortion procedure from start to finish. Don't forget to ask what the *supervising doctor's* credentials are.
3. *How* many *supervised abortions have you performed?* Do not let anyone perform the procedure unless he or she has performed *at least 100 supervised* abortions. Doctors learn how to do abortions by apprenticing with an experienced abortionist. Unless the procedures were supervised, there's no way of knowing whether the "thousands" of abortions the doctor *says* he or she has done were done *properly* or were even successful. Don't fall for "I've been doing abortions for about 10 years now." *A younger doctor who has performed 150 abortions in the span of two months is* more *qualified than an older doctor who hasn't done more than 50 abortions in the last 10 years.*
4. *Is this facility set up to handle any potential complications?* Although major complications are rare in the first trimester, about 3% of all first-trimester abortion procedures result in minor complications. The risks tend to go up as the pregnancy progresses (discussed further below). It's important to find out what happens to you if you're in this 3%. Will you need to be transferred to a hospital?
5. *Do you (or the supervising doctor) have hospital privileges?* If you *do* need to be transferred to a hospital in the event of an emergency during or after the procedure, who will manage your care in the hospital?

This is a concern if you live in an underpopulated area, and are having an abortion done in a small, backwoods-type of abortion clinic. Here's the situation you really want to avoid: the doctor performing the abortion flies in from a larger city to do his or her "abortion rounds" for the week. The doctor does the abortion and leaves. You go home, only to suffer symptoms of a serious bacterial infection (discussed below) or hemorrhage. You call the abortion clinic and find out that the doctor isn't there. The skeleton staff at the clinic is useless. You go to the Emergency unit of your local hospital and tell the doctor on call that you've had an abortion and are now suffering from *X* or *Y* symptoms. The doctor, however, is not only completely untrained in abortion complications but is an *avid* pro-life activist who treats you with clear contempt, and provides you with shoddy, unacceptable care.

6. *Do you provide local or general anesthetics?* For any kind of abortion procedure, local anesthetics are *always* better than general anesthetics. Why? First of all, there are far fewer complications involved with a local. Under a general, the doctor may perform the procedure with less gentleness, which can result in perforating your uterine lining or tearing your cervical opening. There are also the normal risks involved with a general anesthetic, such as respiratory problems, vomiting, and allergies. Second, for a general anesthetic to be administered properly, *an experienced anesthesiologist must be present.* Usually, the only appropriate setting for a general anesthetic is a hospital; unless you're in a good clinic, you might wind up with a cut-rate anesthesiologist who's moonlighting to make a few extra bucks. Finally, abortions performed under general anesthetics *cost* more and can run anywhere from $100 to $1000 extra. Most abortion centers usually include all services in one lump fee—which may also include general anesthesia. If you do have a general anesthetic, make sure you don't drive yourself home.
7. *How can I reach you after the procedure, should I experience any problems or need to ask you a question?* Make sure that you can call the doctor after hours, or at least be provided with an after-hours emergency number should you experience a problem. (Postoperative care is discussed below.)
8. *How much will this cost?* Again, costs vary. Here are some ballpark figures: first-trimester abortions, under local anesthetic (when they're not covered by insurance) should be around $250. The same proce-

dure under a general anesthetic is well over $300. Early mid-trimester procedures (15–16 weeks) done under a local will cost about $500; late second-trimester procedures will cost about $800–$900. If a procedure under a general is done beyond 15 weeks, add $500–$1500 extra to these costs. In Canada, cost is not a factor, as all therapeutic abortions are covered under universal health care.

Once you're satisfied with the abortionist's credentials and the facility, you might want to ask the following:

1. How confidential is the procedure? Does it go into my medical records?
2. How long will it take? How many follow-up appointments are involved?
3. What should I bring with me to the facility?
4. Can I bring a support person along who can stay in the room with me? (partner, friend, parent, etc.)
5. Will there be a nurse and/or counselor present during the procedure?
6. If I don't speak English, is there someone available who speaks the same language as I do to explain follow-up care and the procedure?
7. If I'm HIV positive, are there special arrangements that need to be made?
8. Should I be concerned about pro-life activists picketing the facility? If so, is there an alternate entrance and exit I can use?

Where Should the Abortion be Performed?

According to the National Abortion Federation in Washington, D.C., 90% of all abortions today are being performed in licensed abortion clinics. These clinics are well equipped and also offer counseling services and follow-up appointments. Most of these clinics will be peppered with both board-certified gynecologists and family practitioners. If you are having the abortion done for medical reasons, are having an abortion in the second trimester (discussed below), or are aborting because you're carrying a child with a genetic defect, your abortion will likely be done in the hospital, probably by your prenatal care practitioner or an on-staff gynecologist. Otherwise, you can expect to be referred to an abortion clinic.

What to Expect in a First Trimester Abortion

In North America, about 90% of all abortions are performed during the first trimester; 95% are done before 16 weeks. First-trimester abortions are less traumatic and safer, resulting in fewer complications. The first-trimester procedure revolves around what's called a suction curettage. This procedure is similar to a basic D & C procedure described in chapter 7, but your cervix may not need to be dilated if you're in the very early stages of a pregnancy. Instead, a thin, plastic, strawlike tube is inserted into your cervical canal and the doctor uses a specially designed plastic syringe to manually suck out the uterine contents. If you're in a later stage, your cervix may need to be dilated a little more, and the tube inserted into the cervix is attached to an electric pump that produces a vacuum pressure to suck out the contents of the uterus. Before the procedure is performed, you'll need to be thoroughly examined and assessed by the doctor first.

The Preoperative Assessment

As in many abortion cases, because you're not seeing your regular physician, a complete medical history and physical workup will need to be done. Your abortion doctor will examine you for any chronic conditions, such as heart disease, asthma, thyroid disease, allergies, any congenital diseases or abnormalities, or any history of gynecological problems.

You'll also have your blood and urine taken and will undergo a complete pelvic exam. This will entail a Pap smear and swabbings for gonorrhea and chlamydia.

You will need to have your pregnancy *confirmed* as well. For example, you may think you're pregnant because you've missed your period, but you may not have yet had an official pregnancy test. (Believe it or not, some women have undergone abortion procedures after one or two missed periods, convinced that they're pregnant, only to discover after the procedure that they weren't.)

Once everything checks out, a counselor may come into the examination room to discuss your decision, make sure that you're clear about why you want the abortion, and explore whether you've considered the consequences. The counselor will then explain the procedure to you in detail. You'll be told exactly what to expect during and after the procedure. In some clinics, the doctor may be the one who counsels you and goes over this information. Once the clinic is confident that you understand what you're doing (and are of sound mind and body), you'll probably be switched to another room, where the procedure will be done.

You might also be required to undergo an ultrasound procedure for the doctor to check the condition of your uterus. Usually, the doctor can feel the size and shape of your uterus with his or her hands during a bimanual pelvic exam. Depending on the clinic, you might be given an antibiotic prior to the procedure to prevent an infection.

The Suction Curettage Abortion

If you're not past six weeks in your pregnancy, you'll have a suction curettage, a procedure that has five other names: *aspiration abortion, preemptive abortion, endometrial aspiration, menstrual extraction* (not an accurate label but used anyway), and *menstrual regulation.*

This procedure takes about 15 minutes. You'll probably be given a local anesthetic, but many clinics may tell you that you don't need it. (A local anesthetic is a good idea.) A long, thin tube will be inserted into the cervical canal that leads to the uterus. The doctor will then place a long, flexible, plastic syringe through the tube into the uterus and manually suck out the contents. As the tissue is removed, your uterus will start to contract in an effort to shrink back to its normal size and push out the rest of the contents. Most women will feel cramping comparable to a miserable period. It's rare *not* to feel cramping. Once the tube is removed, the cramps will start to subside, but you'll feel crampy for the next several hours and possibly for a few days. (This is discussed further below.)

Some women may need to have a *curettage* done after the suction. A long, sharp, spoonlike instrument, called a *curette,* is used to scrape out the lining of the uterus. This usually isn't necessary, but it depends on the circumstances and whether the doctor is confident that he or she has removed everything. It's important that no tissue is left behind. If you do need a curettage, your cervix may be dilated further and the curette will be inserted through the cervix while the doctor scrapes out the lining. (This procedure is discussed in chapter 8, and you will need a local anesthetic for this).

If you're 6–16 weeks pregnant, you'll have one of the following procedures, depending on your doctor, the clinic, the advancement of your pregnancy, your health, and so on:

1. *Early uterine evacuation* (EUE). This is the same procedure described above, except that a *wider* tube is inserted into the cervix. Depending on the circumstances, you may need a D & C afterward.
2. *Vacuum aspiration.* A wide tube is inserted into the cervical opening to dilate it, and an electronic pump is used to suck out the uterine contents. Afterward, a standard D & C procedure is performed. A local anesthetic is necessary.
3. *D & C procedure.* You may just have a standard D & C procedure with no suction. This is usually reserved for later pregnancies. You'll still need a local for this.
4. *Dilation and evacuation (D & E).* Generally, once you're beyond 12 weeks, you'll most likely have this, which involves a standard D & C, vacuum suction, and sometimes forceps to take out larger pieces of tissue. The use of forceps really varies depending on your doctor's skill, how well the procedure is going, how pregnant you are, and so on. This is now considered the *standard* second-trimester abortion procedure recommended in North America. It can be performed safely until the 24-week cutoff.

What are the Risks Involved?

Right now, a first-trimester abortion (up to 12 weeks) is considered one of the safest surgical procedures. The risk of *major* complications is low. In fact, there's only a 0.2-0.6% chance of something going dramatically wrong during the procedure. The risk of death is also very low, about less than 1.1 per 100,000 abortions. Meanwhile, 10 out of every 100,000 women die during routine childbirth.

There are several *minor, correctable* complications involved that affect about 3% of all procedures. Hemorrhaging is one of the more common, correctable complications that can take place. This can happen during the procedure or later on when you're at home. The causes of hemorrhaging during the procedure can be due to accidentally tearing (lacerating) the cervix during the procedure, or accidentally puncturing the uterine wall. If tearing is the problem, this usually heals on its own; a larger tear may need stitches. If the uterine wall is perforated accidentally, the problem may just correct itself, depending on where the puncture is. Otherwise, stitches may be necessary, and you may need to be transferred to a hospital for further observation until you heal.

More common reasons for hemorrhaging are caused by leftover, or "retained," tissue in the uterus. Usually, the uterus will contract on its own to get rid of this. But if your uterus doesn't contract enough or at all, drugs can be administered to help the contractions along. If this fails, you may need a second D & C.

Another complication is infection. As discussed in chapter 6, any time your cervix is dilated, bacteria can enter the uterus and cause an infection of some sort. Infections are usually aggravated by a pre-existing, untreated sexually transmitted disease (STD) like chlamydia or gonorrhea, or pre-existing pelvic inflammatory disease (PID), which would be caught in your initial exam. If you do develop an infection, this is easily treated with antibiotics. See chapter 6 for more details.

Another rare but potential problem revolves around a "missed abortion" or "continued pregnancy." Again, this is not likely to happen since your doctor will carefully inspect you to make sure nothing was left over. But in some cases, a woman may be aborting a multiple pregnancy, or one that involves a "double uterus," where one pregnancy is aborted while the other continues uninterrupted. If this is the case, you'll need to repeat the procedure about a week later.

Post-abortal syndrome can also develop. It happens if the uterus doesn't contract properly, or if a blood clot blocks the cervical opening and prevents blood from leaving the uterus. As blood accumulates in the uterus, you may feel abdominal pain, cramping, nausea, and your uterus will be tender and enlarged. These symptoms usually occur about one to two hours after the procedure. You'll need to have the uterus suctioned again or a D & C procedure to get rid of the blood. You may also be given synthetic oxytocin hormone to help stimulate uterine contractions.

Finally, you may have an ectopic pregnancy and not know it. In this case, your pregnancy will be in very early stages, a test will be positive, and you'll undergo an abortion, only to experience ectopic pregnancy symptoms later on, after the procedure. (See chapter 10 for details on ectopic pregnancy.)

What Happens Afterward

Most women will experience some irregular bleeding, cramping, or spotting. This will go on for about two weeks. Some women will continue to feel menstrual-like cramping and bleeding for as long as six weeks. Taking anti-inflammatory medication is helpful.

You might also experience feelings of depression. These feelings will stem from normal grief following the abortion and are not abnormal. It's important to seek post-abortion counseling. Review the postpartum depression section in chapter 10. You'll probably experience feelings that range from blues to bonafide depression. If these feelings don't pass within a couple of weeks, you may need longer-term therapy to fully recover emotionally.

You'll also need to follow certain hygiene guidelines after the procedure, outlined in chapter 6 under "Prevention of PID." In addition, you should refrain from sexual intercourse until your cervix has resumed its normal size.

Your period will return about four to six weeks after the procedure, but this varies depending on how far along you were in your pregnancy at the time of the abortion. Because your lining has been removed and your body is rebalancing its hormones, it will take that long for your menstrual cycle to get back on track. However, you can pregnant immediately after an abortion, so make sure you religiously practice a barrier method of birth control, in conjunction with a male condom, to prevent infection. Review chapter 4 for details on contraception.

The Abortion Pill: RU 486

In time, there may be a much less invasive method to abort in the first trimester through a drug known as *RU 486*, also called the "abortion pill." It was developed by Dr. Etienne-Emile Baulier in 1980, and is an alternative to surgical termination of pregnancy for thousands of women living in countries where the drug has been approved. It also offers the potential for saving the lives of women in countries where access to safe abortion is denied. RU 486 is a real breakthrough in abortion technology.

The pill works by blocking the action of progesterone, which is crucial in order to sustain a pregnancy. In fact, many women miscarry because they have insufficient amounts of progesterone in their system. Without progesterone, the lining of the uterus breaks down and menstruation begins, expelling any fertilized egg. RU 486 is then combined with *prostaglandins,* which induce uterine contractions during labor. In France, England, and Sweden, where the drug is approved, RU 486 combined with prostaglandins was effective in 95% of the women who received it; they all aborted within two to four hours afterward. The countries who approved RU 486 do not make it available to the general public, however. A doctor must administer the drug, and the cutoff is nine weeks after the last period. The advantages of the drug are that it offers access to abortion at an earlier stage of pregnancy, is less expensive than surgical abortion, does not require as much surgical expertise, allows for greater privacy for women, and offers less risk from anesthesia and surgical complications. RU 486 is not available in North America because of continued ethical debate over its use. But recently a London, England, clinic has made RU 486 available to American women who are willing to travel there. It is currently being tested as a legitimate treatment for fibroids and endometriosis.

What to Expect in a Second-Trimester Abortion

Until about five years ago, women who had abortions done beyond 16 weeks were subjected to a horrible, rather nightmarish procedure known as *amnioinduction, induction abortion,* or *induction miscarriage.* After you checked into a hospital, the abortion practitioner inserted a needle into your abdomen (just like amniocentesis), and injected a miscarriage-inducing solution into the amniotic sac (usually a saline solution). The solution killed the fetus by poisoning it. You were then required to wait about 24 hours for labor to set in, and then you literally went into labor, *and gave birth* to the dead fetus. This is the procedure that has perhaps fueled the pro-life activists more than any other. Worse, because an amnioinduction procedure involves childbirth, there are numerous complications involved as well.

In 1994, no woman living *anywhere* in North America needs to subject herself to an amnioinduction procedure. A far safer, cheaper, shorter, and less traumatic *D & E* procedure is now the standard, second-trimester procedure performed, *and it can be done right up until the 24th week of pregnancy.* In fact, the only reason amnioinduction still exists as a procedure at all is because there aren't enough doctors in North America *trained* to do a D & E procedure. If you live in a large city that has plenty of excellent hospitals and facilities, you won't have any trouble getting a D & E in the second trimester. If you live in an underpopulated area, ask your gynecologist or primary care physician for the name of a doctor or clinic that does second-trimester D & Es. If this fails, don't waste your time hunting for an updated abortion clinic. Just call either the National Abortion Federation or the Planned Parenthood Federation of America. Tell them that you need to have a second-trimester D & E and that you're interested *only* in clinics advanced or large enough to perform this procedure. Then, call the clinic to confirm that they indeed do the procedure. Make an appointment and travel to that clinic (probably located in a larger center) to get the D & E done. *The expense of an amnioinduction procedure is* equal to, if not more than, *a two-way bus or train fare and the cost of a D & E procedure.* Don't let anyone try to convince you that a D & E procedure is not appropriate this "late" or that it involves more complications. Amnioinduction is an archaic and cruel procedure that has been abandoned by skilled abortion practitioners.

The D & E Procedure

The D & E procedure you'll undergo at any point in the second trimester is almost identical to the first-trimester procedure, with just a few variations. First, because you'll be further along in your pregnancy, you'll need to have your cervix dilated several hours prior to the procedure. This means that after your preoperative assessment, screening/exam, and counseling session are complete, you'll have a seaweed root (called *laminaria*) inserted into your cervical opening 24 hours before the procedure. Laminaria is used as a natural dilator of the cervix, thought to cause less irritation because it's organic. After the tube is inserted, you'll be sent home, and will feel crampy. You'll report back to the hospital the next day for the procedure. You'll have a fresh dilator (plastic tube or laminaria) inserted into your cervical opening, and the doctor will administer a local anesthetic. You'll have the contents of the uterus suctioned out with the vacuum pump described in the earlier section. Forceps may also be used to help retrieve larger pieces of fetal tissue. You'll feel cramping as the uterine contracts during the procedure. Then a standard D & C procedure is done. The risks and complications experienced after the procedure are virtually identical to those of the first-trimester procedure, and the cramping and bleeding following the procedure are also similar. This entire procedure takes about 20 minutes. (Some sources estimate as little as 10 minutes and as long as 45 minutes.)

Most hemorrhaging after a D & E is caused by retained placental tissue in the uterus. Treatment for complications at this stage is exactly the same as that for first-trimester complications.

If you've had a *second* D & C to control bleeding caused by retained tissue, or to extract blood from the uterus, you might start to notice abnormal bleeding a few weeks later. If this happens, you may need to be put on a progesterone supplement to induce a "withdrawal" bleeding and have your lining shed again. This should take care of the problem. You'll also need to follow the same aftercare guidelines discussed earlier.

Basic information on abortion is difficult to obtain because the woman who *needs* the information is often too ashamed to ask for it. The procedure is also shrouded in mystery for many women, who may choose not to abort because they fear the amnioinduction procedure, which is now outdated. Obviously, preventing unwanted pregnancy in the first place would in turn prevent the need for many abortions. Yet the same factions that are against abortion are also against distributing adequate birth control information in schools! It's equally important to understand your fertility cycle and use fertility awareness techniques in conjunction with contraception to prevent unwanted pregnancy.

The irony about accidental pregnancy is that it typically happens to women who do not want a child. Meanwhile, women who *do* want children often find that getting pregnant is much more difficult than they anticipated. Many of these women will go on to seek assisted conception or adopt a child instead. About 90% of the time, there is a reason for the infertility that can be corrected. Often, the problem has to do with a couple's failure to understand the fertility cycle to begin with. Fortunately, several observation techniques are now available to women so that they can monitor their fertility accurately. There are also home fertility kits on the market that work on the same principles as home pregnancy kits. Using fertility awareness to prevent or plan pregnancy, as well as outlining common reasons for infertility is discussed in the next chapter.

CHAPTER 12

Fertility Awareness and Infertility

The fundamentals of family planning revolve around basic fertility awareness. In our society, *healthy* discomforts of a normal menstrual cycle are often medicated. Women who suffer from normal premenstrual symptoms, such as bloating or premenstrual breast pain, may be put on medications that eliminate their symptoms and, in more extreme cases, halt or alter their cycles. Yet these classic premenstrual symptoms are important clues to the timing of the cycle. To mask these symptoms is to *mask the cycle.* (See chapter 2 for more details.)

This trend in women's health care is contributing to decreased fertility awareness and is creating problems for women on both sides of the fertility battle. Since fewer women are using more natural methods of birth control, they are subjected to certain risks of various contraceptives. Women who *do* want to conceive may find that their natural, "uninduced" cycles are not as predictable or easy to read as they thought. Women need to be *taught* how to read their cycles.

Infertility is a rather broad term. Technically, it means two things: either conception is being *delayed* for some reason, or a pregnancy cannot be *sustained.* Unfortunately, people tend to confuse the word *infertility* with *sterility.* There is a huge difference between the two terms; *infertility* refers to a transient or temporary state, while *sterility* is a permanent state, although it can often be reversed.

When a couple remains infertile after one year of unprotected intercourse, an initial infertility workup is recommended. This is an arbitrary cutoff date chosen because 80% of couples will achieve a pregnancy within 12 months of unprotected intercourse. A more accurate label for many couples who are branded "infertile" might be "delayed fertility," because that's usually what "infertility" *means.*

Currently, about one in seven couples will not conceive after one year of unprotected sex. Ninety percent of the time there is a physical cause behind this delayed conception: 35% involves the man, 35% involves the woman, and 20% involves both partners, while for the remaining 10% of the time, no cause can be found.

When it comes to female-related infertility, 20% is due to an irregular ovulation cycle, accompanied by poor cervical mucus (discussed below). There are replacement hormones or drugs available that can induce ovulation. The remaining 80% of female infertility is due to scarring of the tubes from pelvic inflammatory disease (PID) caused by gonorrhea, chlamydia, and intrauterine devices (IUDs), and from endometriosis. Some of this scarring can be reversed through microsurgical techniques (see chapter 6).

Over 10 million couples in North America are plagued by infertility; this translates into about 15% of couples of childbearing age. It's believed that about 3.5 million couples in North America are definitely sterile; about 3 million are considered subfertile, meaning not as fertile as the average couple, but *not* sterile, while about 1.5 million couples can expect a long wait before conception.

When a couple is sterile, it means that there is a *permanent* physical phenomenon at work preventing pregnancy. Unless corrected through surgery or other therapies, the problem *will* persist. (Correcting permanent problems is discussed further below.) Sometimes the problem is not correctable, as in the case of a woman who has had a hysterectomy, a bilateral oophorectomy, or a bilateral salpingectomy. In these cases, there are some options to pregnancy, including assisted conception techniques. Of course, some men or women deliberately seek out permanent methods of contraception, that *will* render them sterile. These methods are also discussed below.

Infertility is not as concrete as sterility. In many cases it's caused by a combination of factors that, when looked at individually, are not obstacles to conception. For example, virtually every woman is working, subjected to stress. As a result, women can be exhausted and emotionally drained and their *partners* can be exhausted and emotionally drained. On top of this, couples are planning first pregnancies at a much older age than their parents. These factors are not "causes" of infertility but may certainly contribute to delayed fertility or problem pregnancies for many women.

This chapter outlines fertility awareness techniques, covers some of the common obstacles that delay conception, and describes what investigating infertility entails. Usually, there is a logical explanation behind infertility that is easily correctable. When there is a physical problem that is causing one partner to be sterile, the variety of reproductive technologies available can often reverse sterility. What happens when no explanation can be found? This is good news and bad news; while the couple's ability to conceive appears to be in fine form, the frustration of the delay in conception can be maddening. A couple may suffer from irreversible sterility. For both these circumstances, options may need to be seriously looked at. Yet, regardless of how bleak a couple's chances of conception look, *many couples have the opportunity to parent a child!* Parenting without pregnancy, as well as choosing a childfree lifestyle, is discussed as well. Since, it's not possible to cover all of the issues regarding fertility and infertility in a single chapter, please consult my book, *The Fertility Sourcebook,* for the complete story.

Fertility Awareness Techniques

If you're using hormonal contraception or a barrier method, fertility awareness is not necessary to *prevent* conception. However, it is always the first step in *planning* conception. Many menstrual cycles do not consist of an exact number of days. Some women may have a 33-day cycle one month, a 36-day cycle the next, and a 31-day cycle the next. I have cycles that run anywhere between 35 and 45 days, and I *never* know how many days to expect between cycles. And I am *not* an unusual "menstrual cycle statistic" by any means. Cycles like these create problems for women trying to conceive, because there is a very small time frame within our cycle when we actually *can* conceive (see chapter 2).

We are fertile during ovulation, which takes place about 14 days before our period begins. Women with predictable menstrual cycles can easily use a calendar to "catch" the fertile peak in their cycles. For example, a woman with an average 28-day cycle would circle day 14 of the cycle on her calendar, and begin having frequent intercourse between day 12 and day 16. Women with unpredictable cycles or women with irregular cycles will have a much harder time doing this. Fortunately, there are several *other* fertility awareness techniques for women who are not born "calendar girls." You'll get the best results if you combine *all* of these methods.

Charting Your Menstrual Cycle

Of course, there's no way of *knowing* how regular your cycles are until you start to chart them. A classic case for charting exists when women decide to conceive after being on hormonal contraception for years. Often, their regular cycles don't return for *several months*. For other women planning to conceive, charting serves very useful purposes.

First, by charting your cycle, you'll become aware of your body's premenstrual symptoms, which are useful "precursors" to your period and, hence, signs of when your fertile stage has begun or *passed*. For instance, if you suffer from tender breasts roughly a week *before* your period, you might begin to notice a pattern of premenstrual breast pain that can *assist* you in establishing a pattern of fertility. Similarly, symptoms such as mood swings or bloating can be used in this way as well.

Second, charting your cycle will alert you to the problem of an irregular cycle, which could mean that you're ovulating irregularly, or not at all. The various causes of irregular cycles are discussed in chapter 2. Correcting the underlying problem that's *causing* your irregular cycles may prevent delayed conception and save you from needless frustration. Charting is discussed thoroughly in chapter 2, and should be done for at least four cycles before an accurate pattern can be established.

Observing Cervical Mucus

This is a crucial fertility awareness method that any woman can easily get in the habit of doing. It also has the benefit of convenience, unlike the basal body temperature (BBT) method discussed below. This method is sometimes called the Billings method, invented by Evelyn and John Billings, an Australian couple who developed a way of interpreting the *changing consistencies* of vaginal discharge, which is influenced by the cervical mucus bathing the vaginal walls. All you need to do is observe your toilet paper about twice a day, when you wipe yourself before or after going to the bathroom. Or, you can simply insert a finger into your vagina to collect whatever discharge is present.

Here's how it works. After your period finishes, you'll notice several days of no vaginal discharge at all (your "dry days"). Your vagina will still be moist, however, as it always is. Then, your mucus days will begin. The discharge starts out sticky, then gradually becomes creamier, wet, and slippery. Finally, on your mucus peak day, the discharge has the consistency of egg white (some women describe it as snotlike) and will be dripping out of your vagina, very evident when you wipe yourself or take off your underwear. This discharge will also be thinner, transparent, and stretchy, and you should be able to stretch it between two fingers. *This* mucus is your "fertility marker." You will be ovulating either just *before* or just *after* it appears. The mucus will last for just about two days, then it will begin to get thicker and stickier. These are your postpeak days, also known as your luteal phase. This is when premenstrual symptoms will begin to make an appearance. The mucus will remain on the thicker, sticky side until your period starts. Then, the whole phase begins again.

To catch the peak, you'll need to begin having frequent intercourse (every other day) as your mucus days begin, and continue frequent intercourse until your postpeak mucus appears. Mucus usually develops between three to nine days prior to ovulation. So you will probably need to have frequent intercourse for about two weeks. *Warning: This method is useless if you have a vaginal infection or an untreated STD.*

If you don't notice any mucus, this is a problem. Without cervical mucus, sperm can't survive or be transported to the fallopian tubes to fertilize the egg. The mucus also nourishes and protects the sperm, allowing them to live for three to five days. If you don't notice any mucus, this is a sign that you may not be ovulating and may have a hormone deficiency or even a vaginal infection of some sort. You'll need to see your doctor. That being said, it should also be noted that nothing's 100%. You could still conceive, but a lack of mucus will make conception far more difficult.

The LH Test Kit (The Ovulation Home-Test Kit)

It's now possible to pick up a test kit that will detect your LH (luteinizing hormone) surge. This surge triggers ovulation and occurs anywhere from 12 to 36 hours prior to ovulation. This means that you can now accurately pinpoint when you're ovulating 12–36 hours in advance. LH is present in the blood throughout your cycle, but only in small amounts. Just before ovulation, the amount of LH suddenly increases, known as the LH surge. This test can pick up increased levels of LH in your urine up until about 24 hours after your surge. With the aid of a specific kind of antibody, known as *monoclonal antibodies*, these kits can detect even minute amounts of LH in the urine.

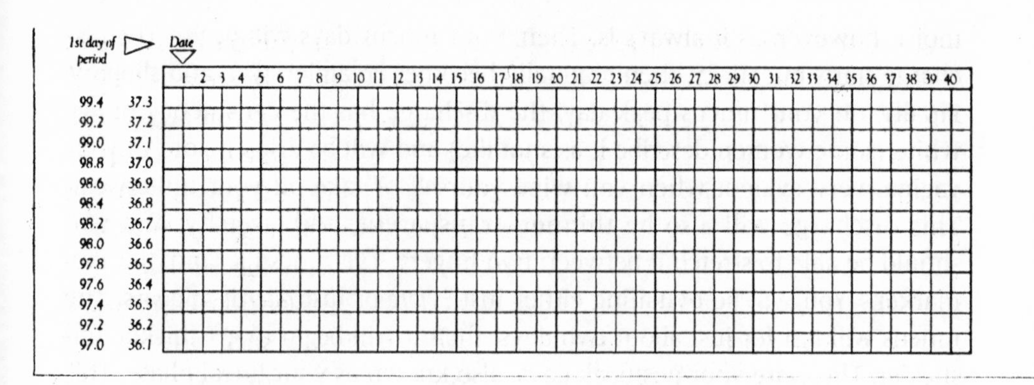
1st day of period
Date
1 2 3 4 5 6 7 8 9 10 11 12 13 14 15 16 17 18 19 20 21 22 23 24 25 26 27 28 29 30 31 32 33 34 35 36 37 38 39 40
99.4 37.3
99.2 37.2
99.0 37.1
98.8 37.0
98.6 36.9
98.4 36.8
98.2 36.7
98.0 36.6
97.8 36.5
97.6 36.4
97.4 36.3
97.2 36.2
97.0 36.1

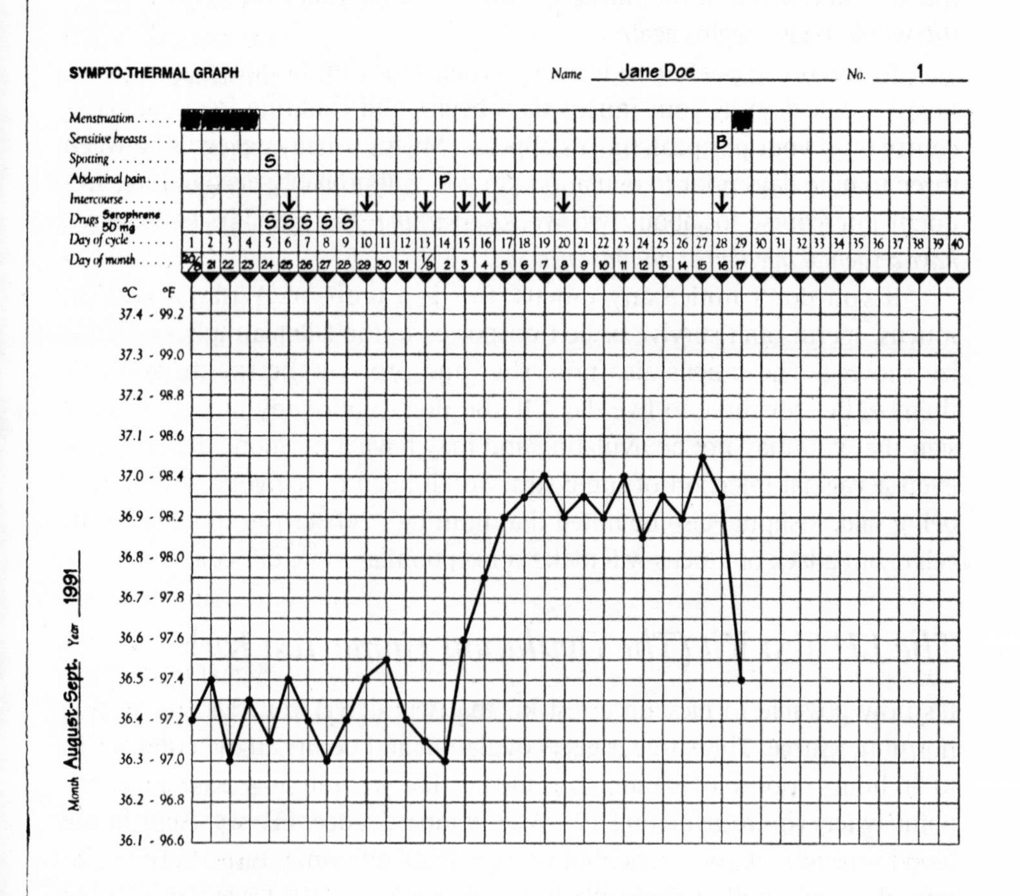
SYMPTO-THERMAL GRAPH
Name Jane Doe
No. 1
Menstruation
Sensitive breasts
Spotting
Abdominal pain
Intercourse
Drugs Serophene 50 mg
Day of cycle
Day of month
S
P
B
S S S S S
1 2 3 4 5 6 7 8 9 10 11 12 13 14 15 16 17 18 19 20 21 22 23 24 25 26 27 28 29 30 31 32 33 34 35 36 37 38 39 40
20/8 21 22 23 24 25 26 27 28 29 30 31 1/9 2 3 4 5 6 7 8 9 10 11 12 13 14 15 16 17
°C °F
37.4 - 99.2
37.3 - 99.0
37.2 - 98.8
37.1 - 98.6
37.0 - 98.4
36.9 - 98.2
36.8 - 98.0
36.7 - 97.8
36.6 - 97.6
36.5 - 97.4
36.4 - 97.2
36.3 - 97.0
36.2 - 96.8
36.1 - 96.6
Month August-Sept. Year 1991

Since the late 1980s, several LH test kits have come on the market. They take anywhere from 10–30 minutes to perform. There are a variety of brands available. You can ask your doctor or pharmacist to recommend one.

All LH test kits operate on the same principle. You buy the tests about 14 days before your next period. Each kit contains a chart that will suggest a good time for you to begin testing, based on the average length of your past periods. Each kit contains either a stick or test pad with a blue reference spot to compare to your test result. Either one will have monoclonal antibodies on them, which will detect any LH. If you're using the stick, you dip the stick into your urine cup and check to see if it changes color; if you're using a test pad, you drop a small amount of your urine onto the pad and see if it turns blue. You then continue testing until the blue becomes darkest, which will mark the surge. All the kits have an 800 number you can call if you have any questions. Before you purchase a kit, go over the instructions carefully with the pharmacist and ask if he or she can show you how to use it. The kits are expensive and can cost anywhere from $60 to $100, depending on how many test sticks or test pads you're supplied with (expect either a six-day or nine-day supply). You can also purchase individual refills, which cost roughly $10 for one refill.

Using the kit along with your mucus observations and basal body temperature chart (discussed below), you should get a very clear picture of your fertility. This kit may also be useful in timing various diagnostic tests.

Basal Body Temperature Chart (Symptothermal Method)

The basal body temperature (BBT) method is a real nuisance, but it's a good way of charting exactly when you're ovulating. It employs an ultrasensitive thermometer that tracks your body's *exact* temperature. A digital thermometer is your best bet. These thermometers are fairly cheap and can be purchased at any pharmacy. Each thermometer comes with a blank graph and a sample graph to show you how to chart your temperature accurately. At the top of the graph are the days of your cycle, from 1 to about 45. Underneath each cycle day is room for the month and actual calendar date. Listed vertically are temperatures from about 99.0°F down to 97.0°F. (In Canada, the readings would be in metric units, from about 39°C to 36°C.)

Each morning, before you get out of bed, you'll need to take your temperature orally or vaginally and chart it on the graph. Here's the problem:

Unless you take your temperature at the same time each morning, the graph won't be accurate! After ovulation, your temperature rises between about 32°F and 32.9°F (about 0.2° to 0.5°C).

After doing about three charts, you should notice a very distinct pattern of ovulation, which will help you time *future* intercourses and tell you whether you are indeed ovulating regularly. However, this method will not tell you *when* to have intercourse on the spot, since the temperature doesn't rise until *after* ovulation. Yet many couples make the mistake of planning their intercourse around this chart. This is a bad idea and creates stress that can interfere with sexual intimacy. The purpose of the chart is to help you plan future intercourses and assist you in observing your own unique fertility pattern.

There is current debate among gynecologists about the accuracy of these charts. Some women don't experience any sharp differences in temperature, yet are ovulating anyway; some women have an even, or "flat," pattern throughout their cycle, yet are still ovulating. If you're one of these, the absence of a pattern should tell you that you *may* not be ovulating, *but you must also observe no change in your cervical mucus, and no LH surge from an LH home test kit to suspect that you're anovulatory.* The next step is to have your doctor perform blood tests that check your hormonal levels, or an *endometrial biopsy* (discussed below and in chapter 8), a test that determines whether you're ovulating or whether you have a hormonal imbalance.

So You're Still Not Pregnant?

If you're practicing fertility awareness and are still not pregnant, there are a variety of factors that may be affecting your conception.

Frequency of intercourse.

Having intercourse once during your fertile period just won't cut it. You need to start having intercourse a good few days before ovulation, and keep up the pace until a couple of days afterward. For optimum sperm counts, don't have intercourse every day; do it every *other* day. In fact, some couples just have intercourse every other day throughout the *entire* cycle, which usually isn't practical for the majority of us who work for a living!

Your lubricant may be the culprit.

Using a sexual lubricant can interfere with the sperms' survival in the vagina. If you're using a lubricant, stop.

Your partner's masturbation habits.

Find out whether your partner masturbates between his bouts of intercourse with you. Men who don't have intercourse every other day tend to go ahead and masturbate privately. This usually isn't any of your business, but if you're timing your intercourse to specific dates, and your partner has masturbated that day or the day before, his sperm count will be significantly lower, resulting in reduced fertility. You'll need to figure out a better schedule for him if his private masturbation is interfering with your fertility. (He most likely will not realize that it's a problem, if in fact, it is.)

The temperature of your partner's crotch.

The testicles hang below the man's crotch for a reason: for the testicles to produce enough sperm, *they need to be a few degrees cooler than body temperature.* If your partner is wearing tight underwear or tight pants all the time, his sperm count could be reduced. Encourage him to wear boxer shorts and looser-fitting pants. Then see what happens. Exposure to heat from other sources, such as hot baths, saunas, whirlpools, hot cars in traffic, or a fever *can* affect fertility as well. In fact, the latter is usually more of a problem than the "boxer" issue.

Your diet.

Starvation diets, purging and binging rituals, and yo-yo dieting *affect ovulation.* If you have difficulty eating regularly or normally, you need to see a nutritionist and get your diet under control. Similarly, if you're obese, your ovulation cycle can also be affected. Unless you're eating balanced meals and are maintaining a *stable* weight, you won't be creating optimum conditions for conception. In addition, how much do you drink? Do you smoke? All of these factors may affect your ability to conceive.

An undiagnosed STD.

Here's a classic scenario: Jane Doe finally meets Mr. Right on her 33rd birthday. They marry on her 34th birthday, and she becomes Jane Doe-Right. After trying to conceive for a year or so, Jane goes to her doctor to find out what's wrong. Her doctor does a routine pelvic exam, screens for STDs, and discovers that Jane has been walking around with chlamydia for some time. Her doctor then examines her new husband, who also has chlamydia (surprise, surprise!). It turns out that his otherwise normal sperm count is being *killed off* by elevated levels of white blood cells produced by the infection. They both get treated with doxycycline, and Jane gets pregnant not too long after.

Your STD history in general.

If you've been treated for chlamydia or gonorrhea in the past, you might have scarring on your fallopian tube. There's a diagnostic procedure that can check this (discussed below). First, make sure your husband undergoes a semen analysis. That way, if he does have a problem, he can be treated before you subject yourself to more invasive procedures.

Your stress level.

In chapter 2, I discussed why stress can cause you to skip a period. In short, it's your body's way of protecting you from a "stressed" pregnancy. By the same token, if you're currently under a lot of stress, your ovulation cycle may become irregular until you de-stress. What could happen is that you chart and observe your period in January, February, and March, pinpoint your cycle, and then just plan intercourse by a calendar each month. You start a new job in May and take on significantly more stress, while trying to conceive in the process. The fact that you're not conceiving creates even more stress. Carefully charting your periods and observing your fertility cycle *each month* will tell you whether you have a problem. If there is a problem, try relaxing for a few weeks (can you take time off?) and see whether your fertility cycle changes.

Are you a DES daughter?

Diethylstilbestrol (DES) was a drug given to pregnant women from about 1941 until the early 1970s. This drug was given to prevent miscarriage but is known to cause a wide range of reproductive and pelvic problems for the offspring of these women. Finding out whether you're a DES daughter and the specific exam you require is discussed in chapter 3.

Environmental and occupational hazards.

There are a variety of chemicals that have been linked to reduced fertility in men and women or labeled dangerous to pregnant and lactating women. Review *The Fertility Sourcebook* for more information.

The Infertility Workup

When you begin your infertility workup, you'll undergo a series of tests that will hopefully pin down the problem. The first tests women encounter in the process are uncomfortable, expensive, and invasive. On the other hand, a man's workup involves a simple semen analysis. All he has to do is ejaculate into a specimen cup and deliver it to a lab. Because of this, *it's crucial that your partner gets his tests done first.* Only when your partner is given a clean bill of health should you begin to schedule your own tests. Some men may be reluctant to get a semen analysis. If this is the case, you're better off waiting for him to agree to the test, rather than continuing with the process. Since this is a *gynecological* sourcebook, I'll cover the steps involved in a female infertility workup in detail, and only briefly discuss the male workup.

Remember the "journey" analogy I used in chapter 8 to discuss the investigation of tumors, irregular bleeding, and cancer therapy? The infertility workup can be viewed in the same way. This is a short journey for some, if a cause for the infertility may be found and corrected immediately; it's a longer journey for others who may need to undergo several tests but ultimately reverse the infertility or correct the problem; and it's a "ride to the end of the line" for some who will go on to conceive through assisted conception techniques. It may also be an endless journey for others, whose infertility may be idiopathic (meaning no known cause), or whose attempts at assisted conception haven't worked.

A *semen analysis* begins both the female and male infertility workup. This should be done *before* you seek out an official infertility specialist. Here's why: An "infertility specialist" per se is not a *true* area of specialization in medicine *yet;* in other words, there is no postgraduate residency program a doctor can enter to become a board-certified "fertility specialist." The doctor that manages your infertility workup will vary depending on *who has the problem.* Male infertility specialists are either *andrologists* (specializing in male hormones and reproduction) or *urologists* (doctors who specialize in male and female urinary tract problems but are particularly knowledgeable in penis and testicle "design"). If your partner has an abnormal semen analysis, he'll be sent for a "male infertility workup." If your partner's tests are normal, you'll then go on, as a couple, to a gynecologist who specializes in *reproductive endocrinology.* This doctor will then manage the female workup. If you and your partner decide to undergo assisted conception procedures (discussed further on), you will need to see a gynecologist who not only specializes in reproductive endocrinology, but also is a qualified *fertility surgeon.* However, many general gynecologists can manage a basic workup and treat less complicated problems.

Semen Analysis

The semen analysis essentially checks for a few things: *sperm count* (20–100 million sperm is normal), the movement or *motility* of the sperm; the shape and maturity of the sperm cells to determine the quality, known as the *morphology;* consistency or *viscosity; volume* (amount of semen produced; about 1 teaspoon is normal), and the *pH balance* (it should be slightly alkaline).

Your partner can either masturbate into a specimen cup (supplied by your lab or doctor) or into a clean glass jar. If the semen is being collected at home (discussed below) you can bring your partner to orgasm by manually petting him. Some labs tell you it's fine to bring your partner to orgasm through oral sex or coitus interruptus (pulling out), but saliva may interfere with the test results. Your partner will need to abstain from ejaculation for at least 48 hours prior to taking the test. For best results, doctors recommend four days.

If your doctor has a laboratory in his or her office building or clinic, you could just send your partner over to the doctor's office, where he can do the test in a bathroom or private room. This is certainly the simplest route. Or, your doctor could give you a requisition form for a semen analysis, and your partner can report to a lab at his convenience and do the test there. However, many men find this test embarrassing and are unable to ejaculate under these conditions. In this case, get a semen analysis requisition from your doctor, find a lab that's not more than an hour away (sperm can survive for at least that long in a cup), and pick up a semen analysis *kit* from that lab (most will have them). Have your partner do the test at home, and then drive the specimen over to the lab as soon as it's collected. It's important to keep the specimen warm. Placing it in front pants pockets, close to your body, tucking it into the waistline of your pants or skirt, or tucking it under your arm are the best ways to transport it. If you spill any of the semen during or after collection, you'll need to repeat the test. Do *not* put the collection in the fridge or freezer overnight.

You should call your doctor's office to find out the results. If the results are normal the male partner may not need any further tests. You'll then proceed to the female workup discussed below.

If the results are abnormal, you'll need to repeat the test at least twice over the next three months before jumping to any conclusions. Fevers, infections, or viruses (including STDs) can affect the sperm count for months afterward. If two collections come back abnormal, your partner will be referred to a urologist and/or andrologist. Many urologists are also andrologists (in the same way that gynecologists may also do gynecologic oncology). It is *this* doctor who proceeds with the male workup. This entails a *sperm antibody test* (some men form antibodies to their own sperm), *hormonal blood tests, testicular biopsy* (a lack of sperm-generating cells within the testicles means that your partner is permanently sterile), a *vasography* (checks the structure of your partner's duct system and locates any obstruction), a *fructose test* (normal seminal vesicles should add fructose to the semen; a negative fructose test indicates that there's a problem with the vas deferens or seminal vesicles), a *hamster egg test*, or *sperm penetration assay* (this test checks whether the sperm can penetrate a hamster ovum; if it can't, in vitro fertilization won't work, and your partner's problem will be investigated further), and a *bovine cervical mucus test* (this test checks the sperm's ability to penetrate cervical mucus from cows).

Your First Official "Infertility" Visit

After a normal semen analysis, your family doctor will refer you to a gynecologist who does reproductive endocrinology (many of them don't). If your gynecologist has been managing the workup so far and is skilled in reproductive endocrinology, you don't need to be referred elsewhere. The good news at this point is that there is a 90% chance that the cause of your infertility will be found either here or in the next series of tests discussed below.

Both you and your partner should see the gynecologist together. You should also bring in your BBT chart and any other calendar/chart you're using to keep track of your cycles. The doctor will begin by basically interviewing both of you. He or she will first take a full medical history of both of you, asking about things like appendicitis and previous surgeries. He or she might then request separate interviews, asking each of you about your relationship, how long you've been together, and how long you've been trying. Your partner will be asked whether he has impregnated a woman in the past; you'll be asked whether you've ever been pregnant yourself or had any abortions. These questions are important. For example, if your partner *has* impregnated a woman in the past, the likelihood of finding a problem with you is greater. Meanwhile, a woman in her mid-to-late 30s or early 40s, who had an abortion in her teens or early 20s, may have been scarred as a result. In the 1970s, abortion technology wasn't what it is today; scarring or damage in the pelvic area may have taken place (see chapter 11). You'll also be asked a great deal about your lifestyle, diet, and weight history. Ovulation irregularities are usually caused by one of three things: excessive weight loss or weight gain, excessive exercise, and emotional stress.

Your doctor will then perform a full pelvic exam on you, screening for STDs, doing a Pap smear, and so on. You'll also have a complete physical.

Your doctor will check your reproductive hormone levels, thyroid hormone levels, your heart, your lungs, and so on. Your doctor may also want to do an ultrasound just to check the shape and condition of your pelvic tract. The idea is to make sure that you don't have any obvious gynecological problems or infections at work.

Your doctor may not notice that you have excessive hair on your face, back, abdomen, or breasts, because you might be *removing* it. But if you're asked whether you have excessive body hair, you should answer truthfully. There is a condition known as *polycystic ovary syndrome,* in which your ovaries have small cysts that interfere with ovulation and hormone production. You'll also be asked about any skin problems, such as acne, and you may also have a history of irregular periods and/or battling with obesity. Obesity, oily skin and acne, irregular cycles, and excessive hair growth are symptoms of polycystic ovary syndrome. If you *do* have this problem, you may not have been ovulating regularly, which you might have noticed already through fertility observation techniques. Your doctor will do some additional blood tests to check for any elevated levles of *androgen,* a male hormone all women secrete in small amounts. You can also have elevated androgen levels and not have polycystic ovary syndrome. If androgen is the problem, you may need to be put on female hormone supplements to offset it. Diagnosing and treating polycystic ovary syndrome is discussed below under hormonal problems. This condition is a classic "textbook" cause of female infertility.

No competent infertility specialist will proceed with the workup without taking a full menstrual and contraceptive history. The doctor will be looking for an IUD history as well as any signs of endometriosis or PID. He or she will also make sure that you've been having regular menstrual cycles throughout the "trying to conceive" period for at least a year, that you've been timing your intercourse correctly, that you've been having intercourse frequently during your ovulation peak, and so on. He or she should ask to see your BBT chart (see above). If you haven't been doing a BBT chart, you'll need to start one. Keep track of your cycles for at least three months, and then review the chart pattern with your doctor before you continue.

Pinpointing a Hormonal Problem

Roughly 30% of all female infertility is caused by a hormonal imbalance of some sort. Depending on what kind of imbalance you have, you'll be plagued with different infertility problems that include irregular ovulation, failure of the embryo to implant in the uterus, poor-quality cervical mucus, or the inability to sustain a pregnancy, causing you to repeatedly miscarry (discussed further on).

When irregular ovulation is cited as the probable culprit, you'll undergo a series of simple blood tests done at various points in your cycle (different hormones peak at different times in your cycle) to find what hormone is either missing, deficient, or exploding from your body. You'll most likely undergo an endometrial biopsy (see below) as well. Sometimes a hormonal imbalance is linked to a specific syndrome, such as polycystic ovary syndrome; sometimes the cause for your hormonal imbalance is idiopathic (meaning unknown). At any rate, you might be able to be treated with fertility drugs, designed to induce ovulation (see below).

Polycystic ovary syndrome.

As discussed above, this is a classic female infertility problem. About 4% of the general female population suffer from this. Here, your estrogen levels are fine, and in fact, your LH levels are higher than usual, working overtime to try to kick-start the cycle. But the higher androgen levels interfere with your FSH (follicle stimulating hormone), which you need to trigger progesterone. So your follicles never develop, and instead turn into small, pea-size cysts on your ovaries. Your ovaries can then enlarge. Because your androgen levels are out of whack, you can develop facial hair, hair on other parts of your body (this happens in 70% of the cases and is called *hirsutism*) or even a balding problem. Acne is a typical symptom because of an increase in androgen. Obesity is another symptom (although women who have a normal weight or are thin can also have this syndrome). Your periods will also be irregular, and you might be at greater risk for developing *endometrial hyperplasia,* discussed in chapter 8.

Now, if this problem was caught earlier on in your menstrual history, you would have simply been put on combination oral contraceptives (OCs) to induce normal withdrawal bleeding and pump your system with normal levels of estrogen and progesterone. Or, you would have been put on progestin, a synthetic progesterone supplement, and would have been instructed to take it about midcycle.

If you were treated earlier on with progestin, you won't experience problems with your cycle unless you go off it for some reason. But women who were treated with OCs for irregular cycles at a very young age may not know *why* they suffered from irregular periods to begin with. When these women go off contraception to conceive, they'll be plagued by the same symptoms that initially warranted oral contraception.

Sometimes, women with normal cycles for many years may develop polycystic ovary syndrome later in life. In this case, they will suddenly develop irregular cycles (called *secondary amenorrhea,* discussed in chapter 2) out of the blue.

To reverse infertility in women with polycystic ovary syndrome, doctors will use the fertility drug *clomiphene citrate* (Clomid or Serophene). Roughly 80% of all "polycystic" women on clomiphene will ovulate; about 50% of them will get pregnant. Clomiphene is discussed further below.

Other factors that affect ovulation include

1. *Prolonged use of OCs.* It usually takes 3–12 months for your cycles to return to normal after going off OCs. Five percent of the women who stop using OCs will not see normal cycles for over a year. In these cases, fertility drugs may be suggested as well.
2. *Hyperprolactinemic.* Fifteen percent of irregular ovulation is caused by secreting too much of the hormone prolactin, which interferes with both ovulation and embryo implantation in the uterus. Thirty percent of the time, women who have too much prolactin will notice milk in their breasts (called galactorrhea) or will notice milk when they squeeze their nipples during breast self-examination (BSE) (see chapter 8). Other symptoms might include decreased vaginal secretions and irregular cycles. This problem is caught by a simple blood test and then followed up by a CAT or MRI scan to check for possible *benign* pituitary tumors (occurring in about 5% of all women who are hyperprolactinemic). The drug bromocriptine (discussed below) is the usual treatment to offset prolactin secretion, to shrink any tumors that exist.
3. *Premature ovarian failure.* This is when your body goes into premature menopause. Your ovaries just "close for business." This is responsible for about 10% of all ovulation problems, and if you're under 30, your doctor may want to do a chromosome test. Diagnosis is fairly easy through blood tests and physical examination. Some causes include a decreased number of eggs at birth (they just get used up earlier), exposure to radiation or chemotherapy, or chromosomal abnormalities. This is not a treatable condition, but you may be put on hormone replacement therapy (HRT) to prevent osteoporosis and menopausal symptoms. (See chapter 13 for more on this.) In this situation, you and your partner have three choices: adoption, surrogate parenting, or childfree living.
4. *A deficiency in GnRH (gonadotropin-releasing hormone).* This hormone triggers the release of FSH and LH from the pituitary gland. Without

this, you won't ovulate. This is treated by replacing the hormone synthetically with GnRH or Pergonal, which contains LH and FSH.

5. *Luteal phase defects.* This is when you don't have enough progesterone to keep your uterus "embryo-friendly." Remember how the follicle bursts and then turns into a corpus luteum, which secretes progesterone? Well, this stage of your cycle is also called the luteal phase. Most women have a luteal phase that lasts 10–14 days. If your luteal phase lasts for less than 9 days, you have a luteal phase "defect." This is diagnosed from a blood test done during your luteal phase (the "serum progesterone test") as well as an endometrial biopsy (see below). You might want to review chapter 2 to recall how a normal cycle should work.

The endometrial biopsy.

The biopsy procedure, discussed in chapter 8, is used to investigate hormonal imbalances that can cause irregular cycles or anovulatory cycles, irregular uterine bleeding, and repeated miscarriages (see below). In each situation, the biopsy is done at different times in the cycle to check for different things, but it's preferable to do it before the bleeding starts. In *this* case, the biopsy is done within the first 18 hours of your period to examine the characteristics of your endometrium: to make sure it's the right consistency and thickness for that time of the month, which will indicate whether you're secreting the right *combination and levels* of hormones. Since some doctors may choose to do the biopsy just before your period, to avoid risking pregnancy, it's important to practice a barrier method of contraception for this cycle. Waiting until you get your period is wiser. The outcome of your endometrial biopsy will determine whether you have a progesterone deficiency, an estrogen deficiency, or even a LH deficiency. Depending on the hormonal imbalance, you may just need a hormone supplement. *Note: If you have symptoms suggesting elevated levels of androgen or possible polycystic ovary syndrome, these factors will be investigated before you have the biopsy and would not necessitate an endometrial biopsy.* In this case, it is also important to check for endometrial hyperplasia.

Fertility Drugs

Your fertility observation charts, blood tests, and/or an endometrial biopsy (see below) will confirm whether you are ovulating regularly or have a lutueal phase defect. To treat you, your doctor may suggest putting you on a drug therapy that induces ovulation or increases your progesterone level during your luteal phase. This is a similar situation to being put on progesterone supplements to induce menstruation. There are four fertility drugs prescribed for ovulation/luteal phase problems:

Clomiphene Citrate (Clomid or Serophene)

With the exception of hyperprolactinemic women, this is the first drug you'll be placed on. This is an *antiestrogen* and induces ovulation by tricking the pituitary into producing FSH and smaller amounts of LH. FSH will cause your ovary to spit out several follicles, which will increase your estrogen levels. Then, when you stop the drug, you'll get your LH surge, which stimulates ovulation and provides you with a nice, "high-quality" luteal phase. This drug is also used for women undergoing *in vitro fertilization* (IVF).

Roughly a million women have used clomiphene by now. It tends to work best in women who ovulate occasionally rather than never, and it may be used to treat an inadequate luteal phase, but it is utterly useless for improving fertility in women who ovulate regularly and who have no menstrual cycle abnormality. Using a 28-day cycle as an example of how it works, you'd start about 50 millligrams of clomiphene on day 5 of your cycle. You'd take it until about day 9 and then go off it. This will induce ovulation about 6–10 days later (or roughly the 15th to 19th day of the cycle). You'll need to keep track of your BBT throughout this process and will probably have your serum progesterone levels taken around this time to monitor whether the drug is working. If you don't menstruate at all, you'll have your period induced by a progesterone supplement before you start the drug treatment. If 50 milligrams don't do the trick, the dosage may be gradually increased to as much as 250 milligrams a day for five or more days per cycle.

Women who shouldn't use clomiphene are those with large fibroids (the drug may stimulate them to grow even larger), those with ovarian cysts (because the drug causes more follicles to ripen, there's a higher risk of developing cysts), and those with liver problems (dysfunctional livers won't absorb and break down the drug properly).

Clomiphene is considered to be a safe drug, *but* it is simply too new to yield any statistics on whether children born to mothers on clomiphene suffer any long-term side effects. What is known is that clomiphene does cause certain immediate side effects on users. For one thing, it can reduce the quality of your cervical mucus, solving one fertility barrier but creating another. And, because it increases estrogen in the body, some women report OC-related symptoms such as nausea, vomiting, vision problems, headaches, insomnia, hot flashes, breast tenderness, and premenstrual-like emotional symptoms. Clomiphene is the cheapest of the fertility drugs. About 60% of all women on clomiphene ovulate, while about 30% do get pregnant within the first three months of treatment. There is also about a 10% chance of conceiving twins if you take the drug, and in fact, the risk of miscarriage *drops* (because the drug also helps the luteal phase, the pregnancy "sticks").

Bromocriptine (Parlodel)

Again, bromocriptine is the drug prescribed for *hyperprolactinemia*. It suppresses your hypothalamus, and hence suppresses prolactin. This won't *cure* your hyperprolactinemia, but it will control it while you take the drug. You'll also need a CAT scan to rule out the possibility of a benign pituitary tumor.

The dosage is pretty low because bromocriptine is extremely potent. You'll start with about 2.5 milligrams once a day, then will eventually graduate to 2.5 milligrams three times daily. Once you get pregnant, you'll be taken off the drug immediately. The side effects can be nasty dizziness, nausea, nasal congestion, low blood pressure, and headaches. The side effects subside with time. The drug is considered safe, but has only been in use for about a decade. So far, it hasn't been known to cause any birth defects, but it's still too new to yield any long-term statistics.

About 90% of women on bromocriptine will ovulate as long as they take it; 65–85% of these women get pregnant. This is a more expensive drug.

Human Menopausal Gonadotropin (Pergonal)

Women who don't respond to clomiphene will move on to HMG. HMG is basically pure FSH and LH hormone. Believe it or not, it's a natural hormone made from the *urine* of postmenopausal women! This is a very expensive drug, costing well over $1000 per cycle. It is an injectable drug that needs to be administered during your "dry days" for about 12 days in a row. Your partner can be trained to administer injections. Your estrogen levels, mucus, and ovaries will be monitored. Then, you'll need to have ultrasounds done to determine the quality, quantity, and maturity of your follicles. If too many follicles develop, the doctor will stop the treatment until the next cycle to avoid a grossly multiple birth. Basically, the HMG dosage is adjusted to the number of follicles developing, estrogen levels, and so on. When the ultrasound reveals mature eggs, you'll be injected with *human chorionic gonadotropin (HCG),* which stimulates LH. Ovulation should occur 24–36 hours later.

This drug regimen is sometimes used in conjunction with clomiphene. Most women who take this will have low estrogen levels. It may also be used on some women undergoing IVF, women with polycystic ovary syndrome, or women with luteal phase defects.

Women who shouldn't take this drug are those with possible pituitary tumors, thyroid disorders, adrenal problems, or ovarian cysts. There are lots of side effects. First, twins occur in 20-40% of all pregnancies that result from HMG. There are also higher risks of miscarriage and premature delivery. In about 5% of HMG cycles, you'll become sort of "estrogen-toxic" due to an overproduction of estrogen in your body (called *hyperstimulation syndrome.*) The side effects include abdominal swelling, ovarian enlargement, and weight gain. In more severe cases, swelling might warrant hospitalization for about two weeks.

In the end, while 75% of women will ovulate with HMG, the pregnancy rate on the drug drastically varies: 20–80% of all HMG cycles will end in pregnancy. The bottom line is that because of the expense, inconvenience, and side effects, this drug should be used as a last resort.

Gonadotropin-Releasing Hormone: Getting Pumped Up

If you have a GnRH deficiency, you'll be put on natural GnRH hormone, but it is administered in a very peculiar way. You'll be provided with a battery-run pump about 3 inches by 4 inches, also used by diabetics for taking measured doses of insulin.

GnRH hormone is placed in a bag inside the pump. One end of the bag is plastic tubing that's attached to the pump; the other end is a needle attached to an arm vein with surgical tape, which is changed every four or five days. You can wear long sleeves to hide the needle, and the pump can be worn in a pocket. Once you start the pump, it automatically pulsates a tiny injection of GnRH into your system every 90 minutes, simulating what your hypothalamus would normally do. Then, your body responds by producing the right amount of hormones necessary for you to ovulate. You'll also need a HCG injection with this.

There are no known side effects to this system, except the inconvenience of the pump. Most women on this system will ovulate after about a week on the pump. However, this is also very expensive.

The Postcoital Test (PCT): Is Your Cervical Mucus "Sperm-Friendly?"

Once your doctor has exhausted ovulation problems, he or she will next suggest the postcoital test. Some doctors may suggest a *hysterosalpingogram*, a test that checks for blockage or scarring of the fallopian tubes (discussed below). If you have a history of chlamydia, gonorrhea, PID, IUD use, previous abortions, ectopic pregnancy, endometriosis, pelvic cancer (this would have to have been caught very early to still have any reproductive organs intact; see chapter 9), or pelvic surgery, this will likely be the next step.

If you haven't had any of these things in your past, your doctor will proceed with the postcoital test, which is less invasive than a hysterosalpingogram and checks for more problems. This test is painless. You'll need to make an appointment with your gynecologist around your mucus peak day. Then, you and your partner will need to have intercourse about 12 hours before the appointment. (Some doctors do it 2–4 hours after, but this isn't the best time, explained below.) The timing depends on your schedule and your doctor's. When you arrive at your doctor's office, he or she will get you into the Pap position, and then insert a syringe high inside your vagina to collect your postcoital mucus. The doctor will insert an instrument into your cervical canal to retrieve mucus. Your cervical opening should also be dilated slightly and will change in color slightly around ovulation. Your doctor will make sure to check for this. The dilated opening allows more sperm through.

This is an important test that reveals the *relationship* between your partner's sperm and your cervical mucus. It tells the doctor how well they're "getting along." The test also tells the doctor about your ovulation cycle. After collecting the postcoital mucus, your doctor places it under a microscope and examines it. The first thing that's checked is the cervical mucus consistency. It should be eggwhite-like, transparent, stretchy (stretching about 6-10 centimeters), have an alkaline pH balance (to match the pH balance of healthy sperm), and be rich in mucin, glycoprotein, and salt. If your mucus is too dry or scanty, or lacking these properties, the sperm will not be able to survive long enough to fertilize the ovum. The doctor will also check for sperm life signs and the number of sperm present. *This is why 12 hours after intercourse is the best time for the test.* Since healthy sperm should be able to survive for *at least* 24 hours after intercourse, if there are no live sperm after 12 hours, there's a big problem. If sperm are absent, or immobilized (live but paralyzed) after 12 hours, this is an indication of mucus rich in sperm antibodies, faulty sperm production, or sometimes just poor intercourse positions. Another reason why this test is best performed 12 hours after intercourse is because it puts far less pressure on you and your partner. The two of you can simply have intercourse the night before. Then, in the morning, you go for the test, or vice versa.

If everything is normal, you'll move on to the next stop: a hysterosalpingogram, to check out your tubes, discussed below.

Roughly 15% of all female infertility problems *are* caused by poor-quality cervical mucus. If *this* is what the postcoital test finds, you may be put on estrogen supplements about 7–10 days before ovulation to try to raise the quality of the mucus. This doesn't work too often, though. A somewhat odd remedy that *has* been known to work is taking *decongestant cough syrup* during the first two weeks of your cycle to increase mucus production throughout the body! In fact, this is considered the "answer" to infertility in some small towns. Some women have reported an increase in the quality and quantity of their mucus by using this method and *have* gotten pregnant as a result. (Sometimes truth really *is* stranger than fiction.) There is no definitive scientific evidence to support the cough syrup cure. In any event, many specialists will tell you to give it a try, because at worst, this peculiar practice is harmless. You'll be asked to repeat the PCT a few times during your mucus "Total Quality Management" effort. If estrogen and cough syrups fail, the only other choice left to you is to have your partner's sperm placed high inside your cervix: this is known as *artificial insemination by husband (AIH)*, although of course, your partner doesn't have to be your husband.

If the PCT results find that the sperm are immobilized or dead, *yet* the semen analysis and cervical mucus is normal, your infertility may be caused by the presence of sperm antibodies, which means a kind of "sperm allergy." With this kind of test result, you'll be asked to repeat the test using the missionary positions-pillow-bicycle routine discussed earlier. If you still get the same PCT result, *immunological infertility* is probably what's going on. For some reason, your own immune system thinks that the sperm is a virus or invader and develops antibodies against it that destroy the sperm. This can be confirmed with further tests on both of you. There is no known effective treatment for this. Some doctors suggest clearing out all sperm from your system, using a condom for the next six months, and then trying again. The theory is that your body may relax once it's rid of its "invader." Then, you can sneak the sperm back during ovulation, and hopefully become pregnant before your immune system has time to destroy the sperm. Another theory is to put you on cortisone treatments to suppress your immune system; this has a very low success rate of about 25%. Otherwise, your only choice is IVF, discussed in the next section.

Looking into the Tubes: Hysterosalpingogram (HSG)

If your ovulation cycle is normal and you've passed your PCT with flying colors, it's time to check out the fallopian tubes. An HSG checks for PID-related *salpingitis,* inflammation of the fallopian tubes due to infection (discussed in chapter 6) or *endometriosis* (discussed in chapter 2). If you have a colorful pelvic history, an HSG will be the first stop for you, and if you pass, you'll then go to the hormonal tests, then to PCT.

This test may be uncomfortable but is not extremely painful unless the tubes are blocked. The pain *is* brief, however. You'll get into a Pap position, and your doctor will place a clamp on your cervix, which is uncomfortable. Then, your doctor injects a dye into the uterus, which should fly through your tubes and is eventually absorbed by your body. An X ray is taken as the dye is injected and can tell whether the dye passed through the tubes' open ends. If the dye passes through, your tubes are open; if it doesn't, your tubes are blocked. If your tubes are blocked, your doctor may want to do a laparoscopy (see chapter 2). Or, he or she may suspect PID and treat you with an aggressive antibiotic regimen (see chapter 6). Because the dye is a foreign substance, to prevent any risk of infection you may need to be on antibiotics for about three days before you take this test. Some doctors recommend that you take anti-inflammatory medication prior to the test to reduce cramping. Laparoscopy will find other structural problems caused by PID, cysts, or endometriosis. Pelvic reproductive surgery is discussed in chapter 6. Treatment for endometriosis is discussed in chapter 2.

Unexplained Infertility

About 10% of couples will not find an identifiable cause of infertility. Of those, 20% will get pregnant each year for three years. While it may be a relief that nothing is "technically wrong with you," it's also a maddening predicament. The situation can create tension in your relationship and may be aggravated by rude or tactless remarks from outsiders.

Assisted Conception

If you've found the cause of your infertility and it cannot be reversed or treated successfully, you may be a candidate for assisted conception. You'll need to find a gynecologist who is trained in two areas: reproductive endocrinology and fertility surgery. Couples with unexplained infertility are also ideal candidates for some of these procedures. Until 1978, couples who couldn't conceive had two choices: adoption or child-free living. In 1978, the first "test tube" baby, Louise Brown, was born. Since then, thousands of children worldwide are born as a result of reproductive technologies that literally assist couples in the conception process. In the 1980s, the ethical implications of various assisted conception techniques were debated; critics argued about the moral issue of children being conceived in a laboratory. Yet essentially, these techniques are no more "immoral" than administering drugs that induce ovulation, correcting anatomical problems surgically, or *preventing* conception through contraceptive technologies. We are now living in an era where the term *family planning* has taken on a futuristic dimension. However, the technology of many of these procedures is by no means a perfect science. There is a high degree of trial and error involved with these techniques, and a very high failure rate as a result. Many couples need to be assisted *repeatedly* before they have a successful pregnancy. Although assisted conception is a wonderful option for couples who can't conceive, it is not a panacea to infertility. The assisted conception process is difficult and stressful and truly requires a committed and emotionally stable couple.

Before you and your partner look into assisted conception, it's important to examine all of your options first. This includes surrogacy (which, although considered by some to be "assisted conception," is actually one of the oldest alternatives to infertility, written about in the Old Testament), adoption, and choosing a life without children. The documentary series *Only Human* reported the results of a survey it conducted on parents of toddlers. Each couple was asked: "If you could turn back the clock and make your decision about children again, would you make the *same* decision, based on what you know *now*?" Over 75% of these couples said no. Seeking the services of a good counselor or therapist is often helpful when you're making this decision; it's difficult to be objective and realistic when you want a child so badly.

Although you may successfully conceive through the techniques discussed below, the risk of miscarriage is high and the rates of successful births are low. Ultimately, you need to weigh these risks against other options. You'll have to gauge whether you're strong enough to weather not only the disappointment and pain of infertility, but the added anxiety of a high-risk pregnancy and the grief of potentially losing a pregnancy you worked so hard to achieve. Miscarriage and the risks involved in an unremarkable pregnancy are discussed in chapter 10; repeated miscarriage is discussed below.

Assisted conception is complicated and involves several steps. To *truly* grasp the nature of each procedure, a degree in molecular biology really helps! Since most of us can't boast this credential, what I've done is provide you with a brief description of each process. If you're considering any of these procedures, you'll need to research far more detailed sources, which I've listed at the back of the book.

In Vitro Fertilization (IVF)

The term *in vitro* means "in glass"; today, "in plastic" is more accurate. This is a process that combines using fertility drugs (clomiphene and, if not successful, HMG) to induce ovulation, removing those eggs via microsurgery and/or ultrasound, and then placing them in a plastic dish and fertilizing them with your partner's sperm.

The process is expensive, stressful, and drawn out. (In the United States, a "good" price is $8000 *per attempt*; in Canada, some of these procedures may not be covered by universal health care.) Bear in mind that successful IVF requires at least two attempts for any kind of success. Even if you are ovulating regularly, you'll be placed on clomiphene to stimulate the production of multiple follicles on your ovary. You may also be placed on HMG. This increases your doctor's chances of obtaining a good, "fertilizable" egg. You'll be monitored closely, and when your eggs are ripe, you'll undergo a microsurgery procedure vaginally with the aid of ultrasound or by laparoscopy where your doctor actually *retrieves* your eggs.

The fertility drugs do tend to create chromosomally imperfect eggs, so you may need to have more than one cycle's worth of eggs retrieved before your doctor finds an acceptable one. When this happens, the egg is "nurtured" in the laboratory until it is mature enough to interact with your partner's sperm. Any other "good" embryos retrieved might be frozen for future attempts, known as *cryopreservation*. At that point, your partner must follow the same rules for a semen analysis and provide the lab with a specimen. The lab then carefully "washes" the sperm, simulating the natural capacitation process sperm naturally undergo when they swim upstream toward the egg. The sperm are placed in the dish with the egg and do their thing. This whole process of growing the eggs, washing the sperm, and fertilizing the egg takes about a week. Meanwhile, your uterus may be helped along by progesterone supplements to help make it "embryo-friendly."

Then, you report back to the hospital and the fertilized eggs are transferred into your uterus either vaginally or through laparoscopy again. *Only 10% of all embryos in IVF transfer well and actually implant themselves within the uterus.* This is a huge drawback that should make you question whether the stress of repeated IVF procedures is worth it. After the embryo transfer is done, you'll report to the clinic about two weeks later for a pregnancy test. If your test is negative, you'll need to decide whether you're going to repeat the process and repeat the fee.

IVF does not carry encouraging success rates. First, bear in mind that only 55% of all pregnancies occurring in normal, fertile couples will result in a live birth. For IVF, only 15–20% of all IVF pregnancies will result in a live birth. The miscarriage rate is higher in IVF pregnancies and ranges from 45 to 60% in women over 40.

In vitro fertilization is obviously not for everyone. There are some specific cases where it is an ideal option:

- *Women who have tubal blockages of some sort.* In this case IVF is tried *after* microsurgery, which can successfully "declog" a fallopian tube. After microsurgery, you should try to conceive for another year or so before you seek out IVF. It's best to discuss with your doctor or therapist the pitfalls and benefits of repeated microsurgery versus repeated IVF attempts. Keep in mind that many centers will go directly to IVF instead of attempting to repair badly damaged tubes. Once you've made your decision, you'll be required to go through a screening process by your selected IVF program/clinic, discussed below.

- *Women with endometriosis.* Again, your doctor will first try to treat your endometriosis through drug therapy and/or microsurgery. If you don't respond and still can't conceive after at least a year, you can seek out IVF.
- *Couples with immunological infertility.*
- *Men with low sperm counts.*
- *Women who don't get pregnant despite fertility drug treatment.*
- *Couples with unexplained fertility.*

Here are some guidelines for making the IVF decision:

1. *Are you familiar with the procedure, the costs involved, and the success rates?* If you can afford only one attempt, you might want to save your money and seek out an alternative. Most couples try once or twice; however, most successes require at least a second attempt. For couples with unexplained infertility, low sperm count, or delayed conception in spite of fertility drugs, taking that money and using it to get away, forget, and relax, just may result in a pregnancy!
2. *Are you prepared to deal with the stress involved?* If you feel stressed now, wait until you begin IVF. You need to be in superb psychological "shape."
3. *Are you prepared to deal with a failed IVF attempt?* Remember, even if you're lucky enough to conceive, the miscarriage rates are high. Can you *really* handle losing this pregnancy? You might want to review chapter 10.
4. *Have you and your partner figured out how many attempts you're willing to go for?* Discuss this with your partner before you seek out IVF. Know your limits in advance, and know when to say "enough is enough."

Review IVF programs with either your reproductive endocrinologist/gynecologist, or your andrologist/urologist. These doctors will be able to refer you to a good program. If this fails, contact RESOLVE, Inc., an infertility organization that has an IVF referral service, and will direct you to a program in your area. The number is 617-643-2424. In Canada, contact the College of Physicians and Surgeons.

Once you've made your decision on an IVF clinic, you'll need to undergo a screening process. For most programs you'll need to meet these basic requirements:

1. *Can you ovulate on your own?* In order for fertility drugs to work best, you'll need to be able to ovulate on your own and just have your ovulation "augmented" by the drugs.

2. *Do you have "accessible ovaries?"* If you have endometriosis growing all over your ovaries, scarring as a result of PID, or numerous fibroids blocking the way, your doctor will have a harder time getting to the eggs.
3. *How old are you?* Your fertility does decline as you age. Most programs have cutoff ages of about 40, but may give priority to women over 35.
4. *Have you had all your prepregnancy screenings done?* You'll need to be screened for certain conditions, such as rubella, before a pregnancy. Check out chapter 10 for more information.
5. *Is your partner's semen analysis normal?* It's hard to believe that some couples haven't checked this out before undergoing IVF, but it happens. In any event, if there are sperm problems, IVF won't work!
6. *Are you willing to go for a psychological workup?* You'd better, because all programs recommend pretreatment counseling first. If you're not psychologically "up to it," IVF will do you no good.
7. *Can you afford it?* You may need to disclose your income and assets to a clinic. They won't attempt IVF if you can't pay for it.

Gamete Intra-Fallopian Transfer (GIFT)

This is a very similar process to IVF but about half as expensive. It carries the same risks, the same success rates, and the same stress. There are three differences, however:

1. You need one good fallopian tube, normal semen, and good PCT results. (Couples with unexplained infertility usually are the best candidates.)
2. Instead of fertilizing the eggs in a laboratory, your mature eggs and your partner's "prewashed" sperm are mixed up in a syringe together and inserted via laparoscopy right into your fallopian tube. Then, you just wait for nature to take its course.
3. You'll need to follow the bed-rest guidelines discussed in chapter 6 after the procedure. More than one try is usually the norm, with a maximum of four tries.

Artificial Insemination

Artificial insemination is not a difficult procedure and is an ideal option for women with cervical mucus problems. What you do need is to be able to ovulate, have an "embryo-friendly" uterus, have a good set of fallopian tubes, and have no other pelvic abnormalities. What you don't necessarily need is your partner's sperm.

Artificial insemination is an option for cervical mucus problems, low sperm count, poor motility, or sperm antibodies. Your partner's sperm is collected semen-analysis style, washed, and injected by syringe either very high into your vagina (this carries only a 13% success rate) or right into your cervix (this carries a 10–25% success rate). Artificial insemination is done only after you've tried to treat your infertility with other means.

Donor insemination (DI) is done when your partner has a zero sperm count or other irreversible problems resulting in abnormal sperm. However, you need to be perfectly fertile yourself, and not on any fertility drugs. Here, someone *other* than your partner provides the sperm. This is basically surrogate parenting in reverse. The child will have the mother's genes only. This, again, is a difficult decision that you'll need to carefully weigh over the alternatives. The donor can be from a sperm bank that has prescreened donors for STDs and all kinds of other problems. Do *not* select your own donor and attempt DI with a turkey baster!

The success rates of DI are higher because there's no infertility problem to reckon with. Success rates range between 40 and 80%. However, because of the stress involved, your otherwise healthy cycles may become irregular. This will correct itself without the use of clomiphene.

Embryo Transfer

Here, a female donor supplies eggs for an IVF procedure. This is when your partner is fertile, but *you* have an irreversible problem that does not respond to treatment. You will need to have a healthy uterus for this and be able to sustain a pregnancy. Your husband's sperm is inseminated into a donor woman who's fertile. When a pregnancy results, your uterus is "prepped" for a pregnancy, and the embryo is transferred to you. This is not a very successful treatment because there's a very high rate of miscarriage or failure to implant the embryo. If it's successful, you'll carry the fetus to term and give birth to a child that is genetically your husband's but not yours.

Host Uterus

When you're ovulating perfectly and your partner is fertile, but your uterus can't successfully sustain a pregnancy, you might want to consider a host uterus. Here, you'll go through an IVF program where your egg and your husband's sperm are fertilized. The embryo is then implanted into the healthy uterus of *another* woman, who will carry your genetic child to term for you. Often, a relative of the woman is selected—sister, mother—who can share the pregnancy experience with you. The success rate is about the same as for IVF, but this technique might work better because the uterus is healthier.

Intravaginal Culture: The New IVF?

This is a very new procedure that was developed in France. It works exactly like IVF, except the egg and sperm are put inside the vagina to fertilize on their own, with a diaphragm put in place to "hold them there." Then the fertilized egg is removed and through laparoscopy is placed directly in the uterus. The vagina is used because it's cheaper than IVF and may yield the same results. This procedure is too new to yield any significant statistics regarding success rates.

Repeated Miscarriage

As discussed in chapter 10, if you've miscarried more than twice, you're prone to what's known as repeated miscarriage. This *is* considered a form of infertility, but in my opinion, labeling repeated miscarriage as infertility, meaning "inability to *conceive*," is inaccurate. Repeated miscarriages have to do with an "inability to *complete* the pregnancy." This is truly a different kind of problem than never even *becoming* pregnant to begin with. Nevertheless, women who suffer from repeated miscarriages will need to undergo a battery of tests under the care of an "infertility specialist"—a reproductive endocrinologist/gynecologist.

The tests are similar to the workup described above: an endometrial biopsy, and an hysterosalpingogram. In most cases of repeated miscarriage, the cause is found; in a few cases, nothing is ever determined to be as the definitive cause, but women who have suffered as many as six or seven miscarriages can go on to have a successful pregnancy.

Some completely preventable causes of miscarriages have to do with undiagnosed STDs. There is no accurate statistic that can tell us how many miscarriages are caused by STDs. That's why it's crucial to have a thorough screening done before you try to conceive. Another cause of some miscarriages that's also not statistically tracked is the effect of certain toxins that include anesthetic gases (on any consent form for a surgical procedure, you'll be informed about a risk of miscarriage). Exposure to lead and mercury are also causes, but usually these toxins are discovered before a second miscarriage.

Some doctors believe that a significant number of repeated, first-trimester miscarriages are caused by a progesterone deficiency; others don't espouse this theory at all. In any event, if your doctor *is* a "believer," the treatment involves daily dosages of natural progesterone in suppository form during the luteal phase of the menstrual cycle. Then, if conception occurs, progesterone suppositories are given daily for the first 12 weeks of pregnancy. Some doctors will also prescribe clomiphene citrate prior to conception, which will increase the amount of progesterone throughout the early stages of pregnancy, and which is associated with lower incidences of miscarriage. Progesterone supplements in suppository or clomiphene form are successful about 80% of the time.

Between 20 and 25% of all repeated miscarriages are due to immunological problems. In some cases, the woman's immune system causes her body to reject the fetus as foreign tissue. (This is also discussed briefly in chapter 5 in the section on pregnancy). This problem can often be solved by injecting white blood cells from the woman's partner into her body before conception, so that her body gets "used to" his cells and therefore "recognizes" the fetus later on as "friendly." Some clinics report about a 70% success rate using this method.

Other immunological causes involve women who produce antibodies that indirectly cause clotting in blood vessels that lead to the developing fetus. The fetus is deprived of nutrients and dies in utero, which triggers an abortion. There are no definitive treatments, but some clinics are looking into combining acetylsalicylic acid (pain relievers), corticosteroids, or anticoagulants such as *heparin*.

About 15% of all repeated miscarriages are caused by a uterine structural problem, where tissue interferes with fetal development. This is usually correctable with surgery, but it depends on the severity of the defect.

Finally, about 3% of repeated miscarriages are caused by an "incompetent cervix," discussed in chapter 10. This problem leads to second-trimester miscarriages. This can be prevented by stitching up the cervix.

While about 5% of repeated miscarriages are caused by chromosomal abnormalities, this is not a "correctable" problem but a "luck of the draw." It is also the cause of most first-time miscarriages that occur in one in six normal pregnancies. Couples need to keep trying until they strike a "good mix" of chromosomes. Fetuses that self-terminate because of genetic abnormalities are discussed more in chapter 10.

A Word About Secondary Infertility

It is possible to be infertile after having one or more biological children. This is known as secondary infertility, while primary infertility is the official label given to couples who have never conceived. Secondary infertility carries unique frustrations because couples can't help saying, "We've reproduced once, why can't we reproduce again?" Couples plagued with secondary infertility will go through the exact workup discussed above. Some of the causes of secondary infertility have to do with:

- *Endometriosis* (see chapter 2)
- *Age.* Sometimes five years can make a big difference in a woman's fertility cycle and a man's sperm count. Many couples have one child and then space out the next one to coincide with their first child's school schedule. For busy career couples, this spacing helps make two children more manageable.
- *Scarring in the pelvic region.* As discussed in Chapter 6, childbirth may put you at risk for a bacterial infection, causing PID. The bacteria can enter your pelvic region through the dilated cervix.
- *Stress.* This can affect ovulation. After having one child, a couple's "workload" and exhaustion level can increase enormously.
- *Strenuous exercise and weight loss.* Many women will overdo it in the gym in a mad scramble to reclaim their figures after childbirth. This can affect ovulation.

Whatever the cause, couples with secondary infertility will need to consider the same options as couples dealing with primary infertility.

Parenting Without Pregnancy

You can still parent a child without experiencing pregnancy and childbirth. In fact, this is often a satisfying solution to many infertile couples and preferable to assisted conception procedures.

Until the incidences of STDs and PID decline, and anovulatory cycles related to financial and emotional stress *decrease,* adoption will continue to be as much a "gynecological" solution as it is a "social" decision. There is considerable stress involved with repeated workups and reversing certain causes of infertility. Many couples will and *should* ask "Is all this worth it for a biological child?" After reviewing their true motivations for wanting a biological child, many couples will *not* pursue infertility testing and assisted conception and decide to love a child that's already here. This is a logical decision, considering how many unwanted children there are who *need* parents! Unfortunately, there are two societal myths that interfere with a couple's decision to adopt: "Biological parents make *better* parents," and "biological children make *better* children." *This just isn't true!*

Until the 1970s, adoptions in North America were handled by public or private agencies that had more babies up for adoption than couples willing to parent them. As a result of more sophistication regarding birth control, the legalization of abortion, and the destigmatizing of parenting a child outside of marriage, there are now more couples seeking to adopt a baby than there are available babies. In the 1990s, more than half of all North American adoptions are independent adoptions (private adoption). This is when birth parents are actively involved in finding an adoptive family. Although public and private agency adoption is still alive and well, the process usually takes longer and involves no contact between the birth parents and adoptive parents.

If you're willing to adopt an older child, a child who is a visible minority (even if you are, too), or a special-needs child, you can expect a child from a public or private agency almost immediately. The average wait in these same agencies for a Caucasian infant is *four to eight years.* The wait is much less through independent adoption.

Open adoption and international adoption are other options. Adoption is a complex topic that cannot be covered fully here. If you are considering adoption as an alternative, there are some excellent agencies that can guide you. See the appendix. Whether you go the adoption or surrogate route, you can combine this decision with continuing your attempt to conceive.

Surrogate Parenting

Surrogacy is a very old custom that goes back to the Old Testament. The first case of surrogacy involved Sarah and Abraham. The infertile Sarah (who probably just needed some clomiphene) "offered up" her handmaid, Hagar, to Abraham. With Abraham's sperm, Hagar conceived and bore him a son, Ishmael. (Unfortunately, Sarah got very jealous and cast Hagar out into the wilderness. Then, she, herself, conceived a child at the age of 100—really pushing back the biological clock!)

Surrogacy today is a little more sophisticated. This is an option if your husband is fertile but you are not. It involves artificially inseminating your partner's sperm into a surrogate womb, creating a child who has your partner's genes but not yours. Surrogate mothers are found by contacting family law practitioners who specialize in adoptions. Surrogacy is considered an offshoot of adoption: "adoption in advance." Less than 1,000 surrogate arrangements have been done in North America but it's predicted to become a booming business in the near future. The lawyer will draw up a contract between you, your partner, and the surrogate mother, addressing issues such as miscarriage. However, if the surrogate changes her mind, the contract is no guarantee that the courts will take your side. You'll also need to pay a fee to the surrogate, which averages between $10,000 and $20,000.

The Oldest Alternative: Child-free Living

Every family seems to have a kindly aunt and uncle who "never had any children." Until you *yourself* struggled with infertility, you probably never wondered *why* they had no children; you just accepted it. Well, if that aunt and uncle are now seniors, they could have adopted from a wide assortment of newborns in the past, *but they didn't.* Today, they probably live comfortably in a small condo somewhere, travel a great deal, enjoy their retirement, and dote on a large selection of nieces and nephews. When they pass on, they'll probably leave their money to their "favorite" niece or nephew and will always be fondly remembered.

Now, compare them to the "other" aunt and uncle with three miserable sons. Everyone in the family knows that these sons scammed their own parents out of their life savings. One son is a stingy businessman who nobody in the family likes, the other is a cocaine addict who sold his father's collector's-edition car to buy more coke, and the third son is a bum and never worked an honest day in his life.

I exaggerate these two lifestyles to point out that there is no guarantee of "happiness" either way. Some couples with children wish they'd never had them; couples with no children may regret it. The decision *itself* is not as important as how *comfortable you are with your choice.*

In the more recent past, a child-free lifestyle was often a *political* decision for many couples. During the 1950s and 1960s, many couples chose this because they feared a nuclear holocaust. By the 1970s, the issue of overpopulation became the motivating factor for the choice. Yet by the 1980s, child-free living had become a symbol of infertility and failure. This is a pity, considering what a liberating lifestyle option it can be. Obviously, you'll need to review your original reasons for wanting children before you make this choice. You'll also need to research the decision by interviewing other couples who are living child-free. Then, interview couples with children and find out how much of their own lives have been sacrificed. Remember, parenting is a selfless, largely self-sacrificing job. Choosing a child-free lifestyle may just be an appealing option in an economically turbulent and difficult world. In the 1990s, many couples are also choosing child-free living as a political choice because they truly feel the world is an environmental disaster area. Whatever your reasons, the decision is, of course, *reversible* anytime you wish.

In chapters 10, 11, and 12, we've focused on the risks we take on during a particular time frame in a woman's gynecological life: *her childbearing years.* The next chapter explores a completely different set of gynecological risks and rules: *the menopausal years.* With the cessation of the menstrual cycle comes new health challenges. The next chapter on menopausal health should be read by women experiencing menopause, women past menopause, women preparing for menopause, and daughters of pre-, peri-, or post-menopausal women.

CHAPTER 13

Menopause 101

Menopause is a recent phenomenon in our society. Several decades ago, women simply died prior to menopause. Only in this century have women ever outlived their ovaries.

Menopause is a Greek term taken from the words *menos*, which means "month," and *pause*, which means "arrest"—the arrest of the menstrual cycle. It is a time in every woman's life when her ovaries slow down, run out of eggs, and get ready to retire. The process involves a complex shutting down of hormones that have nourished the menstrual cycle until this point. As a result, the normal hormonal fluctuations women are used to throughout their menstrual cycles become far more erratic, responsible for the infamous menopausal "mood swings" that have created much of the negative mythology surrounding menopause in our culture.

Nevertheless, natural menopause and *menarche* (the first menstrual period) have a lot in common: They are both *gradual* processes that women ease into. A woman doesn't suddenly wake up to find herself in menopause any more than a young girl wakes up to find herself in puberty. However, when menopause occurs *surgically*—the by-product of an oophorectomy, ovarian failure following a hysterectomy (see chapter 7), or certain cancer therapies—it can be an extremely jarring process. *One out of every three women in North America will not make it to the age of 60 with her uterus intact.* These women may indeed wake up one morning to find themselves in menopause and will suffer far more noticeable and severe menopausal symptoms than women in whom menopause occurs naturally.

Because of surgical menopause, *hormone replacement therapy* (HRT) and *estrogen replacement therapy* (ERT, or "unopposed estrogen") have become hotly debated issues in women's health. The loss of estrogen in particular leads to drastic changes in the body's chemistry that trigger a more aggressive aging process (discussed further below). Replacing these hormones will offset the aging process and is an appropriate therapy for millions of women who are in surgical menopause and who should not be "aging before their time."

But what about women in natural menopause? Are the benefits of HRT as clear? (All women with an intact uterus will receive HRT, meaning progesterone *and* estrogen therapy.) Do all women in natural menopause *want* their natural aging process to be medicated?

In our youth-obsessed culture, the aging female body is associated with negative imagery. Women are encouraged to alter their appearance surgically to "cheat" the natural aging process. They dye their hair, undergo plastic surgery, have collagen injections to hide wrinkles, and spend billions of dollars each year on cosmetics, pills, creams, and fitness/diet products. If aging were perceived as a *positive* experience, perhaps North American women could welcome natural menopause rather than dread or fear it.

The purpose of this chapter is to discuss both the natural and surgical menopausal facts of life, which include the myths of menopause, the symptoms of menopause, the osteoporosis issue, the variety of health problems that women face as they age, and the benefits and risks of HRT and ERT. Hormone therapy is *not* a panacea to aging, nor is it the right decision for every menopausal women. One's age, medical history, and menopausal symptoms all need to be factored into the HRT or ERT decision. As a *gynecological* sourcebook, this chapter will also focus on the new gynecological facts of life for women in menopause: vaginal changes, uterine prolapse, urinary incontinence, sexual and lifestyle changes, gynecological warning signs, the appropriate tests during pre- and perimenopause, and the postmenopausal pelvic exam that must include a Pap smear for all intact uteri.

I've called this chapter "Menopause 101" for a reason: It is an introductory chapter that contains all the basic information, but it should be read in conjunction with more detailed books devoted solely to the subject of menopause. These books are listed in appendix B. As of this writing, *The Menopause Sourcebook* is in the works and will include most of the information discussed below, as well as discussing natural therapies for menopausal symptoms. As with pregnancy and infertility, menopause is an expansive topic that cannot possibly be covered in one chapter.

Natural Menopause

When menopause occurs naturally, it tends to take place anywhere between the ages of 48 and 52, but it can occur as early as your late 30s, or as late as your mid-50s. When menopause occurs *before* 35, it is technically considered premature menopause, but just as menarche is genetically predetermined, so is menopause. For an average woman with an unremarkable medical history, what she eats or does in terms of activity will *not* influence the timing of her menopause. Women who have had chemotherapy, though, or have been exposed to high levels of radiation (such as radiation therapy in their pelvic area for cancer treatment) may go into menopause earlier. In any event, the average age of menopause is 50.

Other possible causes of early menopause include mumps (in small groups of women, the infection causing the mumps has been known to spread to the ovaries, prematurely shutting them down) and specific autoimmune diseases, such as lupus or rheumatoid arthritis (in some of these women, their bodies develop antibodies and attack the ovaries). Smokers also tend to have earlier menopause.

The Stages of Natural Menopause

Socially, the word *menopause* refers to a process, not a precise moment in the life of your menstrual cycle. Medically, the word *menopause* does *indeed* refer to one precise moment: the date of your last period. The events preceding and following menopause amount to a huge change for women both physically and socially. Physically, this process has four stages:

1. *Premenopause.* Although some doctors may refer to a 32-year-old woman in her childbearing years as premenopausal, this is not really an appropriate label. The term *premenopause* ideally refers to women on the cusp of menopause. Their periods have just *started* to get irregular, but they do not yet experience any classic menopausal symptoms such as hot flashes or vaginal dryness. A woman in premenopause is usually in her mid-to-late 40s. If your doctor tells you that you're premenopausal, you might want to ask him or her how he or she is using this term.
2. *Perimenopause.* This term refers to women who are in the thick of

menopause. Their cycles may be wildly erratic, and they are experiencing hot flashes and vaginal dryness. This label is applicable for about four years, covering the first two years prior to the official "last" period to the next two years following the last menstrual period. Women who are perimenopausal will be in the age groups discussed above, averaging to about age 51.

3. *Menopause.* This refers to your final menstrual period. You will not be able to pinpoint your final period until you've been completely free from periods for one year. Then, you count back to the last period you charted, and *that* date is the *date of your menopause. Note: After more than one year of no menstrual periods, any vaginal bleeding is now considered* abnormal.
4. *Postmenopause.* This term refers to the last third of most women's lives, ranging from women who have been free of menstrual periods for at least one year to women celebrating their 100th birthday. In other words, once you're past menopause, you'll be referred to as postmenopausal for the rest of your life. The terms *postmenopausal* and *perimenopausal* are sometimes used interchangeably, but this is technically inaccurate.

Used in a *social* context, nobody really bothers to break down menopause as precisely. When you see the word *menopausal* in a magazine article, you are seeing what's become acceptable medical slang, referring to women who are premenopausal and perimenopausal, a time frame that *includes* the actual menopause. When you see *postmenopausal* in a magazine article, you are seeing another accepted medical slang, which includes women who are in perimenopause and "official" postmenopause.

"Diagnosing" Premenopause or Perimenopause

When you begin to notice the signs of menopause, either you'll suspect the approach of menopause on your own, or your doctor will put two and two together when you report your symptoms. Two very simple tests will accurately determine what's going on and what stage of menopause you're in. Your follicle stimulating hormone (FSH) levels will dramatically rise as your ovaries begin to shut down; these levels are easily checked through one blood test. In addition, your vaginal walls will thin, and the cells lining the vagina will not contain as much estrogen. Your doctor will simply take a Pap-like smear from your vaginal walls—simple and painless—and analyze the smear to check for vaginal "atrophy," the thinning and drying out of your vagina. As I'll discuss below, you'll need to keep track of your periods and chart them as they become irregular. Your menstrual pattern will be an added clue to your doctor about whether you are pre- or perimenopausal.

Recognizing the Signs of Natural Menopause

In the past, a long list of hysterical symptoms has been attributed to the "change of life," but medically, there are really just three classic *short-term* symptoms of menopause: erratic periods, hot flashes, and vaginal dryness. All three are caused by a decrease in estrogen. As for the emotional symptoms of menopause, such as irritability, mood swings, melancholy, and so on, they may or may not be directly related to hormone changes. Some women may find that estrogen therapy improves these symptoms, some may not, and some actually have psychiatric illnesses that require appropriate treatment. Decreased levels of estrogen, however, can make you more *vulnerable* to stress, depression, and anxiety, because estrogen loss affects REM sleep.

Every woman entering menopause will experience a change in her menstrual cycle. Not all women will experience hot flashes or even notice vaginal changes. This is particularly true if a woman is overweight. As discussed in chapter 8, estrogen is stored in fat cells, which is why overweight women also tend to be more at risk for estrogen-dependent cancers. The fat cells convert fat into estrogen, creating a type of estrogen reserve that the body will use during menopause, which can reduce the severity of estrogen loss symptoms. In addition, many women go through menopause without experiencing changes in their moods. The assumption that mood swings always accompany menopause, or that women who suffer from premenstrual syndrome (PMS) will always experience more severe menopausal symptoms, is an absolute myth. It is believed, however, that women who do suffer from PMS are more *likely* to experience mood swings.

Erratic periods.

Every woman will begin to experience an irregular cycle before her last period. Cycles may become longer or shorter with long bouts of amenorrhea. Sometimes she will just stop having her periods, never experiencing an erratic phase in her cycles. Periods may suddenly become light and scanty or heavy and crampy. The impact of suddenly irregular, "wild" cycles can be disturbing because menstrual cycle changes may also signify other problems. It's imperative to chart your periods (see chapter 2) and try to sort out your own pattern of "normal" irregular cycles. Bring your chart to your gynecologist to help confirm your suspicions that you are indeed entering menopause. If you're not entering menopause, you'll need to isolate the cause of your cycle changes, which is discussed in chapter 2. (Irregular cycles are also addressed in chapter 2.)

Of course, since you can go into menopause earlier than you might have anticipated, irregular cycles may not always be on your list of suspected causes behind your sudden cycle changes. Is there any way you can more accurately predict when your own menopause might occur? Yes. Although most women can expect their menopause to occur in their 50s, women who go into earlier menopause will usually have a family history of earlier menopause. Periods will generally become erratic approximately two years before the final period. However, some women may experience a longer premenopausal process than others.

Hot flashes.

Roughly 85% of all pre- and perimenopausal women experience "hot flashes." Hot flashes can begin when periods are either still regular or have just started to become irregular. They usually stop one to two years after your final menstrual period. A hot flash can feel different for each woman. Some women experience a feeling of warmth in their faces and upper bodies; some women experience sweating and chills. Some women feel anxious, tense, dizzy, or nauseous just before the hot flash; some feel tingling in their fingers or heart palpitations just before. Some women will experience their hot flashes during the day; others will experience them at night and may wake up so wet from perspiration that they need to change their bedsheets or nightclothes.

Nobody really understands what causes a hot flash, but researchers believe it has to do with mixed signals from the hypothalamus, which controls both body temperature and sex hormones. Normally, when the body is too warm, the hypothalamus sends a chemical message to the heart to cool off the body by pumping more blood, causing the blood vessels under the skin to dilate, which makes you perspire. During menopause, however, it's believed that the hypothalamus gets confused and sends this "cooling off" signal at the wrong times. A hot flash is not the same as being overheated. Although the skin temperature often rises between 4–8°F, the internal body temperature drops, creating this odd sensation.

Why does the hypothalamus get so confused? The answer is decreasi levels of estrogen. We know this because when synthetic estrogen is given to replace natural estrogen in the body, hot flashes disappear. Some researchers believe that a decrease in luteinizing hormone (LH) is also a key factor, and a variety of other hormones that influence body temperature are being looked at as well. Although hot flashes are harmless in terms of health risks, they are disquieting and stressful. Women in the following categories will experience more severe hot flashes than others:

- *Women who are in surgical menopause* (discussed further below).
- *Women who are thin.* When there's less fat on the body to store estrogen reserves, estrogen loss symptoms are more severe.
- *Women who don't sweat easily.* An ability to sweat makes extreme temperatures easier to tolerate. Women who have trouble sweating may experience more severe flashes.

Just as you must chart your periods when your cycles become irregular, it's also important to chart your hot flashes. Keep track of when the flashes occur, how long they last, and number their intensity from 1 to 10. This will help you determine a pattern for the flashes and allow you to prepare for them in advance, which will help reduce the stress. Report your hot flashes to your doctor, just as you would any changes in your cycle. Symptoms of hot flashes can also indicate other health problems, such as circulatory problems.

Short of taking ERT or HRT (see below), the only thing you can do about your hot flashes is to lessen your discomfort by adjusting your lifestyle to cope with the flashes. The more comfortable you are, the less intense your flashes will feel. Once you establish a pattern by charting the flashes, you can do a few things around the time of day your flashes occur. Some suggestions:

- Avoid synthetic clothing, such as polyester, because it traps perspiration.
- If you have night sweats, use only 100% cotton bedding.
- Avoid clothing with high necks and long sleeves.
- Dress in layers.
- Keep cold drinks handy.
- If you smoke, cut down or quit. Smoking constricts blood vessels and can intensify and prolong a flash.
- Avoid "trigger" foods such as caffeine, alcohol, spicy food, and sugar, and avoid eating large meals. Substitute herbal teas for coffee or regular tea.

...r doctor the benefits of taking vitamin E supplements. ...s vitamin E is essential for proper circulation and produc-...ones.
- Exercis... ...rove your circulation.
- Reduce your exposure to the sun; sunburn will aggravate your hot flashes because burnt skin cannot regulate heat as effectively. (Sun is discussed further below.)

Vaginal changes.

Estrogen loss will also cause vaginal changes. Since the production of estrogen causes the vagina to stay moist and elastic, the loss of estrogen will cause the vagina to become drier, thinner, and less elastic. This may also cause the vagina to shrink slightly in terms of width and length. In addition, the reduction in vaginal secretions causes the vagina to be less acidic. This can put you at risk for more vaginal infections, particularly yeast (see chapter 6). Again, women who are in surgical menopause and women who are physically thinner tend to have more severe vaginal dryness and repeated yeast infections.

As a result of these vaginal changes, you'll notice a change in your sexual activity. Your vagina may take longer to become lubricated, or you may have to depend on lubricants to have comfortable intercourse (see chapter 4 for information on safe lubricants).

Estrogen loss can affect other parts of your sex life as well. Your sexual libido may actually increase because testosterone levels can rise when estrogen levels drop. (The general rule is that your levels of testosterone will either stay the same or increase.) However, women who *do* experience an increase in sexual desire will also be frustrated that their vaginas are not accommodating their needs. First, there is the lubrication problem: More stimulation is required to lubricate the vagina naturally. Second, a decrease in estrogen means that less blood flows to the vagina and clitoris, which means that orgasm may be more difficult to achieve or may not last as long as it normally has in the past. Other changes involve the breasts. Normally, estrogen causes blood to flow into the breasts during arousal, which makes the nipples more erect, sensitive, and responsive. Estrogen loss causes less blood to flow to the breasts, which makes them less sensitive. Finally, since the vagina shrinks as estrogen decreases, it doesn't expand as much during intercourse, which may make intercourse less comfortable, particularly since the vagina is less lubricated.

Surgical Menopause

As discussed in chapter 7, surgical menopause is the result of a bilateral oophorectomy—the removal of both ovaries before natural menopause. Surgical menopause can also be the result of ovarian failure following a hysterectomy (for reasons discussed in chapter 7), or following cancer therapy, such as chemotherapy or radiation treatments.

A bilateral oophorectomy is often done in conjunction with a hysterectomy, or sometimes as a single procedure when ovarian cancer is suspected, for example. Chapters 7, 8, and 9 discuss reasons why an oophorectomy or hysterectomy might be performed. Chapter 7 discusses the hysterectomy and oophorectomy procedures in detail, but does not address the symptoms and treatment of estrogen loss for women in surgical menopause. These are highlighted in the following sections.

Bilateral Oophorectomy Symptoms

If you've had your ovaries removed after menopause, you won't be in "surgical menopause" and won't feel any hormonal differences in your body. If you've had a hysterectomy, though, you may experience some of the structural problems discussed in chapter 7. If you've had your ovaries removed before you've reached natural menopause, you'll wake up from your surgery in *post*menopause. Once the ovaries are removed, your body immediately stops producing estrogen and progesterone. Your FSH will skyrocket in an attempt to "make contact" with ovaries that no longer exist. Unlike women who go through menopause naturally, women wake up after a bilateral oophorectomy in immediate estrogen "withdrawal." It's that sudden: One day you have a normal menstrual cycle, the next day, you have none whatsoever. This can cause you to become understandably more depressed, but you'll also *feel* the physical symptoms of estrogen loss far more intensely than a woman in natural menopause. Your vagina will be *extremely* dry, your hot flashes will feel like sudden violent heat waves that will be very disturbing to your system, and of course, your periods will cease altogether instead of tapering off naturally. The period you had prior to your surgery will have been your last, so you won't even experience pre- or perimenopause, just postmenopause. You'll need to begin ERT *immediately* following surgery to prevent these sudden symptoms.

If you no longer have your uterus, you'll be on estrogen only, or unopposed estrogen. If you still have your uterus, you'll be placed on estrogen and progesterone HRT, for the reasons explained in the HRT/ERT section below. Any short-term menopausal symptoms will be alleviated by HRT/ERT. If there's a question as to whether your symptoms are related to menopause, your doctor will perform a vaginal smear and a blood test to detect your FSH levels. Dosages will vary from woman to woman, so don't compare notes with your friends and wonder why "she's taking only X amount" when you're taking Y amount.

If the blood supply leading to your ovary was not damaged during your surgery (see chapter 7), then you should still be able to produce enough estrogen for your body. If you begin to go into ovarian failure, the symptoms will depend on how fast the ovary is failing; you may experience symptoms more akin to natural menopause, or you may experience sudden symptoms mirroring the surgical menopause experience.

Ovarian Failure from Cancer Therapy

Chemotherapy and radiation treatments that involve the pelvic area may throw your ovaries into menopause. As above, you may experience a more gradual menopausal process, or you may be overwhelmed by sudden symptoms of menopause. This depends on what kind of therapy you've received and the speed at which your ovaries are failing. Before you undergo your cancer treatment, discuss how the treatments will affect your ovaries and what menopausal symptoms you can expect. (Other questions to ask your oncologist are listed in chapter 9.)

Postmenopausal Symptoms

The long-term effects of estrogen loss have to do with traditional symptoms of "aging." One of the key reasons why women will choose HRT or ERT (discussed further below) is to slow down or even reverse these symptoms. Yet it's important to keep in mind that the long-term effects of estrogen loss will not immediately set in after menopause. These changes are subtle and happen over several years. Even women who experience severe menopausal symptoms will not wake up to find that they've suddenly aged overnight; these changes occur gradually whether you experience surgical or natural menopause.

Skin Changes

As estrogen decreases, skin, like the vagina, tends to lose its elasticity; it too becomes thinner because it is no longer able to retain as much water. Sweat and oil glands also produce less moisture, which is what causes the skin to gradually dry, wrinkle, and sag.

Good moisturizers and skin care will certainly help to keep your skin more elastic, but there is one known factor that aggravates and speeds up your skin's natural aging process, damaging the skin even more: *the sun.* If you cut down your sun exposure, you can dramatically reduce visible aging of your skin. Period. The bad news is that much of the sun's damage on your skin is cumulative from many years of exposure. In fact, many researchers believe that when it comes to visible signs of aging, *estrogen loss is only a small factor.* For example, ultraviolet rays break down collagen and elastin fibers in the skin, which causes it to break down and sag. This is also what puts you at risk for skin cancer, the most notorious of which is melanoma, one of the most aggressive and malignant of all cancers.

Other sun-related problems traditionally linked to estrogen loss include "liver spots," light brown or tan splotches that develop on the face, neck, and hands as you age. These spots have *nothing* to do with the liver; they are sun spots caused by sun exposure. They are sometimes the result of HRT, in which case they are called *hyperpigmentation.*

Currently, dermatologists recommend sunblocks with an SPF of at least 15. In fact, sun damage is so widespread in our population that by the late 1990s, sunblock will most likely become part of all North American women's daily cosmetic routine; women will put it on as regularly as they do a daily moisturizer.

The Osteoporosis Issue

Osteoporosis literally means "porous bones" and is perhaps the most feared condition in the postmenopausal community. Unfortunately, osteoporosis is not always preventable and is a classic symptom of aging. Normally, in the life of a healthy, unremarkable woman, by her late 30s and 40s her bones become less dense. By the time she reaches her 50s, she may begin to experience bone loss in her teeth and become more susceptible to wrist fractures. Gradually, the bones in her spine weaken, fracture, and compress, causing upper back curvature and loss of height, known as a "dowager's hump." Osteoporosis is unfortunately more common in women than men because when a woman's skeletal growth is completed, she typically has 15% lower bone mineral density and 30% less bone mass than a man of the same age. Studies also show that women lose more trabecular bone (the inner, spongy part making up the internal support of the bone) at a higher rate than men.

There are three types of osteoporosis women are prone to: *postmenopausal, senile,* and *secondary. Postmenopausal osteoporosis* usually develops roughly 10–15 years after the onset of menopause. In this case, estrogen loss interferes with calcium absorption, and you begin to lose trabecular bone three times faster than the normal rate. You will also begin to lose parts of your *cortical* (the outer shell of the bone), but not as quickly.

Senile osteoporosis affects men and women. Here, you lose cortical and trabecular bone because of a decrease in bone cell activity that results from aging. Hip fractures are seen most often with this kind of osteoporosis. The decrease in bone cell activity affects your capacity to rebuild bone in the first place, but is also aggravated by low calcium intake.

In *secondary osteoporosis,* an underlying condition causes bone loss. These conditions include chronic renal disease, hypogonadism (an underactivity of the sex glands), hyperthyroidism (an overactive thyroid gland), some forms of cancer, gastrectomy (removal of parts of the stomach which interferes with calcium absorption), and the use of anticonvulsants.

Currently, it's estimated that 30 million North American women over the age of 45 are affected by osteoporosis, while more than 500,000 postmenopausal women in the United States alone will have an osteoporosis-related fracture each year. These fractures usually involve the spine, hip, or distal radius. This might sound like a pretty bleak picture, but there are certainly things we can do to help offset and combat osteoporosis and possibly even prevent it altogether.

What causes bone loss?

Our bones are always regenerating. This process helps to maintain a constant level of calcium in the blood, essential for a healthy heart, blood circulation, and blood clotting. About 99% of all the body's calcium is in the bones and teeth; when blood calcium drops below a certain level, the body will *take* calcium from the bones to replenish it. But by the time we reach our late 30s, our bones lose calcium faster than it can be replaced. The pace of bone calcium loss speeds up for "freshly postmenopausal" women who are three to seven years beyond menopause. The pace then slows once again, but as we age, the body is less able to absorb calcium from food. One of the most influential factors affecting bone loss is estrogen; it slows or even halts the loss of bone mass by improving our absorption of calcium from the intestinal tract, which allows us to maintain a higher level of calcium in our blood. And, the higher the calcium levels in the blood, the less chance you have of losing calcium from your bones to replenish your calcium blood levels. In men, testosterone does the same thing for them regarding calcium absorption, but unlike women, men never reach a particular age when their testes *stop* producing testosterone. If they did, they would be just as prone to osteoporosis as women.

But estrogen alone cannot prevent osteoporosis. A long list of other factors affects bone loss. One of the most obvious is calcium in our diet. Calcium is regularly lost to urine, feces, and dead skin. We need to continuously account for this loss in our diet. The less calcium we ingest, the more we force our body into taking it out of our bones. Exercise also greatly affects bone density; the more we exercise, the stronger we make our bones. The bone mass we have in our late 20s and early 30s will affect our bone mass at menopause.

Several physical conditions and external factors help to weaken our bones, contributing to bone loss later in life:

- *Heavy caffeine and alcohol intake.* These are diuretics; they cause you to lose more calcium in your urine.
- *Smoking.* Research shows that smokers tend to go into earlier menopause, while older smokers have 20–30% less bone mass than nonsmokers.
- *Women in surgical menopause who are not on ERT.* Losing estrogen earlier than you would have naturally increases your bone loss.
- *Antacids containing aluminum and corticosteriods.* These interfere with calcium absorption.
- *Diseases of the small intestine, liver, and pancreas.* These prevent the body from absorbing adequate amounts of calcium from the intestine.
- *Lymphoma, leukemia, and multiple myeloma.*
- *Chronic diarrhea from ulcerative colitis or Crohn's disease.* This causes calcium loss through feces.
- *Surgical removal of part of the stomach or small intestine.* This affects absorption.
- *Hypercalciuria.* This is a condition where one loses too much calcium through the urine.

- *Early menopause (before age 45).* The earlier you stop producing estrogen, the more likely you are to lose calcium.
- *Lighter complexions.* Women with darker pigments have roughly 10% more bone mass than women with fairer pigments because the former produce more *calcitonin,* the hormone that strengthens bones.
- *Low weight.* Women with less body fat store less estrogen, which makes the bones less dense to begin with and more vulnerable to calcium loss.
- *Women with eating disorders (yo-yo dieting, starvation diets, binge/purge eaters).* When there isn't enough calcium in the bloodstream through diet, the body will take what it needs from the bones. These women also have lower weight.
- *Family history of osteoporosis.* Studies show that women born to mothers with spinal fractures have lower bone mineral density in the spine, neck, and midshaft.
- *High-protein diet.* This contributes to a loss of calcium through the urine.
- *Women who have never been pregnant.* They haven't experienced the same bursts of estrogen in their bodies as women who have been pregnant.
- *Amenorrhea in childbearing years* (typically affects women athletes who do endurance activities). Studies show that women with amenorrhea have 20–30% less bone mineral content than those with regular cycles, which is associated with faster bone resorption seen with estrogen deficiency.
- *Athletes.* Athletes have a low percentage of body fat needed for menstruation (see above), while excessive exercise releases B-endorphin, which researchers believe may suppress estrogen circulation.
- *Lactose intolerance.* Since so much calcium is in dairy foods, this allergy is a significant risk factor.
- *Teenage pregnancy.* When a woman is pregnant in her teens, her bones are not yet fully developed and she can lose as much as 10% of her bone mass unless she has an adequate calcium intake of roughly 2000 milligrams a day during the pregnancy and 2200 milligrams a day while breastfeeding.
- *Scoliosis.*

Preventing osteoporosis.

As boring and repetitive as it may sound, the best way to prevent osteoporosis is to ingest more calcium and thus increase your bone mass. This boils down to eating right and exercising. It's not enough to just take calcium supplements or eat high-calcium foods; you need to cut down on diuretic foods such as caffeine and alcohol. How much is "enough"? According to the National Institutes of Health Consensus Panel on Osteoporosis, premenopausal women require roughly 1000 milligrams of calcium a day; for perimenopausal or postmenopausal women already on HRT or ERT, 1000 milligrams a day; and for peri- and postmenopausal women not taking estrogen, roughly 1500 milligrams a day. For women who have already been diagnosed with osteoporosis, the panel recommends 2500 milligrams of calcium a day. Foods rich in calcium include all dairy products (an 8-ounce glass of milk contains 300 milligrams), fish, shellfish, oysters, shrimp, sardines, salmon, soybeans, tofu, broccoli, dark green vegetables (except spinach, which contains oxalic acid, preventing calcium absorption). It's crucial to determine how much calcium you're getting in your diet *before* you start any calcium supplements; too much calcium can cause kidney stones in people who are at risk for them.

In addition, not all supplements have been tested for absorbency. Dr. Robert Heaney, in his book *Calcium and Common Sense*, suggests that you test absorbency yourself. Drop your supplement into a glass of warm water and stir. If the supplement doesn't dissolve completely, chances are it won't be absorbed by your body efficiently. A calcium supplement is just that—a supplement—and should not replace a high-calcium diet. If your recommended calcium intake is about 1000–1500 milligrams a day, you should get only 400–600 milligrams from calcium supplements. Your diet should make up the remainder.

As for exercise, good activities are walking, running, biking, aerobic dance, or cross-country skiing. These are considered good ways to put more stress on the bones, increasing their mass. Carrying weights is also a good way to increase bone mass.

Diagnosing osteoporosis.

If you are at high risk for osteoporosis, to detect it early you'll need to undergo a bone density scan. In the past, CAT scans were used, but since they involve such high levels of radiation, they are considered outdated. Today, a procedure known as *absorptiometry* is used, which involves the use of a radioactive substance.

Absorptiometry is either *single-photon* or *dual-photon*. These tests measure bone density by "counting" how much radioactivity is absorbed by the bone. In single photon, the radioactive substance is directed at your forearm bone, while a detector literally counts the amount of radiation that passes through the bone, determining its density. The amount of radiation absorbed by your bone is directly proportional to how much bone you have; the more radiation absorbed, the more bone mass there is. Your forearm is used because it's surrounded by soft, uniform, thick tissue. Using single-photon is cheaper and involves less radiation, but it is not effective in showing the bone density of either your hip or spine. With dual-photon absorptiometry, two beams of a radioactive substance are directed at your bone, measuring density in all areas; this is a more costly screening that isn't as widely available as a single photon.

What about regular X rays? By the time osteoporosis shows up on a regular X ray, it is already quite advanced. Nevertheless, before you consent to a bone density screening, if you've had any X rays done in the last three years which show any bone, request for them to be reviewed for any signs of bone loss. Early bone loss will not show up, but if bone loss is detected from a regular X ray, you can save yourself the time and expense of further screenings and explore other treatment or diagnostic options with your doctor. If you've already been diagnosed, there are some treatments that can help prevent it from advancing any further, but there's no way to replace the bone that you've lost. You'll need to be careful about breaking or fracturing your bones. An excellent resource for anyone with osteoporosis is the National Osteoporosis Foundation in Washington, D.C., 202-223-2226. This foundation publishes an excellent periodical with continuous treatment updates.

Treating osteoporosis.

During and after menopause, estrogen supplements are considered one of the most effective methods of preventing bone loss. Again, estrogen helps the intestinal tract absorb calcium more efficiently, but it also helps *keep* calcium in the bones. It's important to note, though, that estrogen doesn't help your body rebuild bones; it simply helps strengthen the bones already in your body. If you have had a hysterectomy, you will need ERT only. If you still have your uterus, you will need to be placed on both estrogen and progesterone supplements (HRT) to prevent the development of endometrial hyperplasia, discussed in chapter 8. Otherwise, you'll need to have regular diagnostic screenings (via transvaginal ultrasound or endometrial biopsy) to make sure your uterine lining is normal. Both ERT and HRT are discussed in more detail in the next section. Studies show that women who start estrogen therapy within a few years of menopause tend to maintain their bone density levels and have fewer hip and wrist breakages than women who are not on ERT. In fact, one of the greatest reasons for saying yes to ERT or HRT is that the longer you delay hormone replacement, the more your bones will deteriorate. Then, when you do decide on the therapy, you'll derive fewer benefits. The current recommendation for "prophylactic" estrogen therapy is to begin estrogen supplements within six years of menopause. However, if you take estrogen as a preventive treatment for osteoporosis, you'll need to be on it for life. Once you go off the therapy, bone loss *will* resume. The bottom line is that estrogen therapy doesn't cure osteoporosis; it simply helps to prevent it from advancing.

Dosages of estrogen vary from woman to woman. It depends on your age, menopausal history, weight, height, and countless other factors. Currently, most doctors will put you on the lowest possible dose of estrogen, which might average at roughly .625 milligrams daily. But research at the Kaiser Permanente Medical Center and University of California Medical Center in San Francisco revealed that .3 milligrams of estrogen daily will slow bone loss if taken in conjunction with 1500 milligrams of calcium daily. The best way to make sure that you're taking the right amount of estrogen is to first determine whether you're in a high-risk group for osteoporosis (outlined above), and then work with a qualified nutritionist on creating a reasonable high-calcium diet and exercise regimen that you can stick to. Then, balance your estrogen needs with your risk group and calcium intake. Studies show that when estrogen is started at the beginning of menopause, the rate of osteoporosis-related fractures can be decreased by approximately 50%. Estrogen can be administered through patches, vaginal creams, or in pill form (see below).

Calcitonin supplement is another treatment for osteoporosis. This is a hormone produced in the thyroid gland, which conserves calcium in the bone, slowing bone loss. Calcitonin decreases in the body as you age, and women produce less calcitonin than men. This hormone was approved for use as treatment by the FDA in 1984, and it is given as a daily injection, along with 1500 milligrams of calcium and 400 IUs of vitamin D. This is currently an expensive treatment, but a cheaper form of calcitonin that you would inhale is being developed. Salmon calcitonin is used instead of the human form; this synthetic form is more potent and longer lasting than human calcitonin. Calcitonin is used as an *alternative* to estrogen. It also helps to relieve skeletal pain.

Etidronate disodium, a chemical compound that slows down the resorption of bone, has recently become a new treatment for osteoporosis. In the past this compound was used to treat other bone diseases. Studies have shown that women taking etidronate showed a 5% increase in the bones in their spines. This treatment should be used only when vitamins and calcium have not proven helpful, and should be administered under strict medical supervision.

Calcitrol is another treatment. It's the body's "working form" of vitamin D, which helps increase calcium absorption in the body. The vitamin D we get from food or sun is changed into calcitrol by the liver and kidneys. Again, the body makes less calcitrol as we age. As a treatment, calcitrol increases calcium absorption and decreases fractures in osteoporosis patients. One study showed that patients on calcitrol had 50–75% fewer spinal fractures.

Finally, researchers are looking into the use of anabolic steroids to strengthen bones; synthetic parathyroid hormone to maintain the balance of calcium in the body (the parathyroid gland, not to be confused with the thyroid, maintains our levels of calcium); and *thiazides*, diuretics that reduce the amount of calcium lost through urine.

All About Hormone Replacement Therapy

HRT, estrogen *and* progesterone (the progesterone is given to women after menopause who still have their uterus to prevent hyperplasia), or ERT, estrogen only (given to women after surgical menopause who no longer have a uterus), is both a "prophylactic" therapy and a "cure" for menopausal symptoms. Designed to replace the estrogen lost after menopause, its benefit is twofold: (1) It prevents or even reverses the long-term consequences of estrogen loss (osteoporosis, skin changes, vaginal thinning, dryness, and a list of other ailments) and (2) it treats the short-term symptoms of menopause such as hot flashes and vaginal dryness.

You have the choice of taking HRT or ERT as either a *short-term therapy* or a *long-term therapy.* There are some risks involved with HRT and ERT that you'll need to weigh against the benefits.

The Benefits

What exactly is estrogen responsible for in our bodies? In addition to protecting our bones and maintaining our reproductive organs, estrogen also helps to maintain appropriate levels of high-density lipoprotein (HDL), which keeps our arteries clear of plaque, preventing them from clogging and causing heart attacks and strokes. By raising HDL, known as "good" cholesterol, the low-density lipoproteins (LDL) that cause fatty substances to *collect* in the arteries (causing arteriosclerosis) drop. LDL is known as "bad" cholesterol. Estrogen also helps protect us from rheumatoid arthritis. It's our ovaries, of course, that make estrogen, but other sources of estrogen come from androstenedione (a hormone) and testosterone, which are converted by our tissues into a form of estrogen called *estrone*, a weaker form of estrogen than the kind our ovaries produce. Obese women have estrone in greater amounts. Although this may prevent severe menopausal symptoms, estrone is *not* considered a potent enough form of estrogen to protect against osteoporosis or heart disease.

Thirty years ago, menopausal women, regardless of whether they still had a uterus, were placed on pure estrogen hormone without any progesterone. This is known as "unopposed estrogen therapy," because in a natural cycle the progesterone "opposes" the estrogen and counterbalances high estrogen levels. This created several problems. First, women experienced side effects similar to those of early oral contraceptives (OCs): nausea, dizziness, bloating, and so on. Second, women who went into menopause naturally tended to develop endometrial hyperplasia, which often became uterine cancer (see chapters 8 and 9).

Today, all women who have gone through menopause naturally, and who decide to go on HRT, will be given estrogen *and* progesterone. The progesterone, of course, triggers the uterine lining to shed regularly, which prevents endometrial hyperplasia. Estrogen and progesterone *together* also mirror the normal menstrual cycle and help prevent the side effects normally felt with solo estrogen. Estrogen levels now are much lower than they were in the past; current HRT doses are about 10 times lower than those of the average combination OC.

If you're in surgical menopause, you won't *need* any progesterone because you're no longer at *risk* for endometrial hyperplasia. But because your menopausal symptoms will be more severe, your need for estrogen may be greater. Again, since the estrogen doses are so much lower now, you probably won't experience any short-term side effects from the estrogen.

What to Expect in the Short Term and Long Term

Generally, HRT/ERT will begin to relieve your estrogen-loss menopausal symptoms within days of starting the therapy. Your hot flashes will disappear, your vagina will become moist again and will lubricate on its own during sex, and your vagina's acidic environment will be restored, preventing yeast and other vaginal infections from plaguing you. If you change your mind and go *off* the therapy, your symptoms may return in a far more severe form.

In the long term, your HDL levels will be maintained, and you won't experience any severe bone loss, which can put you at risk for fractures and breakages.

As for heart disease, roughly half a million North American women die of heart disease every year. Heart attack statistics are much lower in premenopausal women than in postmenopausal women. In the premenopause age group, men outperform women by a vast degree. However, 10–15 years after menopause, women equal men in terms of heart attacks. To date, most of the research shows that estrogen will *protect* women from heart disease. Out of 19 major studies done before 1991, 11 showed that estrogen reduced the risk of heart disease *by 50% or more*. One study, interestingly, involved giving estrogen to men: Their risk of heart disease dramatically *increases* with estrogen. No one knows why this is, but if men were able to derive the same heart protection from estrogen as women, heart attack mortality statistics would probably decrease dramatically.

It's also important to review these studies in the proper context. Women who take estrogen are usually healthier and more willing to make *other* lifestyle adjustments that will lower their risk, such as changing diet and quitting smoking.

Animal research reveals that progesterone added to HRT *may* have the *opposite* influence on HDL that estrogen has. If you decide to go on HRT for strictly the heart benefit, you might want to have your cholesterol level checked before you start. This will establish a "baseline," and then you can get your levels checked after you're on HRT for about three months. If there's no improvement in your cholesterol levels, you may want to review your decision with your doctor.

However, the heart benefits seen with estrogen are true only if the estrogen is taken orally or in patches. In order for the estrogen to work its magic with HDL, it needs to be metabolized in the liver.

Finally, estrogen will not counteract a poor diet and lifestyle. If you smoke, drink excessively, are under tremendous stress, eat copious amounts of the wrong foods (you know the ones), or come from a heart attack family, don't expect estrogen alone to shield you from heart disease.

If your decision for going on ERT or HRT is based on cosmetic reasons ("Gee, I won't get any wrinkles with hormone therapy!") you're in for a big surprise: hormone/estrogen replacement therapy *does not prevent wrinkles*. Estrogen can cause you to retain water, which can make your skin puffier, making your wrinkles less noticeable. However, the majority of women have wrinkles because of heredity, excessive or cumulative sun exposure, smoking, and drinking excessive amounts of alcohol. Estrogen can also cause skin dryness, rashes, and permanent brown blotches on your skin (harmless skin decoloration known as hyperpigmentation).

Estrogen therapy will not prevent weight gain, another myth that has been passed down through the estrogen folklore. Weight gain has to do with our metabolisms slowing down as we age, something that estrogen cannot prevent or reverse.

Some women may want to take estrogen to keep their breasts full and shapely; this is not a good reason to go on HRT. Although estrogen promotes cell growth in the breasts, while the retention of body fluid can make breasts swell and fuller, your breasts can also become more tender and painful. But taking HRT to keep your breasts full is not recommended because of the health risks.

HRT/ERT and Depression

Many women may experience feelings of depression as they enter menopause. While mood swings, as discussed above, are caused by peak levels of FSH in the body during menopause, most of the menopause "blues" women experience is rooted in the psychological fear of aging and the stress of menopausal symptoms such as hot flashes. If you're taking HRT because you think it will cure any depression you're experiencing, you're mistaken. Estrogen therapy will relieve night sweats, insomnia, and any anxiety related to your menopausal symptoms. Since you'll be calmer and better rested, you'll be able to *cope* with daily stress more effectively and positively. But if you are depressed to the extent where you can't function normally, you need to seek out counseling or support groups with other women who have experienced menopause.

Although estrogen may have a mild antidepressant effect, some HRT "recipes" may mix in antidepressant medication or tranquilizers, which may help relieve depression. Doctors sometimes prescribe these HRT recipes if their patients seem depressed or anxious. While this is a common practice, *it's not appropriate!* If you *do* need these drugs, it's better to take them separately—*independent* of your estrogen—under a *psychiatrist's* supervision, not a gynecologist's. Tranquilizers can cause dizziness, confusion, and drowsiness.

Make sure you know what you're getting in your estrogen pills before you take them.

One final note: Often, depression seems to just "vanish" once HRT or ERT is started. This vanishing act has *nothing to do with estrogen;* it has to do with time and the positive psychological placebo effect estrogen therapy often has.

The Risks

The risk we hear most regarding the estrogen issue is uterine cancer (see chapters 8 and 9). Well, in the 1990s, this is no longer a risk! In the past, unopposed estrogen was given to women who still *had* a uterus and women without one. If you don't have a uterus, there is no risk of uterine cancer. But what about women who still had their uterus? A funny thing happened: Doctors *forgot* about the uterus, ignoring the fact that the female body is very smart. When it detects estrogen in the body, it says, "Oh, look—estrogen again! Better start preparing the endometrium for a baby!" And guess what? There's no progesterone to trigger the lining to shed, and certainly no baby, so the lining just keeps growing until you wind up with endometrial hyperplasia and eventually uterine cancer. When the uterine cancer rate began to increase in uterus "owners" on unopposed estrogen, the medical community realized its mistake, remembered the uterus and the importance of progesterone, *and today will not administer unopposed estrogen to any woman with a uterus* unless she's aware of the risks and goes for regular endometrial biopsies.

For the record, women in natural menopause who take nothing have a 1 in 1,000 risk of uterine cancer; women with a uterus on unopposed estrogen increase their risk to anywhere from 4 to 8 in 1,000. What if you were on unopposed estrogen in the past and still have your uterus? This is still in debate. It seems that once you go off the estrogen, your uterine cancer risk drops. However, a Boston University School of Medicine study of 1,217 women revealed that the risk of cancer may not drop until you've been off estrogen for as long as 10 years.

With HRT and the progesterone added to the estrogen therapy, the risk of uterine cancer decreases: It's lower in women on HRT than in women on nothing!

Breast Cancer and HRT.

The media have had a field day with this one, so let's keep it simple:

Out of the roughly 100 reliable studies done on the effect of HRT/ERT on breast cancer, one-fourth of the studies conclude that there's no difference; one-fourth will conclude that HRT contributes to a rise in breast cancer; another one-fourth will conclude that the risk of breast cancer actually decreases; and the remainder will conclude that "it depends." If you average every single study result, it turns out that the risk of breast cancer increases anywhere from 1.08% to 1.80% in women on HRT or ERT. To be safe, any woman who is considered at high risk for breast cancer, or who has a history of breast cancer, may not be able to take ERT or HRT—but this is *still* in debate.

It's crucial that everything you read about HRT and breast cancer is understood in its proper context. For example, in the general population, one in 8–10 women not taking hormones will get breast cancer. *The majority of these women will be over 50 and hence peri- or postmenopausal.* We just don't know whether the enormous increase in breast cancer statistics in this age group have to do with estrogen, women living longer, women on HRT, women on HRT who smoke, women on HRT who are obese, women on HRT who have a family history of breast cancer, and so on.

To illustrate the confusion regarding breast cancer and HRT/ERT, two studies done on the long-term risks of breast cancer, published in the *American Journal of Epidemiology*, revealed opposite results. Both studies agreed that short-term use of estrogen (less than 15 years) *didn't* increase the risk. The first study compared 1,686 postmenopausal women who had breast cancer to 2,077 women without breast or gynecological cancer. Between 1980 and 1986, no increased risk was found for breast cancer. Meanwhile, the second study showed that using estrogen for 15 or more years *doubled* the risk. But the risk of breast cancer increases as you age anyway! The women who developed breast cancer at double the normal rate were all over 65. The results are conflicting.

The risks you don't read about.

It might interest you to know that you can *triple* your chances of developing gallbladder disease on ERT or HRT. However, gallbladder disease is easily treated by removing the gallbladder.

If you have fibroids (see chapter 7), they may grow larger on HRT. Just be prepared.

Estrogen also causes fluid retention. This has been known to exacerbate *existing* conditions such as asthma, epilepsy, pre-existing heart disease, kidney disease, and sometimes migraine headaches.

Estrogen may also alter blood sugar metabolism. This is currently in debate, however. If you're diabetic, review the pros and cons with your doctor before you decide to take either ERT or HRT. In the past it was felt that women with diabetes should not take estrogen, but this opinion is being reexamined.

Forms of HRT and ERT

You can take estrogen in a number of ways. The most common estrogen product is called *Premarin,* conjugated equine estrogen (conjugated horse estrogen). Premarin uses a synthesis of various estrogens derived from the urine of pregnant horses. Premarin literally means "pregnant mare's urine." Premarin comes in either pills or vaginal creams. Other common synthetic forms of estrogen include *micronized estradiol* (Estrace), *ethinyl estradiol* (Modicon, Norinyl), *esterified estrogen* (Estratab), and *quinestrol* (Estrovis). Estraderm is the patch, which is transdermal estradiol.

As a short-term therapy, you may need only the vaginal cream to help with vaginal dryness or bladder problems. As a long-term therapy, you'll need the pill form if you want to protect yourself from heart disease. Estrogen can also be "worn." In this case, it's placed in a small plastic patch around the size of a silver dollar, worn on the abdomen, thighs, or buttocks, and changed twice weekly.

Some women also have an allergic reaction to the skin patch and get a rash. If you're one of them, you can investigate taking the estrogen in other forms.

You can also have estrogen injected. Each shot lasts between three to six weeks, but this is expensive and inconvenient.

Women react differently to Premarin or other synthetic forms of estrogen; some do better than others on different chemical recipes. If you don't do well on Premarin, for example, see if estradiol is better for you, or vice versa. Don't just give up and go off HRT or ERT altogether; explore all the estrogen possibilities. Dosages are discussed below.

Progesterone.

Synthetic progestins (a family of progesterone drugs that include natural progesterone) are norethindrone (Ortho-Novum) or *norethindrone acetate* (Norlutate). Progestin is *medroxyprogesterone* (Provera, Cycrin, Amen) and is taken in separate tablets along with estrogen. Together, the estrogen and progestin you take is called HRT. HRT can be administered two ways: *cycli-*

cally or *continuously*. Taking HRT cyclically is very similar to taking an OC because the hormones more closely mirror a natural cycle. The first day you start will be day 1 of the calendar month. You take estrogen from day 1 to day 25; you then add the progesterone from day 14 to day 25. Then you stop all pills and bleed for two or three days, just as you would on a combination OC. This vaginal bleeding is called withdrawal bleeding, which is lighter and shorter than a normal menstrual period. In fact, if the bleeding is heavy or prolonged for some reason, this is a warning that something's not right, and you should get it checked. This is one of the most common prescribed schedules, but others are available and may be recommended.

In addition, you may experience breakthrough bleeding—spotting during the first three weeks after you begin HRT. This kind of bleeding is, again, similar to what happens on a combination OC. This bleeding usually goes away after a few months, but report it anyway. You may need to switch to a lower dose of estrogen or take a higher dose of your progestin. Once your miniperiod of withdrawal bleeding is finished, you simply start the cycle again. Many women can't tolerate cyclical HRT because they feel as though they should be *rid* of their periods by now and not have to deal with pads and tampons ever again.

When HRT is taken continuously, you simply take one estrogen pill and one progestin pill each day. When you do it this way, the progesterone *counteracts* the estrogen; no uterine lining is built up, so there's no withdrawal bleeding.

The appropriate dosages.

Every woman requires a different dosage of estrogen and progestin. You will always be placed on the *lowest* possible dosage of either one, and you may have the dosage increased gradually if necessary. If your estrogen dosage is too high, you'll experience side effects similar to those seen with estrogen OCs: headaches, bloating, and so on.

So before you determine how much estrogen you'll need, it's crucial to first determine how much your body is *still* producing; this really depends on your weight, menopausal symptoms, and a hundred other things. Breakthrough bleeding is a common side effect, however.

Estrogen tablets come in dosages of 0.3, 0.625, 0.9, or 1.25 milligrams. Dosages also depend on why you're taking estrogen. For women who are in a high-risk category for osteoporosis, the most common starting dosage is 0.625 milligrams. But for women who just want short-term relief from their menopausal symptoms, such as hot flashes, starting at 0.3 milligrams is more usual. If you forget to take your estrogen tablet one day, don't worry about it. You will not need to double up the way you would with birth control pills. It's important, however, that once you begin the estrogen, you continue to take it daily without a noticeable break (more than two days). Studies show that when you stop your estrogen, you can suffer from far more severe hot flashes and insomnia than you did before you started the estrogen.

If you're not taking estrogen orally and are on the vaginal estrogen cream, you can use the cream for about three weeks on and one week off. Women who opt for the vaginal cream have decided on estrogen for short-term relief of vaginal dryness and thinning, as well as relief from urinary incontinence, another postmenopausal problem. But vaginal cream does not relieve hot flashes or offer any protection for osteoporosis or heart disease. Using the vaginal creams occasionally, the way you would lubricant, will do you no good. Again, every woman is different. Make sure you discuss with either your doctor or pharmacist how much estrogen you're getting per application.

As for skin patches, they contain either 4 or 8 milligrams of estrogen. The 4-milligram patch releases .05 milligrams of estrogen daily; the 8-milligram patch releases twice that amount. You'll need to change the patch twice a week. Some doctors recommend that you wear the patch for three weeks, and then take a one-week break from the patch before you start again. Obviously, you'll need to discuss this with your doctor and decide what's right for you. Again, women who take the patch will not derive any HDL benefits, but they will be protected from bone loss and menopausal symptoms. In fact, the patch delivers a more continuous flow of estrogen than the pills because there is no fluctuation in dosage.

The androgen strain.

ERT or HRT sometimes contain androgens (male hormones). Doctors will prescribe androgens to improve your libido, if you're experiencing problems. This may be appropriate, but it's important to *know what you're getting!* If your androgen dosage is too high, you can develop male features, such as increased body hair, a deeper voice, and shrinking breasts. These symptoms do not magically vanish once you go off the androgens. Some studies also show that added androgens may have a negative effect on blood cholesterol, actually *increasing* heart disease risk. This may explain why men on estrogen derive no HDL benefits.

Common side effects.

If you're taking *cyclical* progestins with your estrogen because you still have your uterus, bleeding is *not* a side effect! The whole point of adding progestin to your estrogen is to trigger withdrawal bleeding and shed your uterine lining routinely. However, if you're taking continuous progestins with your estrogen, bleeding is not the norm, and it should be checked into.

Common side effects of estrogen will be fluid retention, because estrogen will decrease the amount of salt and water excreted by kidneys. Your legs, breasts, and feet will swell.

Nausea is another common side effect, also seen with OCs. This happens during the first two or three months of your therapy and should just disappear on its own. Some women find that taking their dosages at night (for pills) may remedy this. Decreasing the dosage is also an option.

Some other side effects reported include headaches, skin color changes (called *melasma*) on the face, more cervical mucus secretion, liquid secretion from breasts, change in curvature of the cornea, jaundice, loss of scalp hair, and itchiness. Many women suffer no side effects at all.

A minor side effect is a vitamin B_6 deficiency, seen with OCs. Symptoms of this deficiency are vague and include fatigue, depression, loss of concentration, loss of libido, or insomnia. This is easily remedied by taking a vitamin B_6 supplement.

Are You an HRT or ERT Candidate?

Some women make better HRT or ERT candidates than others. Here's a guide that may help you make the decision:

- *Do you suffer from severe hot flashes that don't respond to natural remedies?*
- *Are your vaginal changes causing painful intercourse, urinary tract infections, or vaginitis, which does not respond to natural remedies, such as more stimulation of the clitoris during sex, or sexual lubricants?*
- *Are you in a high-risk category for endometrial cancer (overweight, hypertensive, diabetic)?* If so, taking progestin to trigger withdrawal bleeding will lower your risk.
- *Are you in a high-risk group for heart attacks or strokes?* If so, ERT or HRT will lower your risk.
- *Are you in a high-risk group for developing osteoporosis?* Again, ERT or HRT will lower your risk.

Those who shouldn't be on ERT or HRT are the following:

- *Women with (a history of) endometrial cancer.* These women should not be on any estrogen.

- *Women with breast cancer.* You shouldn't be on either ERT or HRT if you have (a history of) breast cancer. However, tamoxifen, discussed in chapter 9, does protect you from heart disease.
- *Women who have had a stroke.* Neither ERT or HRT is recommended.
- *Women who have a blood-clotting disorder.* Neither ERT or HRT is recommended.
- *Women with undiagnosed vaginal bleeding.* Neither therapy is recommended.
- *Women with liver dysfunction.* You can be on the estrogen patch or vaginal cream to relieve your menopausal symptoms, but you shouldn't take any pills.

If you have one or more of the conditions below, you still may be able to take HRT or ERT but you should discuss this *thoroughly* with your doctor.

- diabetes
- sickle cell disease
- high blood pressure
- migraines
- uterine fibroids
- a history of benign breast conditions such as cysts or fibroadenomas
- endometriosis
- seizures
- gallbladder disease
- a family history of breast cancer
- a past or current history of smoking.

Here are some commonly asked questions:

Q. *What if I begin my estrogen therapy while I'm still perimenopausal and still getting my period? Will estrogen delay or reverse menopause?*

A. Estrogen won't interfere with your natural menopause because your ovaries *will* run out of eggs with or without hormone treatment.

Q. *What if I just take progesterone?*

A. Progestin alone can relieve up to 80% of your menopausal symptoms, especially hot flashes, but it won't affect your vaginal changes.

Q. *Can I go on and off hormone therapy the way I can with OCs?*

A. You shouldn't go on and off estrogen because it may cause either irregular uterine bleeding or hyperplasia. Moreover, any protection from bone loss or heart disease is negated by going on and off.

Which Specialists Should You Seek Out?

If you decide to go on HRT or ERT, you may need to seek out an *endocrinologist*. Many gynecologists are trained in this area; many aren't. Review chapter 3 and make sure you *interview* your gynecologist about his or her credentials regarding endocrinology. Otherwise, any family doctor or gynecologist can refer you to a reproductive endocrinologist, who may also be a gynecologist.

If you develop bladder problems, you'll need to seek out a urologist. Many gynecologists are trained in urology as well, or you can be referred to one by either your family doctor or gynecologist.

All pre-, peri-, and postmenopausal women should seek out a separate nutritionist to plan an appropriate diet and vitamin supplement program. This is particularly important if you're not taking any estrogen. Appropriate calcium levels can really help prevent fractures due to bone loss.

If you're not planning to go on HRT or ERT, you should seek out a *qualified* herbologist or doctor trained in naturopathy. There are a variety of herbs and foods that can relieve menopausal symptoms and prolong your health in other areas.

If you seem to be suffering from a hodgepodge of different health problems (more common after age 65), and you're balancing many different kinds of medications, you may need to seek out a *gerontologist*, a doctor who specializes in managing health care for older persons.

Finally, you need to continue to see your primary care physician. As discussed in chapter 3, an appropriate primary care physician is a family practitioner, general practitioner, or internist. A gynecologist, urologist, endocrinologist, or even a gerontologist is *not* an appropriate primary care physician; these doctors are specialists, and although you may be seeing them often, they should not replace your primary care doctor.

The Choice Is Yours

Many women will decide against either HRT or ERT because they will want to experience menopause naturally. Some women may want to take hormonal therapy in the short term to relieve more severe symptoms of menopause. Some women who are in their 30s or 40s and in surgical menopause may feel it's more *natural* to replace the estrogen in their bodies they would have normally still produced. And many women will want to take advantage of the estrogen benefits, wishing to prevent bone loss and heart disease as aggressively as they can. There is no right or wrong decision, but there *is* one great sin no woman should commit: *deciding in ignorance!* Whatever you decide, you should make an *informed* decision and truly weigh all the risks and all benefits. This is easier said than done.

The first thing you'll need to do is put together a "family tree" health history. Does osteoporosis run in your family? (Do you recall your mother and/or grandmothers shrinking as they aged? Did they suffer from repeated fractures in their hips, backs, wrists, and so on?) Does heart disease, stroke, uterine or breast cancer run in your family?

The next thing you'll need to do is analyze your *current* health. What is your own medical history? How healthy are you *now?* Do you exercise? Have you been good to yourself calcium-wise? Do you smoke? Do you take drugs? Do you drink excessively? How *severe* are your menopausal symptoms? Have you reached menopause naturally or surgically?

The final step is making a separate appointment with your doctor to *specifically* discuss HRT or ERT. It's crucial that you feel comfortable and positive about your decision.

Other Postmenopausal Problems

As you age, there are several health problems that might plague you. From a *gynecological* perspective, the two most common problems have to do with urinary incontinence and uterine prolapse.

Urinary Incontinence

Urinary incontinence means involuntary urination. This tends to plague women who do a lot of sitting, had several children, have repeated UTIs (see chapter 6), have diabetes, have diseases that affect the spinal chord or the brain such as Parkinson's disease, multiple sclerosis, or Alzheimer's disease, have (a history of) bladder cancer, or have had major pelvic surgery such as a hysterectomy. The muscles of your pelvic floor and abdomen get weaker and your urinary apparatus drops down. On top of this, less estrogen causes the urethra to thin and change, similar to the vaginal changes you experience.

Chapters 1 and 6 discuss *how* the bladder and female urethra work. When we're younger, we have tremendous control over one particular muscle: *pubococcygeal.* This muscle controls the vaginal opening as well as the urinary opening. Normally, when we feel the urge to urinate, we hold it in until we get to the right place. When we get to the toilet, urine doesn't come out immediately. We relax slightly, then urinate. This "relaxing" that takes place prior to urination is the relaxing of the pubococcygeal muscle, which also enables us to stop and start our streams. Anyone who's had to have a urinalysis has probably mastered this technique.

Urinary incontinence is categorized into one of four groups: *stress incontinence, urge incontinence, overflow incontinence,* or *irritable bladder.* Stress incontinence is when urine leaks out during a sudden movement, such as a sneeze or cough or even uncontrollable laughing. This can happen to women of all ages and is considered the most common form of incontinence. You may be in the habit of "holding it in" or simply have aged.

Urge incontinence refers to a sudden, sometimes painful urge to urinate that is so unexpected and powerful you may not always be able to make it to the toilet.

Overflow incontinence occurs in only a small percentage of overall incontinence problems. With no warning, urine suddenly overflows after you change your position (from sitting to standing or vice versa, for example). You may lose just a few drops of urine or enough to require a maxipad. Sometimes these episodes are followed by the urge to urinate a few minutes later, but when you try, nothing comes out. This is a neurological problem where the bladder doesn't contract and empty well. It therefore overflows.

An irritable bladder is a mishmash of all three incontinence symptoms and UTIs. You'll need to see a urologist to sort out what's causing your bladder to behave so erratically. You may have *interstitial cystitis* (see chapter 6).

Treating incontinence.

Estrogen is very helpful as a treatment for incontinence because it restores the "luster" of your urethra just as it restores the vagina. Estrogen has the same beneficial effect whether in pill, cream, or patch form.

The *Kegel exercise* is also very helpful in strengthening the pubococcygeal muscle. The Kegel exercise is a very convenient exercise that you can do in any position, anywhere, anytime: in an elevator, on the subway, in a movie theater, while you're cooking, eating, or lying down. All you do is isolate the muscle that stops and starts your urinary stream. To isolate it, you can also insert your finger into your vagina and try to squeeze your finger with your vaginal opening. Once you've isolated the muscle, just squeeze it five times, then count to five, or squeeze 10 and count 10. The key is to keep the muscles in shape. It's *that* simple, and it really helps. You can also do general exercises to firm up your abdomen and pelvis in conjunction with your Kegel exercises.

Being more conscious of your diet and medications is also important. For example, sedatives, tranquilizers, and certain drugs for high blood pressure or heart disease can trigger bouts of incontinence. Ask your pharmacist. Some drugs or foods are diuretics and will cause you to urinate more frequently. Caffeine and alcohol are classic diuretics. Fruit juice and spicy foods can also irritate the bladder.

Overweight women are also more likely to experience incontinence because the weight exerts more pressure on the bladder, causing the muscles and urethra to overwork themselves. Try losing weight and see if your bladder function resumes.

More invasive treatments for incontinence involve surgery that lifts and tightens the pelvic floor, or the use of *pessaries*, a stiff, doughnut-shaped rubber device (which needs to be fitted and sized) that fits into the top of the vagina and holds it up slightly. This raises the neck of the bladder and helps reposition it.

Some women may choose to live with the problem and wear bladder control products.

Uterine Prolapse: Is It Me, or Is the Sky Falling?

This problem only affects women who still have a uterus. Basically, the problem has to with the uterus sagging or sinking and literally falling down as one ages. When you experience a uterine prolapse, you may feel as though something is "falling out." You may also experience a heaviness in your lower abdomen; constant lower back pain and pressure; menstrual-like cramps that seem to worsen after long intervals of standing; difficulty with penetration during intercourse; constipation combined with the urge to "bear down"; *and urinary incontinence.*

The uterus can fall down a little, called a "straight line" prolapse, or the entire length of the vagina can fall. In more severe cases, the cervix protrudes between the labia, which could interfere with intercourse. This is dangerous because the cervix can get infected through contact with urine or feces.

Because the uterus supports or rests on a variety of other organs, a uterine prolapse can be associated with prolapse of other pelvic organs, such as:

- *Cystocele.* This is a falling bladder. You may feel as though you can't empty your bladder completely and may have UTIs or stress incontinence.
- *Urethrocele.* In this case, the muscles supporting the urethra separate, and the urethra sags into the vagina.
- *Rectocele.* Here, the rectum falls into the vagina, causing constipation. Your stools may also pack into a "pouch," forming a bulging rectum.
- *Enterocele.* This is when the small intestine falls into the back of the vagina.

What causes prolapse?

Pregnancy and childbirth are major contributors. The uterus and tissue expand to such an extent that they lose their elasticity and ability to retain normal positions. During labor, the muscles in the vagina and perineum can be torn. Nonmuscle tissue, ligaments, and fascia may not have the resiliency to retain their normal position and shape. Women who have had 10 kids or more (not seen as much today as in the past) often have internal tearing that destroys their pelvic configuration.

Obesity and poor nutrition is another cause. Poor nutrition prevents tissue from getting enough blood and nutrients. In obese women, fat hangs inside the abdomen like an extra organ pushing directly on the pelvis, uterus, and bowels, or pushing the intestines into the pelvis, ruining normal bowel function. The constant pressure from this extra fat tears the tissue and damages elasticity.

Estrogen loss after menopause causes the mucosal tissue of the ligaments and fascia to thin and weaken (just like the vagina). In this case, hormone therapy can alleviate the problem, combined with good nutrition and exercise.

Occasionally, a large fibroid can push down on the uterus and vaginal wall, causing a prolapse. The fibroid may also put pressure on the bladder and stretch tissues. Finally, simple aging—heredity and gravity—may be the culprit.

Treatment.

Most doctors will recommend a hysterectomy (usually the vaginal procedure). For premonepausal patients who desire fertility, there may be alternatives. Reconstructive surgery can often correct the problem. Check out chapter 7 and contact Hysterectomy Educational Resources and Services (HERS) (see Appendix A) to find out about alternatives to hysterectomy in this case. In some instances, HRT or ERT may help with urinary incontinence, but cannot repair prolapse. Before you decide on treatment, find out why your uterus is falling. Weight loss may improve the situation as well. Some options include a pessary. This is worn like a diaphragm and may be ideal if you're elderly or too frail for surgery.

Routine Exams and Tests After Menopause

You're never too old to discontinue having routine pelvic exams and Pap smears. Even if you no longer have your uterus, you may still have your *cervix*, which is not immune to cervical cancer. Ovaries, vaginas, and vulvas also need to be routinely checked for signs of cancer or infections. And, of course, no one disputes the fact that *the risk of breast cancer increases with age.*

The Routine Postmenopausal Physical

Whether you're on HRT, ERT, or neither, you'll need to have a complete physical on an annual basis. (Review chapter 3 for a discussion of doctor-patient relationships and what to expect in a pelvic exam.) This exam must include:

- a breast and pelvic exam that includes a bimanual exam (if you've had a mastectomy, the remaining breast and chest wall still need to be examined);
- a Pap smear and/or vaginal swab for detecting infections;
- a mammogram (annual mammograms begin anywhere from age 40 to 50, depending on your doctor's recommendations and your risk category);
- an ovarian ultrasound if you're in a high-risk group, and possibly a CA-125 blood test if you're in a high-risk group for ovarian cancer;
- a blood pressure test;
- a complete blood count, including cholesterol, calcium levels, and your cardiac lipid profile;
- if you're not on HRT—a bone density screening either from a recent X ray or bone densitometry (wrist X ray), or from the scans discussed above (this may be spread out longer than annually and depends on your osteoporosis risk group, whether you're taking calcium, whether you're on estrogen, and so on);

- a stool check for blood, which may be a sign of gastrointestinal cancer;
- a urinalysis to make sure your bladder is functioning normally; and
- a thyroid function test (this gland affects your entire metabolism and other parts of your body; thyroid problems are common after menopause and sometimes can be misdiagnosed as menopausal symptoms).

The Red Flags

Unless you're taking HRT *cyclically*, any vaginal bleeding or spotting after your menopause is now considered abnormal. You'll need to get this investigated. Review chapter 8. This discusses the appropriate tests you'll need and some of the causes of benign conditions, as well as symptoms of pelvic cancers.

Other red flags include persistent coughing, headaches, dizziness, lumps, swellings, leg pain, yellow skin or eyes, vision changes, or difficult breathing.

If you decide to start HRT or ERT, you'll need to have your blood sugar, thyroid function, and calcium and phosphorus levels checked before starting HRT. Once you begin your hormone therapy, you should have a follow-up visit to your doctor a few weeks into it; after that, you should have a pelvic exam, vaginal smear (to detect how thin your vaginal walls are), breast exam, and urinalysis. You should also have your FSH, cholesterol, blood pressure, and hemoglobin checked.

You should be doing monthly breast self-exams (see chapter 8), keeping a health log that charts how you feel, and staying alert to "red flags." Never adjust your medications without first discussing it with your doctors.

The Absolute Last Word

If you're like me, this might be the first chapter you're reading in this book! Anything you need to know about you'll find in the index. You can use this book as a quick reference or read it all at once. I've carefully cross-referenced chapters and topics so that you can flip to just one section and then refer to other chapters that touch on the subject in more detail or in another perspective. I've also added two appendices that list other sources of information for each subject, and other titles you might want to read. Again, this is a book that will grow *with* you. Use it, read it, and take it with you to your gynecologist, family doctor, or other specialist. Feel free to discuss and debate various chapters you come across with your doctor, friends, partner(s), daughter(s), mother, or grandmother(s). And *don't* be afraid to get "permission from the author or publisher" to photocopy information and pass it on to a friend! That's what this book is all about—crucial information! Good luck and good health.

Bibliography

Chapter 1

The Boston Women's Health Book Collective, *The New Our Bodies, Ourselves* (1992, Simon and Schuster, New York).

DeMarco, Carolyn, M.D., *Take Charge of Your Body: A Woman's Guide to Health* (1990, The Last Laugh, Winlaw, British Columbia, Canada).

Long, Michelle, M.D., primary care physician, interviewed 1993.

Love, Susan M., M.D., with Karen Lindsey, *Dr. Susan Love's Breast Book* (1991, Addison-Wesley, New York).

Schapira, Laurie Layton, *The Cassandra Complex: Living with Disbelief: A Modern Perspective on Hysteria* (1988, Inner City Books, Toronto, Ontario, Canada).

Chapter 2

The Boston Women's Health Book Collective, *The New Our Bodies, Ourselves* (1992, Simon and Schuster, New York).

Chuong, C. James, Earl B. Dawson, and Edward R. Smith, "Vitamin E in Premenstrual Syndrome," *Nutrition Research Newsletter,* Volume 10, January 1991.

Cumming, David C., Ceinwen E. Cumming, and Dianne K. Dieren, "Menstrual Mythology and Sources of Information," *American Journal of Obstetrics and Gynecology,* Volume 164, February 1991.

DeMarco, Carolyn, M.D., *Take Charge of Your Body: A Woman's Guide to Health* (1990, The Last Laugh, Winlaw, British Columbia, Canada).

"Evening Primrose Oil and PMS," *Nutrition Research Newsletter,* Volume 10, February 1991.

Hufnagel, Vicki, M.D., *No More Hysterectomies* (1989, New American Library, New York).

Intent: A Newsletter for Women with Endometriosis, The Endometriosis Network of Toronto, Inc., Volume 3.1, Spring 1993.

Kennedy, Stephen, "Endometriosis," *The Lancet,* Volume 339, June 20, 1992.

Lander, Debra, M.D., F.R.C.P. (C), psychiatrist, interviewed 1993.

Long, Michelle, M.D., primary care physician, interviewed 1993.

Montgomery, Ann, "Truth About Tampons Needs to Be Told," *Ottawa Citizen,* September 1, 1992.

Osofsky, Howard J., "Efficacious Treatment of PMS: A Need for Further Research," *The Journal of the American Medical Association,* Volume 264, July 18, 1990.

Reid, Robert L., M.D., F.R.C.S., "Understanding Premenstrual Syndrome," Synphasic Education Series pamphlet.

Shaw, Robert W., "Treatment of Endometriosis," *The Lancet,* Volume 340, November 21, 1992.

Shuttle, Penelope, and Peter Redgrove, *The Wise Wound: Menstruation and Everywoman* (1986, Paladin Grafton Books, London, England).

"What Is Endometriosis?" Endometriosis Association, Education Support Research Pamphlet, Milwaukee, Wisconsin, 1992.

Chapter 3

The Boston Women's Health Book Collective, *The New Our Bodies, Ourselves* (1992, Simon and Schuster, New York).

Cain, Joanna M., M.D., and Albert R. Jonsen, Ph.D., "Specialists and Generalists in Obstetrics and Gynecology: Conflicts of Interest in Referral and an Ethical Alternative," *The Jacobs Institute of Women's Health,* Volume 2, No. 3, Fall 1992.

Chez, Ronald A., M.D., and Franklin J. Apfel, M.D., M.H.S., "Women's Health Care: Rights and Responsibilities," *The Jacobs Institute of Women's Health,* Volume 2, No. 3, Fall 1992.

Dawson, Heather R., M.D., C.C.F.P., family physician, interviewed 1992.

Dewitt, Don, M.D., "Family Physicians, Pap Smears and Colposcopy," *American Family Physician,* January 1992.

Long, Michelle, M.D., primary care physician, interviewed 1993.

Malesky, Gail, and Charles B. Inlander, *Take This Book to the Gynecologist with You: A Consumer's Guide to Women's Health* (1991, Addison-Wesley, New York).

Malesky, Gail, and Charles B. Inlander, "Book Extra: What You Should Know About Pap Tests," *People's Medical Society Newsletter,* Volume 10, April 1991.

Maurer, Janet, M.D., *How To Talk To Your Doctor,* (1986, Simon and Schuster, New York).

Maurer, Janet, M.D., lecture, 1992.

Chapter 4

"Advisory Panel Recommends Approval of Female Condom," *AIDS Weekly*, December 21, 1992.

"All About Norplant," *Patient Care*, March 15, 1992.

The Boston Women's Health Book Collective, *The New Our Bodies, Ourselves* (1992, Simon and Schuster, New York).

Buchignani, Walter, "Thinner, Stronger, Safer: Female Condom Due in Canada This Year," *Toronto Star*, February 7, 1992.

Bullough, Vern L., and Bonnie Bullough, *Contraception: A Guide to Birth Control Methods* (1990, Prometheus Books, Buffalo, New York).

Burkman, Ronald T., M.D., *Handbook of Contraception and Abortion* (1989, Little, Brown, Boston).

DeMarco, Carolyn, M.D., *Take Charge of Your Body: A Woman's Guide to Health* (1990, The Last Laugh, Winlaw, British Columbia, Canada).

"Depo-Provera Contraceptive Injection," Factsheet, The Upjohn Company, Kalamazoo, Michigan.

Farr, Gaston, et al, "Contraceptive Efficacy and Acceptability of the Female Condom," *American Journal of Public Health*, Volume 84, No. 12, December 1994

"Female Condom Nears Approval," *AIDS Weekly*, May 3, 1993.

"Female Condom Is Awkward, Comical, California Scientists Say," *AIDS Weekly*, April 5, 1993.

"Female Condom May Empower Voluntary Sex Workers (Thailand)," *AIDS Weekly*, January 25, 1993.

Flattum-Riemers, Jan, M.D., "Norplant: A New Contraceptive," *American Family Physician*, July 1991.

"Frequency of Condom Use Among Female Adolescents" (Tips from Other Journals), *American Family Physician*, June 1992.

Gollub, Erica L., Ph.D., and Zena A. Stein, "Commentary: The New Female Condom - Item 1 on a Woman's AIDS Prevention Agenda," *American Journal of Public Health*, Volume 83, No. 4, April 1993.

—, et al, "Short-Term Acceptability of the Female Condom Among Staff and Patients at a New York City Hospital," *Family Planning Perspectives*, Volume 27, No. 4, July/August 1995

Hatcher, Robert A., M.D., et al., *Contraceptive Technology, 1990–1992*, 15th revised edition (1990, Irvington Publishers, New York).

Heaton, Caryl J., D.O., and Mindy A. Smith, M.D., M.S., "The Diaphragm," *American Family Physician,* May 1989.

"Is Depo-Provera Safe? Despite Government Approval the Controversy Continues," *Ms. Magazine,* January/February 1993.

Margolis, Dawn, "After a 20-year Delay, a New Birth Control Method Hits the Market: Contraceptive Injection," *American Health,* March 1993.

Memon, Farhan, "Female Condom," *Now Magazine,* February 4–10, 1993.

"Oral Contraceptives and Venous Thromboembolism," *American Journal of Nursing,* Volume 10, No. 9, September 1986.

Powell, Marion, M.D., F.R.C.P.(C), "Birth Control and the Pill," Synphasic Patient Education Series Pamphlet.

Raeburn, Paul, "The Female Condom," *Glamour,* February 1995.

"Reality (WPC-333): A Condom for Women to Wear," Media Factsheets, distributed by City of Toronto, Department of Public Health, 1993.

Rispin, Phillipa, "Female Condom Rates High in Trials," *Dimensions,* June 8, 1989.

Segal, Marian, "Norplant: Birth Control at Arm's Reach," *FDA Consumer Magazine,* Department of Health and Human Services, May 1991.

Stehlin, Dori, "Depo-Provera: The Quarterly Contraceptive," *FDA Consumer Magazine,* March 1993.

Szarewski, Anne, and John Guillebaud, "Contraception: Current State of the Art," *BMJ,* Volume 302, May 25, 1991.

Trussell, James, et al, "Comparative Contraceptive Efficacy of the Female Condom and Other Barrier Methods," *Family Planning Perspectives,* Volume 26, No. 2, March/April 1994.

Chapter 5

AIDS and HIV Infection: Psycho-Social Issues: Information for Professionals, booklet, Ministry of Health, Ontario, July 1988.

"AIDS in the '90s: The New Facts of Life," Canadian Public Health Association Pamphlet, Health and Welfare Canada, February 1991.

The Boston Women's Health Book Collective, *The New Our Bodies, Ourselves* (1992, Simon and Schuster, New York).

"Candidiasis," *Treatment Issues for Women Living With HIV and AIDS,* No. 2, Spring 1993, Voices of Positive Women, Toronto, Canada.

Hatcher, Robert A., M.D., et al., *Contraceptive Technology, 1990–1992,* 15th revised edition (1990, Irvington Publishers, New York).

"HIV Often Undetected in Women by Emergency Room Staff (New York)," *AIDS Weekly*, March 22, 1993.

"Human Papilloma Virus and Cervical Cancer Issues for Women with HIV and AIDS," *Treatment Issues*, No. 1, November 1992, Voices of Positive Women, Toronto, Canada.

MacDonald, Kelly S., M.D., F.R.C.P.(C), infectious disease specialist, interviewed 1993.

"Minorities, Women Are Fastest Growing AIDS Populations," Volume 8, *AIDS Alert*, February 1993.

"More Women Diagnosed with AIDS, Different Symptoms Emerging," Volume 7, *AIDS Alert*, July 1992, (AIDS Guide for Health Care Workers).

Richardson, Diane, *Women and AIDS* (1988, Routledge, Chapman and Hall, New York).

"Special Edition Women's Treatment Issues," *Treatment Issues: The Gay Men's Health Crisis Newsletter of Experimental AIDS Therapies*, Volume 6, No. 7, Summer/Fall 1992, distributed by the Gay Men's Health Crisis, New York.

Treatment Issues for Women Living with HIV and AIDS, No. 4, August 1993, Voices of Positive Women, Toronto, Canada.

Voices: A Newsletter for Women Living with HIV/AIDS, Volume 1, No. 4, March 1993, Voices of Positive Women, Toronto, Canada.

Women and AIDS: Choices for Women in the Age of AIDS, booklet, Health and Welfare Canada, 1990.

"Women and AIDS: What You Need to Know Now," *Flare Magazine*, March 1993.

Chapter 6

The Boston Women's Health Book Collective, *The New Our Bodies, Ourselves* (1992, Simon and Schuster, New York).

"Definition, Symptoms and Causes of PID," The Vancouver Women's Health Research Collective Booklet, 1983.

DeMarco, Carolyn, M.D., *Take Charge of Your Body: A Woman's Guide to Health*, (1990, The Last Laugh, Winlaw, British Columbia, Canada).

Dorland's Illustrated Medical Dictionary, 26th Edition (1981, W. B. Saunders Co., Philadelphia).

Garber, Gary, M.D., F.R.C.P., "What You Should Know About Sexually Transmitted Diseases (STDs)," Synphasic Patient Education Series Pamphlet.

Hatcher, Robert A., M.D., et al., *Contraceptive Technology, 1990–1992*, 15th revised edition (1990, Irvington Publishers, New York).

"Hepatitis B Information Sheet," Bay Centre for Birth Control, 1993.

Johnson, Mary Anne G., M.D., "Urinary Tract Infections in Women," *American Family Physician*, February 1990.

MacDonald, Kelly S., M.D., F.R.C.P.(C), infectious disease specialist, interviewed 1993.

Long, Michele, M.D., primary care physician, interviewed 1993.

"Preventing PID (Pelvic Inflammatory Disease)," City of Toronto, Department of Public Health Pamphlet.

Schaaf, V. Mylo, Eliseo J. Perez-Stable, and Kenneth Borchardt, "The Limited Value of Symptoms and Signs in the Diagnosis of Vaginal Infections," *Archives of Internal Medicine*, September 1990.

"STD, Sexually Transmitted Diseases," Health and Welfare Canada Booklet, 1991.

Washington, A. Eugene, M.D., M.Sc.; Willard Cates Jr., M.D., MPH; and Judith N. Wasserheit, M.D., MPH; "Preventing Pelvic Inflammatory Disease," *Journal of the American Medical Association*, Volume 266, No. 18, November 13, 1991.

Washington, A. Eugene, M.D., M.Sc.; Sevgi O. Aral, Ph.D., Wolner-Hanssen, M.D., DMS; David A. Grimes, M.D., King K. Holmes, M.D., Ph.D., "Assessing Risk for Pelvic Inflammatory Disease and Its Sequelae," *Journal of the American Medical Association*, Volume 266, No. 18, November 13, 1991.

"Watch Where You Sit," Research at Eastern Virginia Medical School on the connection between vinyl seats and yeast infections, *The Edell Health Letter*, Volume 9, November 1990.

Chapter 7

The Boston Women's Health Book Collective, *The New Our Bodies, Ourselves* (1992, Simon and Schuster, New York).

DeMarco, Carolyn, M.D., *Take Charge of Your Body: A Woman's Guide to Health* (1990, The Last Laugh, Winlaw, British Columbia, Canada).

Dorland's Illustrated Medical Dictionary, 26th Edition (1981, W. B. Saunders Co., Philadelphia).

Goldfarb, Herbert A., M.D., with Judith Greif, *The No-Hysterectomy Option: Your Body—Your Choice* (1990, Wiley, New York).

HealthFacts, Volume 15, No. 139, December 1990. Subject: post-operative effects of hysterectomy. Editor, Maryann Napoli, published by the Center for Medical Consumers, Inc., 327 Thompson Street, New York.

HealthFacts, November 1992, Subject: fibroid surgery. Editor, Maryann Napoli, published by the Center for Medical Consumers, Inc., 327 Thompson Street, New York.

Hufnagel, Vicki, M.D., *No More Hysterectomies* (1989, New American Library, New York).

Malesky, Gail, and Charles B. Inlander, *Take This Book to the Gynecologist with You: A Consumer's Guide to Women's Health* (1991, Addison-Wesley, New York).

Mesner, Sandy, M.D., primary care physician, Women's College Hospital Cancer Detection Centre, Toronto, interviewed 1993.

Chapter 8

"Breast Cancer," Canadian Cancer Society Pamphlet, May 1988.

"Breast Cancer: Your Best Protection . . . Early Detection," Canadian Breast Cancer Foundation Pamphlet, Toronto, Ontario.

DeMarco, Carolyn, M.D., *Take Charge of Your Body: A Woman's Guide to Health* (1990, The Last Laugh, Winlaw, British Columbia, Canada).

Goldfarb, Herbert A., M.D., with Judith Greif, *The No-Hysterectomy Option* (1990, Wiley, New York).

Hufnagel, Vicki, M.D., *No More Hysterectomies* (1989, New American Library, New York).

Hunter, D.J., et al., "A Prospective Study of Selenium Status and Breast Cancer Risk," *Journal of the American Medical Association*, Volume 264, September 5, 1990.

Love, Susan M., M.D., *Dr. Susan Love's Breast Book* (1991, Addison-Wesley, New York).

"Major Advance Reported in Identifying Cause of Breast Cancer (DNA damage)," Pacific Northwest Research Foundation, *Cancer Weekly*, October 14, 1991.

Mesner, Sandy, M.D., primary care physician, Women's College Hospital Cancer Detection Centre, Toronto, interviewed 1993.

Olson, Linda K., M.D., "Interpreting the Mammogram Report," *American Family Physician*, Volume 47, No. 2, February 1, 1993.

Polevoy, Michael, "High-tech Cancer Tests," *American Health*, September 1992.

Popkin, David, M.D., C.M., F.R.C.S.(C), F.A.C.O.G., "Understanding Cervical and Other Cancers," Synphasic Patient Education Series Pamphlet.

"Studies Show New Way to Diagnose Breast Cancer (Magnetic Resonance Imaging, Israel)," *Cancer Weekly,* April 12, 1993.

Chapter 9

"Breast Cancer: Your Best Protection . . . Early Detection," Canadian Breast Cancer Foundation Pamphlet, Toronto.

Chittoor, Sreeni R., M.D., and Sandra M. Swain, M.D., "Adjuvant Therapy in Early Breast Cancer," *American Family Physician,* August 1991.

Cukier, Daniel, M.D., and Virginia E. McCullough, *Coping with Radiation Therapy: A Ray of Hope* (1993, Lowell House, Los Angeles).

Dollinger, Malin, M.D., Ernest H. Rosenbaum, M.D., and Greg Cable, *Everyone's Guide to Cancer Therapy: How Cancer is Diagnosed, Treated and Managed Day to Day* (1992, Somerville House Publishing, Toronto).

Field, Dean Arden, M.D., and Sandra Miller, M.D., "Cosmetic Breast Surgery," *American Family Physician,* February 1992.

"From Abnormal Pap to Hysterectomy: Diagnostic Tests Are Often Omitted," *HealthFacts,* Volume 17, August, 1992.

Goldfarb, Herbert A., M.D., with Judith Greif, *The No-Hysterectomy Option* (1990, Wiley, New York).

Hand, Roger, et al., "Staging Procedures, Clinical Management, and Survival Outcome for Ovarian Carcinoma," *Journal of the American Medical Association,* Volume 269, March 3, 1993.

Hufnagel, Vicki, M.D., *No More Hysterectomies* (1989, New American Library, New York).

"Hysterectomy Prevalence, Cervical Cancer Deaths," *Journal of the American Medical Association,* Volume 267, No. 7, February 19, 1992.

"Information for Patients: Radiation Therapy," Ontario Cancer Institute/Princess Margaret Hospital, 1992.

Lemon, Betty, B.Sc., and Cary Greenberg, BA.Sc., "Nutrition Guide for People with Cancer," Department of Nutrition at Ontario Cancer Institute, The Princess Margaret Hospital, and the Canadian Cancer Society.

"Loop Electrosurgical Excision Procedure Used for Treating Cervical Cancer," *Cancer Weekly,* December 30, 1991.

Love, Susan M., M.D., *Dr. Susan Love's Breast Book* (1991, Addison-Wesley, New York).

"Major Advance Reported in Identifying Cause of Breast Cancer," *Cancer Weekly*, October 14, 1991.

Mesner, Sandy, M.D., primary care physician, Women's College Hospital Cancer Detection Centre, Toronto, interviewed 1993.

"Ovarian Cancer: Today's Treatment, Tomorrow's Hope," *FDA Consumer*, Volume 26, December 1992.

"What You Need to Know About Breast Cancer," the Burlington Breast Cancer Support Services, Inc., Booklet, June 1991.

Chapter 10

"10 Great Reasons to Breast-Feed," Ministry of National Health and Welfare, Ministry of Supply and Services, pamphlet, Canada, 1990.

Adams Hillard, Paula, M.D., "Coping with Morning Sickness," *Parents' Magazine*, Volume 65, August 1990.

The Boston Women's Health Book Collective, *The New Our Bodies, Ourselves* (1992, Simon and Schuster, New York).

"Breast Cancer: Pregnancy Advisable?" *Nursing 89*, June 1989.

"Breast Versus Bottle," *Flare Magazine*, November1993.

Brennan, Barbara, M.D., F.R.C.S.(C), "Prenatal Testing: Remove Some of the Guesswork," *Expecting: A Pregnancy Guide*, Family Communications, Inc., Volume 44, No. 4, Fall/Winter 1992.

Casiro, O., M.D., F.R.C.P.(C), "Fetal Alcohol Syndrome: Alcohol and Pregnancy Don't Mix," *Expecting: A Pregnancy Guide*, Family Communications Inc., Volume 44, No. 4, Fall/Winter 1992.

DeMarco, Carolyn, M.D., *Take Charge of Your Body: A Woman's Guide to Health* (1990, The Last Laugh, Winlaw, British Columbia, Canada).

Eisenberg, Arlene, Heidi E. Murkoff, and Sandee E. Hathaway, *What to Expect When You're Expecting* (1991, Workman Publishing, New York).

"Exercise During Pregnancy," *American Family Physician*, Volume 42, No. 3.

Freed, Gary L., M.D., MPH, "Breastfeeding: Time to Teach What We Preach," *Journal of the American Medical Association*, Volume 269, No. 2, January 13, 1993.

Gander, Rosemary, "Guidelines: For a Healthy Pregnancy," *Expecting: A Pregnancy Guide*, Family Communications, Inc., Volume 44, No. 4, Fall/Winter 1992.

Green, Debra, and Joanne Malin, "When Reality Shatters Parents' Dreams," *Nursing 88*, February 1988.

Hamblin, Gail, R.N., "Normal Discomforts: How to Cope," *Expecting: A Pregnancy Guide,* Family Communications, Inc., Volume 44, No. 4, Fall/Winter 1992.

Hamilton, Emily, M.D., F.R.C.S.(C), "What Pregnancy Means for You and Your Baby," Synphasic Patient Education Series.

Hanvey, Louise, BN, MHA, "Delivery Decisions: Check Out Your Choices," *Expecting: A Pregnancy Guide,* Family Communications, Inc., Volume 44, No. 4, Fall/Winter 1992.

Kuboniwa, Faith, R.N., BN, SC, "Vaginal Birth After a Caesarean Section," *Expecting: A Pregnancy Guide,* Family Communications, Inc., Volume 45, No. 2, Spring/Summer 1993.

Lakusiak, Ellen, "Nutrition Matters," *Expecting: A Pregnancy Guide,* Family Communications, Inc., Volume 44, No. 4, Fall/Winter 1992.

Lander, Debra, M.D., F.R.C.P.(C), psychiatrist, interviewed 1993.

Lazar, Matthew, M.D., F.R.C.P.(C), F.A.C.P., pediatrician/ neonatal specialist, interviewed 1994.

Levy, Nancy, "Labor and Birth Guide," *Expecting: A Pregnancy Guide,* Family Communications, Inc., Volume 44, No. 4, Fall/Winter 1992.

Love, Susan, M.D., with Karen Lindsey, *Dr. Susan Love's Breast Book* (1991, Addison-Wesley, New York).

"Multivitamin Supplements and Morning Sickness (Vitamins and Minerals)," *Nutrition Research Newsletter,* Volume 11, November/December 1992.

"One Out of 500 Miscarriages from Amniocentesis," *The Doctor's People Newsletter,* Volume 3, October 1990.

Stevenson-Smith, Fay, "After the Birth (Recovering From Childbirth)," *Parents' Magazine,* Volume 68, March 1993.

Watson-MacDonell, Jo, R.N., BScN, "Episiotomy," *Expecting: A Pregnancy Guide,* Family Communications, Inc., Volume 44, No. 4, Fall/Winter 1992

West, Karen, R.N., "Pregnancy's Progress," *Expecting: A Pregnancy Guide,* Family Communications, Inc., Volume 44, No. 4, Fall/Winter 1992.

Chapter 11

The Boston Women's Health Book Collective, *The New Our Bodies, Ourselves* (1992, Simon and Schuster, New York).

Burkman, Ronald T., M.D., *Handbook of Contraception and Abortion* (1989, Little, Brown, Boston).

Lander, Debra, M.D., F.R.C.P.(C), psychiatrist, interviewed 1993.

Policar, Michael, M.D., F.A.C.O.G., Vice President, Medical Affairs, Planned Parenthood Federation of America, interviewed 1993.

Powell, Marion, M.D., "RU 486: The Abortion Pill," *Health Talk*, Volume 2, No. 1, Women's College Hospital and the Regional Women's Health Centre, Toronto, Canada, April 1993.

Chapter 12

Bain, Jerald, M.D., F.R.C.P.(C), Andrologist/Endocrinologist, interviewed 1994.

Burkman, Ronald T., M.D., *Handbook of Contraception and Abortion* (1989, Little, Brown, Boston).

Chihal, H. Jane, M.D., Ph.D., and Sister Mary Madonna Baudier, M.D., "Polycystic Ovary Syndrome," *American Family Physician*, April 1985.

DeMarco, Carolyn, M.D., *Take Charge of Your Body: A Woman's Guide to Health* (1990, The Last Laugh, Winlaw, British Columbia, Canada).

Gorman, Christine, "How Old Is Too Old?" *Time*, September 30, 1991.

Harkness, Carla, *The Infertility Book: A Comprehensive Medical and Emotional Guide* (1987, Volcano Press, San Francisco).

Hey, Valerie, Catherine Itzin, Lesley Saunders, and Mary Anne Speakman, eds., *Hidden Loss: Miscarriage and Ectopic Pregnancy* (1989, The Women's Press Ltd., London, England).

Jones, Deborah, "Recurrent Miscarriages: News About Causes and Treatments," *Chatelaine Magazine*, November 1993.

Khatamee, Masood, M.D., F.A.C.O.G., Executive Director, Fertility Research Foundation, New York City, interviewed 1993.

Raab, Diana, R.N., BS, *Getting Pregnant and Staying Pregnant: A Guide to Infertility and High-Risk Pregnancy*, (1987, Sirdan Publishing, Montreal).

Seibel, Machelle, M.D., F.A.C.O.G., Associate Professor, Obstetrics and Gynecology, Harvard Medical School, Chief, Division of Reproductive Endocrinology and Infertility, Director, In Vitro Fertilization Program, Beth Israel Hospital, Boston, *Infertility: A Comprehensive Text* (1990, Appleton and Lange, a division of Prentice Hall, Norwalk, Connecticut).

Chapter 13

The Boston Women's Health Book Collective, *The New Our Bodies, Ourselves* (1992, Simon and Schuster, New York).

Beard, Mary K., M.D., F.A.C.O.G., and Lindsay R. Curtis, M.D., F.A.C.O.G., *Menopause and the Years Ahead* (1988, Fisher Books, Tucson, Arizona).

Casper, Robert F., and Alcide Chapdelaine, "Estrogen and Interrupted Progestin: A New Concept for Menopausal Hormone Replacement Therapy," *American Journal of Obstetrics and Gynecology*, Volume 168, April 1993.

Colditz, Graham A., Kathleen M. Egan, and Meir J. Stampher, "Hormone Replacement Therapy and Risk of Breast Cancer: Results of Epidemiologic Studies," *American Journal of Obstetrics and Gynecology*, Volume 168, May 1993.

"A Complex Question of Odds: Hormones Versus No Treatment," *Health-Facts*, Volume 18, January 1993.

DeMarco, Carolyn, M.D., *Take Charge of Your Body: A Woman's Guide to Health* (1990, The Last Laugh, Winlaw, British Columbia, Canada).

Doepel, Laurie K., "Looking at Menopause's Role in Osteoporosis," *Journal of the American Medical Association*, Volume 254, No. 17, November 1, 1985.

Doress, Paula Brown, Diana Laskin Seigal, and the Midlife and Older Women Book Project, in cooperation with the Boston Women's Health Collective, *Ourselves Growing Older* (1987, Simon and Schuster, New York).

"Estrogen Replacement Therapy and Breast Cancer Risk," *Cancer Researcher Weekly*, May 10, 1993.

Finucane, Fanchon F., "Decreased Risk of Stroke Among Postmenopausal Hormone Users: Results from a National Cohort," *Journal of the American Medical Association*, Volume 269, June 2, 1993.

George, Susan, M.D., F.R.C.P.(C), F.A.C.P., endocrinologist, interviewed 1993.

Henkel, Gretchen, *Making the Estrogen Decision* (1992, Lowell House, Los Angeles).

Hufnagel, Vicki, M.D., *No More Hysterectomies* (1989, New American Library, New York).

"Hysterectomy and a Woman's Sex Life," *The Women's Letter*, January 1991.

Lindsay, Robert, "Prevention and Treatment of Osteoporosis," *The Lancet*, Volume 341, March 27, 1993.

"Menopause," Women's College Hospital and Regional Women's Health Centre Booklet, Toronto, 1992.

Palferman, T. G., "That Oestrogen Replacement for Osteoporosis Prevention Should No Longer Be a Bone of Contention," *Annals of the Rheumatic Diseases,* Volume 52, January 1993.

Pearson, Cynthia, "FDA Waffles on Premarin Decision," *The Network News,* Volume 15, July/August 1990.

Perry, Susan, and Katherine O'Hanlan, M.D., *Natural Menopause: The Complete Guide to a Woman's Most Misunderstood Passage* (1992, Addison-Wesley, New York).

"Postmenopausal Osteoporosis and Preventative Measures," *American Family Physician,* Volume 45, No. 3, March 1992.

"Postmenopausal Osteoporosis and Synthetic Calcitrol," *American Family Physician,* Volume 43, No. 3, March 1990.

Randall, Lee, "Is HRT for Me?," *Weight Watchers Magazine,* Volume 26, February 1993.

Rappaport, Daniel, M.D., F.R.C.P.(C), radiologist, interviewed 1993.

"Replacement Therapy for Reducing Cardiovascular Disease," *The Western Journal of Medicine,* May 1993.

"Short-term Estrogen Therapy Does Not Increase Breast Cancer Risk," Johns Hopkins School of Public Health, *Cancer Weekly,* March 2, 1992.

Utian, Wolf, M.D., Ph.D., North American Menopause Society, Cleveland, Ohio, interviewed 1993.

Wardlaw, Gordon M., Ph.D., R.D., "Putting Osteoporosis in Perspective," *Journal of the American Dietetic Association,* Volume 93, No. 9, September 1993.

Webber, Gail, menopause educator, interviewed 1993.

APPENDIX A

Where to Go for More Information

Because of the volatile nature (regarding funding and resources) of many health or nonprofit organizations, some of the following addresses and numbers may have changed since this list was compiled. I apologize for any inconvenience. The following list is organized alphabetically by subject.

Abortion

American Civil Liberties Union (ACLU)
Reproductive Freedom Project
132 West 43rd Street
New York, NY 10036
212-944-9800

Civil Liberties and Public Policy Program
Hampshire College
Amherst, MA 01002
413-549-4600. ext. 645

Committee to Defend Reproductive Rights (CDRR)
25 Taylor Street, Suite 704
San Francisco, CA 94102
415-647-2694

Faulkner Centre for Reproductive Medicine
1153 Centre Street, First Floor, Centre House
Boston, MA 02130
617-983-7300

Federation of Feminist Women's Health Centers
6221 Wilshire Boulevard, Suite 419-A
Los Angeles, CA 90048
503-344-0966

International Women's Health Coalition
24 East 21st Street
New York, NY 10010
212-979-8500

National Abortion Federation (NAF)
1436 U Street, NW
Washington DC 20009
202-667-5881

National Black Women's Health Project (NBWHP)
1237 Ralph David Abernathy Boulevard, SW
Atlanta, GA 30310
404-758-9590

National Organization for Women (NOW) Action Center
1000 16th Street, NW, Suite 700
Washington, DC 20036
202-331-0066

National Women's Health Network
1325 G Street, NW
Washington, DC 20005
202-347-1140

Native American Women's Health Education Resource Center
P.O. Box 572
Lake Andes, SD 57356
605-487-7072

AIDS (United States)

National toll-free hotline: 1-800-342-AIDS (2437)
Hours: Mon.-Fri., 8:30 a.m.-5:30 p.m.

ACT UP (AIDS Coalition to Unleash Power)
135 West 29th Street, Suite 10
New York, NY, 10001
212-564-2437

AIDS Project
22 Monument Square, 5th Floor
Portland, ME 04101
207-774-6877

AIDS Project New Haven
850 Grand Avenue, Room 206
New Haven, CT 06511
203-624-0947

AIDS Services of Austin
P.O. Box 4874
Austin, TX 78765
512-451-2273, Spanish: 512-472-2001

Aliveness Project
730 East 38th Street
Minneapolis, MN 55407
612-822-7946

AWARE (Association for Women's AIDS Research and Education)
San Francisco General/Ward 84
995 Potrero Avenue
San Francisco, CA 94110
415-476-4091

Blacks Educating Blacks About Sexual Health Issues (BEBASHI)
1233 Locust Street, Suite 401
Philadelphia, PA 19107
215-546-4140

Cascade AIDS Project
620 SW 5th Avenue, Suite 300
Portland, OR 97204
503-223-5907

Chicago Women's AIDS Project
5249 North Kenmore
Chicago, IL 60640
312-271-2242

Colorado AIDS Project
1576 Sherman Street
Denver, CO 80203
303-837-0166
Toll-free outside Denver: 800-333-2437

Community Health Awareness Group
3028 East Grand Boulevard
Detroit, MI 48202
313-872-2424

DC Women's Council on AIDS
Sistercare Support Network
715 8th Street
Washington, DC 20003
202-544-8255

Feminist Women's Health Center
580 14 Street, NW
Atlanta, GA 30318
404-874-7551

Gay Men's Health Crisis (GMHC)
254 West 18th Street
New York, NY 10011
212-807-7035/Hotline: 212-807-6655
(A superb organization!!)

Health Information Network
Women and AIDS
P.O. Box 30762
Seattle, WA 98103
206-784-5655

Life Force: Women Fighting AIDS
165 Camden Plaza East, #310
Brooklyn, NY 11201
718-797-0937

National AIDS Hotline
800-342-AIDS
Spanish: 800-344-7432
TTY: 800-243-7889

Native American Women's Health Education Resource Center
P.O. Box 572
Lake Andes, SD 57356
605-487-7072

New York City AIDS Hotline
212-447-8200
Hours: Mon.-Sat., 9:00 a.m.-9:00 p.m.

NO/AIDS Task Force
1407 Decatur Street
New Orleans, LA 70116
504-945-4000

People of Colour Against AIDS Network
1200 South Jackson, Suite 25
Seattle, WA 98144
206-322-7061

The Positive Women
P.O. Box 34372
Washington, DC 20043
202-898-0372

Prevention Point Research Group
P.O. Box 170028
San Francisco, CA 94117
415-861-6710

PROTOTYPES—WARN (Women and AIDS Risk Networks)
5601 West Slauson Avenue, Suite 200
Culver City, CA 90230
310-641-7795

San Francisco AIDS Foundation
25 Van Ness Street, Suite 660
San Francisco, CA 94102
415-864-4376
Hotline: 800-863-AIDS

Simon House
16260 Dexter Avenue
Detroit, MI 48221
313-863-1400

Sisterlove Women's AIDS Project
1432 Donnelly
Atlanta, GA 30310
404-753-7733

St. Louis Efforts for AIDS
5622 Delmar Boulevard, Suite 104E
St. Louis, MO 63112
314-367-8400

Topeka AIDS Project
1915 SW 6th Street
Topeka, KS 66606
913-232-3100

University of California San Francisco
AIDS Health Project
P.O. Box 0884
San Francisco, CA 94143
415-476-6430

Women's AIDS Project
8235 Santa Monica Boulevard, Suite 201
West Hollywood, CA 90046
213-650-1508

Women's AIDS Network
c/o San Francisco AIDS Foundation
333 Valencia Street, 4th Floor
San Francisco, CA 94103
415-864-4376
(They get calls from all over the world!)

Women's Health Project
Nelson Tebedo Clinic
4012 Cedar Springs
Dallas, TX 75219
214-521-5124

Women and AIDS Resource Network (WARN)
30 Third Avenue, Suite 513
Brooklyn, NY 11217
718-596-6007

Resources for Teenagers:
Adolescent AIDS Program
Montefiore Medical Center
111 East 210th Street
Bronx, NY 10467
718-920-2179

Hetrick-Martin Institute
2 Astor Place, 3rd Floor
New York, NY 10013
212-674-2400

Teens and AIDS Hotline
800-234-TEEN

Resources for Treatment:
AIDS Treatment Data Network
259 West 30th Street
New York, NY 10001
212-268-4196

Fenway Community Health Center
7 Haviland Street
Boston, MA 02115
617-267-0900

Project Inform
1965 Market Street
San Francisco, CA 94103
800-822-7422

Whitman-Walker Clinic
1407 S Street, NW
Washington, DC 20009
202-797-3500

AIDS (Canada)

AIDS Committee of Toronto (ACT)
P.O. Box 55, Station F
Toronto, Ontario M4Y 2L4
416-340-2437

Canadian AIDS Society
701-100 Sparks Street
Ottawa, Ontario K1P 5B7
613-230-3580

Centre for AIDS Services of Montreal
202-1168 Ste. Catharine West
Montreal, Quebec H3B 1K1
514-954-0170

Community AIDS Treatment Information Exchange
324-517 College Street
Toronto, Ontario M6A 1A8
416-944-1916

Positive Women's Network
c/o Pacific AIDS Resource Centre
1107 Seymour Street
Vancouver, British Columbia V6B 5S8
604-893-2200

Voices of Positive Women
P.O. Box 471, Station C
Toronto, Ontario M6J 3P5
416-324-8703 / FAX: 416-324-9701
(An excellent source of information.)

Cancer

(For information on breast cancer, mammography, pelvic and other cancers, see also DES Daughters and Pap Smears below.)

American Cancer Society
19 West 56th Street
New York, NY 10019
212-586-8700

Breast Cancer Action
P.O. Box 460185
San Francisco, CA 94146
415-922-8279

Attention Canadians:
Burlington Breast Cancer Support Services, Inc.
Burlington Mall, 777 Guelph Line
Burlington, Ontario L7R 3N2
905-634-2333/FAX: 905-634-2110
(This is the best support group in the country!)

Foundation for Alternative Cancer Therapies
P.O. Box 1242
Old Chelsea Station
New York, NY 10113
212-741-2790

National Alliance of Breast Cancer Organizations (NABCO)
9 East 37th Street, 10th Floor
New York, NY 10016
212-889-0606

National Cancer Institute
Office of Cancer Communications
Building 31, Room 10A24
9000 Rockville Pike
Bethesda, MD 20892
Hotline: 800-4-CANCER

National Coalition for Cancer Survivorship
1010 Wayne Avenue, 5th Floor
Silver Spring, MD 20910
301-650-8868

Women's Community Cancer Project
c/o Women's Center
46 Pleasant Street
Cambridge, MA 02139
617-354-9888

Contraception

American Civil Liberties Union
Reproductive Freedom Project
132 West 43rd Street
New York, NY 10036
212-944-9800

Female Condom Information Line: 1-800-274-6601

Planned Parenthood Federation of America
(listed in your local phone book)

Attention Canadians:
The Bay Centre for Birth Control
790 Bay Street, 8th Floor
Toronto, Ontario
416-351-3700
(Also provides counseling on abortion, adoption, prenatal care—again, the best place in the country!)

DES Daughters

The DES Cancer Network
DES Action USA
1615 Broadway
Oakland, CA 94612
510-465-4011

Eating Disorders

Anorexia Nervosa and Related Eating Disorders, Inc.
P.O. Box 5102
Eugene, OR 97405
503-344-1144

National Eating Disorders Organization (NEDO)
445 East Granville Road
Worhtington, OH 43084
614-436-1112

Endometriosis

Endometriosis Association
8585 North 76th Place
Milwaukee, WI 53223
800-992-3636 (for the U.S., Puerto Rico, the Virgin Islands, and the Bahamas.)

St. Charles Medical Center
Endometriosis Treatment Program
2500 NE Neff Road
Bend, OR 97701-6015
800-446-2177

Attention Canadians:
The Endometriosis Network
Toronto Information Line
416-591-3963

General Gynecological Health

American Medical Women's Association (AMWA)
801 North Fairfax, Suite 400
Alexandria, VA 22314
703-838-0500

Center for Medical Consumers and Health Care Information
237 Thomson Street
New York, NY 10012
212-674-7105

Concord Feminist Health Centre
38 South Main Street
Concord, NH 03301
603-225-2739

The Federation of Feminist Women's Health Centers (FFWHC)
633 East 11th Avenue
Eugene, OR 97401
503-344-0966
(They have several clinics on file they can refer you to.)

Lyon-Martin Women's Health Clinic
1748 Market Street, Suite 201
San Francisco, CA 94102
415-565-7667

National Black Women's Health Project (NBWHP)
1237 Ralph David Abernathy Boulevard, SW
Atlanta, GA 30310
404-758-9590

Women's Health Information Center
Boston Women's Health Book Collective
Information Line: 617-625-0271

Hysterectomies

Hysterectomy Educational Resources and Services (HERS)
422 Bryn Mawr Avenue
Bala-Cynwyd, PA 19004
215-667-7757

Infertility/Adoption (also see Endometriosis)

Adopted Families of America
3333 Highway 100 N
Minneapolis, MN 55432
612-535-4829

Compassionate Friends
P.O. Box 3696
Oak Brook, IL 60522-3696
708-990-0010
(Support after miscarriage or death of a child.)

Concerned United Birthparents (CUB)
2000 Walker Street
Des Moines, IA 50317
515-262-2334

Fertility Research Foundation
877 Park Avenue
New York, NY 10021
212-744-5500

National Adoption Information Clearinghouse
11426 Rockville Pike
Rockville, MD 20852
301-231-6512

North American Council on Adoptable Children
970 Raymond Avenue, Suite 106
St. Paul, MN 55114-1149
612-644-3036

Pregnancy and Infant Loss Centre
1421 East Wayzata Boulevard, Suite 30
Wayzata, MN 55391
612-473-9372

Resolve, Inc.
1310 Broadway
Somerville, MA 02144
617-623-0744

Infertility Awareness Association of Canada (IAAC)
774 Echo Drive, Room 523,
Ottawa, Ontario
K1S 5N8
613-730-1322
Fax: 613-730-1323
1-800-263-2929

Menopause

American Association of Retired Persons (AARP)
Program Department
601 E Street, NW
Washington, DC 20049
202-434-2277

American Health Care Association
1201 L Street, NW
Washington, DC 20005
202-842-4444

National Women's Health Network
1324 G Street, NW
Washington, DC 20005
202-347-1140

North American Menopause Society (NAMS)
University Hospitals of Cleveland
2074 Abington Road
Cleveland, OH 44106
216-844-3334

Older Women's League
666 Eleventh Street, NW, Suite 700
Washington, DC 20001
202-783-6686

Menstruation

Society for Menstrual Cycle Research (SMCR)
10559 North 104th Place
Scottsdale, AZ 85258
602-451-9731

Osteoporosis

National Osteoporosis Foundation
1150 17th Street NW, Suite 500
Washington, DC 20036
202-223-2226

Pap Smears

American Society for Colposcopy and Cervical Pathology
c/o American College of Obstetricians and Gynecologists
409 Twelfth Street, SW
Washington, DC 20024
202-638-5577

Pelvic Inflammatory Disease (PID)

The Canadian PID Society
Box 33804, Station D
Vancouver, BC V6J 4L6
604-684-5704
(One of the best places in North America—Americans feel free to call!)

Pregnancy and Childbirth

American Academy of Husband-Coached Childbirth (AAHCC)
P.O. Box 5224
Sherman Oaks, CA 91413
818-788-6662

American College of Obstetricians and Gynecologists
409 Twelfth Street, SW
Washington, DC 20024
202-638-5577

American College of Nurse-Midwives
818 Connecticut Avenue NW, Suite 900
Washington, DC 20006
202-728-9860

American Foundation for Maternal and Child Health
439 East 51st Street, 4th Floor
New York, NY 10022
212-759-5510

American Gynecological and Obstetrical Society
c/o James R. Scott, M.D., OBGYN Dept., Room 2B200
University of Utah
50 North Medical Drive
Salt Lake City, UT 84132
801-581-5501

Childbirth Education Association
P.O. Box 5
Richboro, PA 18954-0005
215-357-2792

Childbirth Without Pain Association
20134 Snowden
Detroit, MI 48235-1170
313-341-3816

Healthy Mothers, Healthy Babies Coalition
409 Twelfth Street, SW, Room 309
Washington, DC 20024-2188
202-863-2458

Informed Homebirth
P.O. Box 3675
Ann Arbor, MI 48106
313-662-6857

International Association of Parents and Professionals for Safe Alternatives in Childbirth (NAPSAC)
Route 1, Box 646
Marble Hill, MO 63764
314-238-2010

International Cesarean Awareness Network
P.O. Box 276
Clarks Summit, PA 18411
717-585-4226 (I CAN)

International Childbirth Education Associates (ICEA)
P.O. Box 20048
Minneapolis, MN 55420
612-854-8660

La Leche League International and
Breastfeeding Reference Library and Database
1400 N. Meacham Rd.
Schaumburg, IL 60173-4840
708-519-7730/Fax 708-519-0035

Maternity Center Association
48 East 92nd Street
New York, NY 10128
212-369-7300

National Association of Childbearing Centers (NACC)
3123 Gottschall Road
Perkiomenville, PA 18074
215-234-8068

Positive Pregnancy and Parenting Fitness
51 Saltrock Road
Baltic, CT 06330
203-822-8573

Read Natural Childbirth Foundation
P.O. Box 150956
San Rafael, CA 94915
415-456-8462

Sexually Transmitted Diseases (STDs)

American Social Health Association (ASHA)
P.O. Box 13827
Research Triangle Park, NC 27709
919-361-8400

Centers for Disease Control
Division of STD/HIV Prevention
Atlanta, GA 30333
404-639-3311

Herpes Advice Center
The Stanford Building
51 East 25th Street
The sixth and seventh Floors
New York, NY 10010
(212) 213-6150

Public Health Department
STD Division (State level)
(listed in your local phone book)
National Herpes Hotline
919-361-8488

Urinary Incontinence

Continence Restored, Inc.
785 Park Avenue
New York, NY 10021
212-879-3131

The Simon Foundation
P.O. Box 815
Wilmette, IL 60091
1-800-23-SIMON

Help for Incontinent People (HIP)
P.O. Box 544
Union, SC 29379
803-579-7900
After hours: 803-427-5434

Special note to Canadians: Although AIDS resources for Canada are listed separately and appendix A is peppered with Canadian resources, the United States outperforms Canada in terms of organizations and resources. For *any* subject listed below, the best places to call in Canada are:

in Toronto:
Women's College Hospital
Regional Women's Health Centre
790 Bay Street, 8th Floor
Toronto, Ontario, M5G 1N9
416-586-0211
(This is the best women's health center in the country.)

in Vancouver:
Vancouver Women's Health Collective
1675 West 8th Avenue, Suite 219
Vancouver, British Columbia V5L 2Y7
604-736-5262
in Montreal:
Montreal Health Press
Box 1000
Station G
Montreal, Quebec, H2W 2N1
514-282-1171

Nationally, Canadians can contact the Consumer Health Information Service, a joint project of the Faculty of Library and Information Science, University of Toronto, Consumers' Association of Canada, Metropolitan Toronto Reference Library, the Toronto Hospital, and the Centre for Health Promotion, University of Toronto, at 789 Yonge Street, Toronto, Ontario, M4W 2G8; outside Toronto: 1-800-667-1999; in Toronto: 416-393-7056, FAX 416-393-7181.

You can also contact your local branch of the Canadian Cancer Society (listed in the White or Yellow Pages. Also note the Burlington Breast Cancer Services, Inc., listed in the "Cancer" section.

All the above numbers will put you in touch with the closest resource in your area. And, all the United States resources welcome calls from Canada!

APPENDIX B

Books That Might Interest You

Abortion

Abortion: A Doctor's Perspective, A Woman's Dilemma, Don M. Sloan with Paula Hartz (1992, D.I. Fine, New York).

Abortion and Women's Health: A Turning Point for America?, Rachel Benson Gold (1990, Alan Guttmacher Institute, New York).

Abortion: Choice and Conflict, Oliver Trager, ed. (1993, Facts on File, New York).

Understanding Abortion, Mary Pipes (1986 Women's Press, London).

A Woman's Book of Choices: Abortion, Menstrual Extraction, RU486, Rebecca Chalker and Carol Downer (1992, Four Walls Eight Windows, New York).

AIDS/STDs

A Book About Sexually Transmitted Diseases, Donna Cherniak (1988, Montreal Health Press). Revised in 1991 as *STD Handbook.*

Dr. Neumann's Guide to the New Sexually Transmitted Diseases, Hans H. Neumann (1987, Acropolis Books, Washington, D.C.).

Promoting Safer Sex: Prevention of Sexual Transmission of AIDS and Other STDs, Maria Paalman, ed. (1990, Swets and Zeitlinger, Rockland, Massachusetts).

Safe Sex: A Doctor Examines the Realities of AIDS and Other STDs, Joe S. McIlhaney (1991, Baker Book House, Grand Rapids, Michigan).

Safe Sex: What Everyone Should Know About Sexually Transmitted Diseases, Angelo T. Scotti (1987, PaperJacks, Toronto, New York).
Sexually Transmitted Diseases, Marjorie Little (1991, Chelsea House Publishers, New York).
Sexually Transmitted Diseases: You May Have One But You Don't Know It, Antonio Novak Feliciano (1992, Vantage Press, New York).

Breastfeeding

Breastfeeding: Getting Breastfeeding Right for You, Mary Renfrew, Cloe Fisher, and Suzanne Arms (1990, Celestial Arts, Berkeley, California).
The Breastfeeding Sourcebook, M. Sara Rosenthal (1995, Lowell House, Los Angeles).
Dr. Susan Love's Breast Book, Susan Love, M.D., with Karen Lindsey (1991, Addison-Wesley, New York).
The Experience of Breast Feeding, Sheila Kitzinger (1987, Penguin, New York).
The Nursing Mother's Companion, Kathleen Huggins (1990, Harvard Common Press, Boston, Massachusetts).

Cancer

Breast Cancer
Breast Cancer in the Life Course: Women's Experiences, Julianne S. Oktay and Carolyn A. Walter (1991, Springer Publishing, New York).
Dr. Susan Love's Breast Book, Susan Love, M.D., with Karen Lindsey (1991, Addison-Wesley, New York).
My Breast: One Woman's Cancer Story, Joyce Wadler (1992, Addison-Wesley, New York).
Relative Risk: Living with a Family History of Breast Cancer, Nancy Baker (1991, Viking, New York).
Textbook of Mammography, Audrey K. Tucker, ed. (1993, Churchill Livingstone, New York).

Living with Cancer
Body and Soul: The Other Side of Illness, Albert Kreinheder (1991, Inner City Books, Toronto).
Cancer and Hope, Judith Garrett Garrison (1989, CompCare, Minneapolis).

Cancer as a Turning Point: A Handbook for People with Cancer, Their Families and Health Professionals, Lawrence LeShan (1989, Dutton, New York).

The Cancer Conqueror: An Incredible Journey to Wellness, Greg Anderson (1990, Andrews and McMeel, Kansas City, Missouri).

Cancer Stories: Creativity and Self-Repair, Esther Dreifuss-Kattan (1990, Analytic Press, Hillsdale, New Jersey).

Choices: Realistic Alternatives in Cancer Treatment, Marion Morra and Eve Potts (1987, Avon, New York).

Diagnosis Cancer, Wendy Schlessel Harpham (1992, W.W. Norton, New York).

From Victim to Victor, Harold H. Benjamin (1987, Jeremy P. Tarcher, Los Angeles).

I Don't Know What to Say: How to Help and Support Someone Who is Dying, Robert Buckman (1988, Key Porter Books, Toronto).

Life After Life, Jill Ireland (1988, Jove Books, New York).

Living as a Woman After Cancer, Jacquelyn Johnson (1987, NC Press, Toronto).

Love, Medicine and Miracles, Bernie S. Siegel (1989, Harper & Row, New York).

Minding the Body, Mending the Mind, Joan Borysenko (1987, Addison-Wesley, New York).

My God, I Thought You'd Died, Claude Dosdall and Joanne Broatch (1986, Seal Books, Toronto).

No Cure for Cancer, Denis Leary (1992, Anchor Books, New York).

1 in 3: Women With Cancer Confront an Epidemic, Judith Brady, ed. (1991, Cleis Press, Pittsburgh).

Peace, Love and Healing, Bernie S. Siegel (1989, Harper & Row, New York).

The Road Back to Health: Coping with the Emotional Side of Cancer, Neil A. Fiore (1984, Bantam, New York).

The Race Is Run One Step at a Time, N. Brinker and C. E. Harris (1990, Simon and Schuster, New York).

Triumph, Marion Morra and Eve Potts, (1990, Avon, New York).

Twelve Weeks in Spring, June Callwood (1986, Lester and Orpen Dennys, Toronto).

Understanding Cancer, J. Laszlo (1987, Harper & Row, New York).

Cancer Treatment

The American Cancer Society Cookbook, Anne Lindsay (1988, William Morrow and Co., New York).

Cancer Treatment, Charles M. Haskell, ed. (1990, W. B. Saunders, Chicago).

Coping with Radiation Therapy: A Ray of Hope, Daniel Cukier and Virginia E. McCullough (1993, Lowell House, Los Angeles).

Everyone's Guide to Cancer Therapy: How Cancer is Diagnosed, Treated and Managed Day to Day, Malin Dollinger, Ernest H. Rosenbaum, and Greg Cable, (1992, Somerville House Publishing, Toronto).

The Facts About Chemotherapy, Paul R. Reich and Janice E. Metcalf (1991, Consumers Union of the United States, Inc.).

Head First, Norman Cousins (1989, Penguin Books, New York).

Managing the Side Effects of Chemotherapy and Radiation, Marilyn J. Dodd (1987, Prentice Hall Press, New York).

Ovarian Cancer

Cancer of the Ovary, Maurice Markman and William J. Hoskins, eds. (1993, Raven Press, New York).

Caregiving

In Sickness and In Health: How to Cope When Your Loved One Is Ill, Earl A. Grollman (1987, Beacon Press, Boston).

Doctor-Patient Relationships

Malpractice—How Doctors Manipulate Women, Robert Mendelsohn (1981, Contemporary Books, Chicago).

Social Change and Women's Reproductive Health Care: A Guide for Physicians and Their Patients, Nada Logan Stotland (1988, Praeger, New York).

Table Manners: A Guide to the Pelvic Examination for Disabled Women and Health Care Providers, booklet (Planned Parenthood Education Department—call 415-441-5454).

Take This Book to the Gynecologist with You: A Consumer's Guide to Women's Health Gail Malesky (1991, Addison-Wesley, New York).

Women and Doctors: A Physician's Explosive Account of Women's Medical Treatment and Mistreatment in America Today and What you Can Do About It, John M. Smith (1992, Atlantic Monthly Press, New York).

Endometriosis

An Atlas of Endometriosis, Robert W. Shaw (1993, Partheon Publishing, Carnforth).

Living with Endometriosis, Kate Weinstein (1987, Addison-Wesley, New York).

Fertility and Infertility

Fertility Awareness: How to Become Pregnant When You Want to and Avoid Pregnancy When You Don't, Regina Asaph Pfeiffer (1984, Prentice Hall, Englewood Cliffs, New Jersey).

The Fertility Sourcebook, M. Sara Rosenthal (1995, Lowell House, Los Angeles).

The Infertility Book: A Comprehensive Medical and Emotional Guide, Carla Harkness (1987, Volcano Press, San Francisco).

Infertility: Women Speak Out About their Experiences of Reproductive Medicine, Renate D. Klein, ed. (1989, Pandora Press, London).

Men, Women and Infertility: Intervention and Treatment Strategies, Aline P. Zoldbrod (1993, Lexington Books, New York).

Never to Be a Mother: A Guide for All Women Who Didn't—or Couldn't—Have Children, Linda Hunt Anton (1992, Harper and Row, San Francisco).

Not Pregnant Yet: Infertile Couples in Contemporary America, Arthur L. Greil (1991, Rutgers University Press, New Brunswick, New Jersey).

General Health

The Bodywise Woman: Reliable Information About Physical Activity and Health, by the staff and researchers of the Melpomene Institute for Women's Health Research (1990, Prentice Hall, New York).

Damned If We Do: Contradictions in Women's Health Care, Dorothy H. Brown (1991, Allen and Unwin, North Sydney, Australia).

The New Our Bodies, Ourselves, Boston Women's Health Collective (1992, Simon and Schuster, New York).

Ourselves Growing Older, Paula Brown Doress and Dian Laskin Siegal (1987, Simon and Schuster, New York).

Women and Health Patricia Smyke (1991, Zed Books, Atlantic Highlands, New Jersey).

Women, Health, and Medicine, Agnes Miles (1991, Open University Press, Philadelphia).

Women's Encyclopedia of Health and Emotional Healing, Denise Foley (1993, St. Martin's Press, New York).

Hysterectomies

The Castrated Woman: What Your Doctor Won't Tell You About Hysterectomy, Naomi Miller Stokes (1986, Franklin Watts, New York).

Hysterectomy: Before & After—A Comprehensive Guide to Preventing, Preparing for, and Maximizing Your Health After Hysterectomy, Winnifred Cutler (1988, Harper & Row, New York).

The No-Hysterectomy Option: Your Body—Your Choice, Herbert A. Goldfarb with Judith Greif (1990, Wiley, New York).

No More Hysterectomies, Vicki Hufnagel (1989, New American Library, New York).

Menstruation

The Menstrual Cycle: Physiology, Reproductive Disorders and Infertility, Michel Ferrin, (1993, Oxford University Press, New York).

Menstrual Health in Women's Lives, Alice J. Dan and Linda L. Lewis, eds. (1992, University of Illinois Press, Chicago).

Menstruation, Health and Illness, Diana Taylor and Nancy Woods, eds. (1991, Hemisphere Publishing, New York).

No More Menstrual Cramps and Other Good News, Penny Wise Budoff (1980, Putnam, New York).

Menopause

An Atlas of Menopause, Malcolm I. Whitehead (1993, Partheon, Carnforth).

The Change: Women, Aging and the Menopause, Germaine Greer (1991, Hamish Hamilton, London).

Making the Estrogen Decision, Gretchen Henkel (1992, Lowell House, Los Angeles).

Managing Your Menopause, Wulf H. Utian and Ruth S. Jacobowitz (1990, Prentice Hall, Englewood Cliffs, New Jersey).

The Meanings of Menopause: Historical, Medical and Clinical Perspectives, Ruth Formanek, ed. (1990, Analytic Press, Hillsdale, New Jersey).

Menopause: A Guide for Women and the Men Who Love Them, Winnifred Cutler, Carlos-Ramaon Garcia, and David A. Edwards (1983, W. W. Norton, New York).

Menopause, A Well Woman Book, Montreal Health Press, (1990, Second Story Press, Montreal, Canada).

The Menopause Sourcebook, Gretchen Henkel (1994, Lowell House, Los Angeles).

Menopause, Naturally: Preparing for the Second Half of Life, Sadja Greenwood (1989, Volcano Press, San Francisco).

Menopause: The Woman's View: A Change for the Better, Anne Dickson and Nikki Henriques (1987, Grapevine, Northamptonshire, England).

Menopause Without Medicine: Feel Healthy, Look Younger, Live Longer, Linda Ojeda (1992, Hunter House, Alameda, California).

No More Hot Flashes and Other Good News, Penny Wise Budoff (1983, Putnam, New York).

Transformation Through Menopause, Marian Van Eyk McCain (1991, Bergin and Garvey, New York).

Venus After Forty: Sexual Myths, Men's Fantasies and Truths About Middle-Aged Women, Rita M. Ransohoff (1987, New Horizon Press, New York).

Women of the 14th Moon: Writings on Menopause, Dena Taylor and Amber Coverdale Sumrall, eds. (1991, Crossing Press, Freedom, California).

Natural Therapies

Holistic Medicine, Kenneth R. Pelletier (1987, Delta, New York).

Homeopathy for Women, Rima Handley (1993, Thorsons).

Osteoporosis

Osteoporosis: What It Is, How to Prevent It, How to Stop It, Betty Kamen and Si Kamen (1984, Pinnacle Books, New York).

Pregnancy, Childbirth, and Parenting

First-Time Motherhood: Experiences from Teens to Forties, Ramona T. Mercer (1986, Springer Publishing, New York).

Mamatoto: A Celebration of Birth, The Body Shop (1991, Virago Press, London).

Parents at Risk, Ramona T. Mercer (1990, Springer Publishing, New York).

Pregnancy, Childbirth and the Newborn, Penny Simkin (1991, Meadowbrook, Deerhaven, Minnesota).

Pregnancy and Parenting, Phylliss Noerager Stern, ed. (1989, Hemisphere Publishing, New York).

The Birth Partner: Everything You Need to Know to Help a Woman Through Childbirth (1989, Harvard Common Press, Boston).

The Complete Book of Pregnancy and Childbirth, Sheila Kitzinger (1989, Alfred Knopf, New York).

The Different Faces of Motherhood, Beverly Birns and Dale F. Hay (1988, Plenum Press, New York).

The Midwife Challenge, Sheila Kitzinger, ed. (1991, Pandora Press, Hammersmith, London).

The Mother Zone, Marni Jackson (1991, MacFarlane, Walter and Ross, Toronto).

The Pregnancy Sourcebook, M. Sara Rosenthal (1994, Lowell House, Los Angeles).

What to Expect When You're Expecting, Arlene Eisenberg, Heidi E. Murkoff and Sandee E. Hathaway (1991, Workman Publishing, New York).

What to Expect in the First Year, Arlene Eisenberg, Heidi E. Murkoff, and Sandee E. Hathaway (1989, Workman Publishing, New York).

Wise Woman Herbal for the Childbearing Year, Susan S. Weed (1986, Ash Tree Publishing, Woodstock, New York).

Woman to Mother: A Transformation, Vangie Bergum (1989, Bergin and Garvey, Granby, Massachusetts).

Your Baby and Child from Birth to Age Five, Penelope Leach (1993, Knopf, New York).

Note: For questions and recommendations about childbirth, pregnancy, parenting books, family planning, and other related topics, contact:

Birth and Life Bookstore
P.O. Box 70625
Seattle, WA 98107
206-789-4444

Parentbooks
201 Harbord Street
Toronto, Ontario M5S 1H6
416-537-8334/FAX: 416-537-9499

Premenstrual Syndrome (PMS)

Premenstrual Syndrome, L. H. Gise, ed. (1988, Churchill Livingstone).

Self-Help for PMS, Michelle Harrison (1985, Random House, New York).

PMS Self-Help Book, A Woman's Guide to Feeling Good All Month, Susan Lark (1984, PMS Self-Help Center, Los Altos, California)

Curing PMS The Drug-Free Way, Moira Carpenter (1985, Century Publishing, London, England).

PMS, Gilda Berger (1986, NC Press, Toronto). Aimed at teenage women with PMS.

Controlling PMS, Robert Wilson (1988, Fitzhenry and Whiteside, Toronto).

Index

D

E

F

I

M

R

S

T

U

V

W

Y